ALLE ZEIT WACH
1842

Prognosis of Coronary Heart Disease Progression of Coronary Arteriosclerosis

International Symposium
Held in Bad Krozingen
October 22–23, 1982

Edited by H. Roskamm

With 94 Figures and 80 Tables

Springer-Verlag
Berlin Heidelberg New York Tokyo 1983

Professor Dr. H. Roskamm
Benedikt Kreutz Rehabilitationszentrum
für Herz- und Kreislaufkranke Bad Krozingen e.V.
Südring 15, 7812 Bad Krozingen

ISBN-13:978-3-642-69054-9 e-ISBN-13:978-3-642-69052-5
DOI: 10.1007/978-3-642-69052-5

Library of Congress Cataloging in Publication Data. Main entry under title: Prognosis of coronary heart disease - progression of coronary arteriosclerosis. Bibliography: p. Includes index. 1. Coronary heart disease - Prognosis. I. Roskamm, H. (Helmut), 1933–. [DNLM: 1. Coronary disease. WG 300 P964]
RC685.C6P74 1983 616.1'23075 83-14662

2119/3140-5 4 3 2 1 0

Preface

The papers presented in this book were held at the International Symposium on "Prognosis of Coronary Heart Disease – Progression of Coronary Arteriosclerosis" on October 22 and 23, 1982 in Bad Krozingen, FRG on the occasion of the 10th anniversary of the Rehabilitationszentrum Bad Krozingen.

The symposium was sponsored and supported by the European Society of Cardiology and the Pharma Schwarz Co. The scientific committee was composed of F. Loogen (Düsseldorf), P. G. Hugenholtz (Rotterdam), and the editor of this book.

To all of these and to my co-workers many thanks.

Bad Krozingen, August 1983 H. Roskamm

Table of Contents

List of Contributors*

* The address of each first mentioned author is indicated below the according contribution heading

[1] Page, on which contribution commences

Prognosis of Patients with Coronary Heart Disease Evaluated Using Data Obtained by Invasive Methods

W. Steinbrunn and P. R. Lichtlen

Cardiology Section, Department of Medicine, University Hospital, 8091 Zürich, Switzerland

Studies on the natural history of coronary disease have established that the angiographic appearance of coronary and left ventricular anatomy and function (Obermann et al. 1972; Humphries et al. 1974; Bruschke et al. 1973a, b; Webster et al. 1974; Burggraf and Parker 1975; Nelson et al. 1975; Hammermeister et al. 1979; Harris et al. 1979) are reliable predictors of survival. However, the value of several of these studies has been questioned because of their retrospective character, the relatively small number of patients, the short follow-up, the lack of comparison with an age- and sex-matched normal population, and the selection for coronary surgery of a considerable proportion of the original population that underwent angiography. Furthermore, most of these studies do not provide any information regarding the quality of life experienced by surviving patients.

The present study, although not entirely freed of these strictures, provides more meaningful information in view of the long follow-up period. All survivors were followed up for periods ranging from 7 to 13 years after angiography. The mortality for the study group was compared with the mortality for an age-matched general population. Furthermore, recruitment of patients began in 1965 and ended in 1971, a time when relatively few myocardial revascularization procedures were being performed at the University Hospital of Zurich. It can be assumed that the study population is representative of the coronary patients studied at that time. Finally, it is noteworthy that surviving patients were also analyzed with regard to their "quality of life" at an average of 9.3 years after angiography.

Methods

Patient Population

The study was based on 644 consecutive coronary angiograms performed in the laboratory of the University Hospital of Zurich by one of us (P.R.L.) between September, 1965 and September, 1971. The indications for angiography were angina pectoris or myocardial infarction with or without angina. We also used it to evaluate the necessity of revascularization procedures (Vineberg's internal mammary implantation, patch grafts, vein grafts) and to confirm the clinical diagnosis of coronary artery disease. A total of 369 patients manifested significant obstructions ($\geq 50\%$ reduction of lumen diameter) of at least one major coronary artery (right coronary artery, left anterior descending branch, left circumflex branch) but no other cardiac disease. Of the 369 patients, 114 (31%) underwent myocardial revascularization procedures within 12 months as a consequence of angiography and were therefore excluded from this study. Two patients with selective right coronary injections only were eliminated, as were three cases where contact was lost from the beginning.

Accordingly, the study group consisted of 250 patients, 238 men and 12 women, with a mean age of 49.2 years (range: 28–72 years) at the time of angiography. Ten patients (9 men, 1 woman) underwent coronary artery bypass surgery 14 months–9.3 years (mean 3.7 years) after the first angiogram. This group and the group of the 11 other woman were too small to warrant the detailed analysis performed on the remaining patients, the 229 unoperated men. Fifteen patients (6%) were lost to follow-up after an observation time ranging from 3 months to 7 years (mean 2.3 years). These patients are included in the study as "withdrawn alive."

Data Collection

Selective coronary arteriography was performed in at least two oblique projections (RAO 15–40° and LAO 40–60°) by the Sones technique in 247 patients and by the Judkins technique in three. The extent of coronary artery disease was classified on a three-vessel scale (right coronary artery, left anterior descending, and left circumflex branch).

In 173 of these 229 patients complete studies with adequate left ventricular visualization at cineangiocardiography were available. They were separated into two groups: group I consisted of 61 patients for whom coronary artery bypass surgery would have been possible according to currently accepted criteria, and group II was comprised of 112 patients for whom surgery was not advisable.

Current anatomical indications for the bypass operation are: proximal lesion of 50% or more in one or more coronary arteries, with distal segments suitable for grafting and which are perfusing myocardium presumed to be viable on the basis of documented contraction of LV segments and absence of an electrocardiographic Q-wave in the area in question.

Left ventriculograms were performed in a 30° RAO projection as a routine starting in 1968 in 173 of the 229 patients after the coronary angiogram. Wall motion was defined as normal, hypokinetic (reduced contraction), akinetic (absent contraction), or dyskinetic (paradoxical movement) in one or more of three left ventricular wall segments (anterior, apical, inferior). Ejection fractions were calculated using the area-length method (Dodge et al. 1960) from 134 ventriculograms, where border recognition was easily ascertained in the absence of premature beats.

The cinefilms were interpreted at the time of the study by one of us (P.R.L.) and during reevaluation by the other (W.S.), independently. In the absence of concurrence a third cardiologist reviewed the films. Only four angiographic studies were not available for review; in these instances diagrams and a description of the findings recorded at the time of catheterization were utilized.

Follow-up data concerning symptoms, medication, functional disability using NYHA criteria, working status or retirement, and "quality of life" (whether satisfied with their present situation) were obtained from patients and/or physicians with the aid of questionnaires and telephone interviews beginning in September 1978. Data on deaths were gathered from attending physicians, relatives, and hospital records. Minimum follow-up observation was 7 years, maximum follow-up 13 years (average 9.3 years).

Data Analyses

The aim of the study was to compare the mortality and the survival rate of our 250 patients with the expected mortality for the general Swiss population (according to the 1968/1973 Swiss Population Mortality Table, 1976). The survival data were calculated from the date on which coronary angiography was performed up to September 30, 1978.

The detailed analysis of the mortality data was confined to the homogeneous group of 229 unoperated male patients measuring the relative mortality - mortality ratio (MR) - and the absolute excess mortality, i.e., extra death rate per 1000 per year (EDR) (Levinson and Singer 1976).

The MR, expressed as a percentage, compares the observed mortality with the one expected; i.e., *MR* = *100* × *(observed deaths/expected deaths)*. The mortality of a group of patients with an MR of 100% is identical with the mortality of the general population of the same age and at the time this study was conducted.

The EDR represents the absolute number of additional deaths per year per 1000 patients exposed to risk during follow-up observation; i.e., *EDR* = *1000* × *(observed - expected deaths)/exposure years*. MR and EDR are commonly used in life insurance medicine for assessing mortality. They have the merit of rendering manifest even small departures from the expected mortality.

For comparison with other reports on this subject annual mortality (AM), expressed as a percentage, is included: *average AMR* = *100* × *(observed deaths/exposure years)*. Upper and lower confidence limits for confidence levels of 95%, assuming a Poisson distribution, were determined to assess the statistical significance of MRs (Lew and Singer 1976).

Results

Mortality Data for Entire Group (n = 250)

Although the entire group is heterogeneous, including as it does both men and women and both operated and nonoparated patients, its mortality is briefly reviewed to provide basic data for the clinical follow-up observations. There were 86 patients with single-vessel, 81 with double-vessel, and 83 with triple-vessel disease. Of these 250 patients, 13 had lesions of the left main coronary artery in addition. Five had isolated left main lesions and hence were counted as having two-vessel disease; the remaining eight exhibited concomitant right coronary disease and were therefore classified as having three-vessel diasease (Fig. 1).

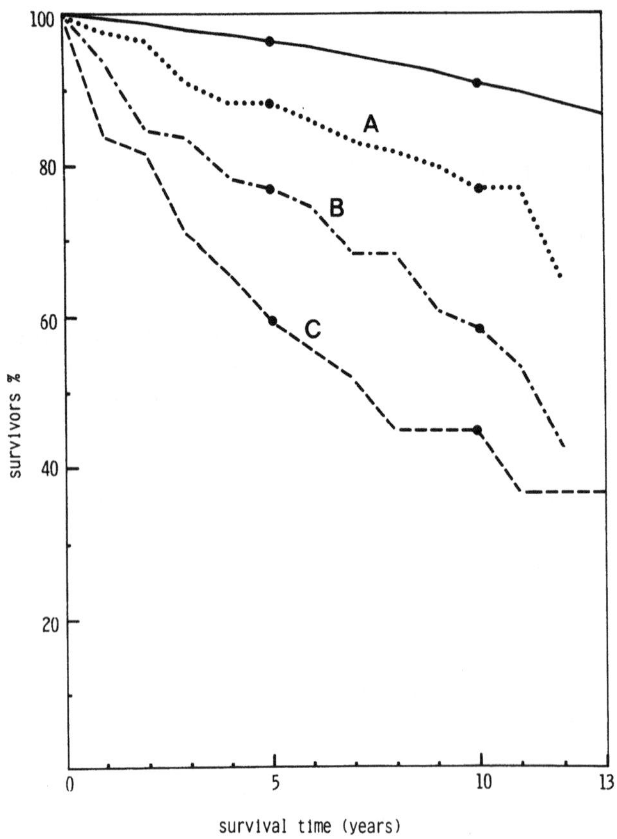

Fig. 1. Cumulative survival curves for 250 patients with coronary artery obstructions of 50% or more in one (*A*, $n=86$), two (*B*, $n=81$), or three (*C*, $n=83$) vessels and cumulative survival curve *(solid line)* of the normal Swiss male population (according to the 1968/1973 Swiss Population Mortality Table; mean age 49 years at start of follow-up observation)

The overall exposure of the 250 patients totaled 1752 person-years. There were 15 patients (6%) lost to follow-up, but of the 140 (56%) alive 7–13 years (mean: 9.3 years) after arteriography, 131 were interviewed; seven were not included because they had undergone coronary surgery, and two could not be contacted.

Of the 250 patients, 95 (38%) died in the course of the follow-up period - 90 men and five women. Of these 95 deaths, 88 (92.6%) were related to the underlying cardiac disease. Of the 88 cardiac deaths, 56 (64%) were sudden, 26 occurring within 2 h of the onset of symptoms; in 30 patients death occurred in the absence of witnesses and the diagnosis of sudden cardiac death was therefore assumed. Among the 39 nonsudden deaths, 29 were due to acute myocardial infarction and ten were noncardiac; however, three of these ten were due to fatal bleeding during anticoagulant therapy, and these have been included in the 88 cardiac deaths.

Figure 1 shows the survival data related to the extent of coronary artery disease. At the end of 5 years the cummulative survival rates for one-, two-, and three-vessel disease were 89%, 77%, and 59% respectively, and at the end of 10 years 77%, 59%, and 45% respectively. The cumulative survival rate for the general population at the age of 49 years was 96.5% at 5 years and 91% at 10 years.

Mortality Data for Group of Nonoperated Male Patients

The exposure of the study group of 229 nonoperated male patients was 1604 person-years (7 years per patient). The average follow-up of the survivors was 9.3 years. Eighty-eight deaths were observed during that period compared with 19.97 deaths expected according to the Swiss Population Mortality Table, resulting in an MR of 441% and in an EDR per 1000 of 42. Of the 79 cardiac deaths, 54 (68%) were sudden. The MRs decreased significantly (see confidence limits, Table 1) with increasing age at time of entry into the study and with increasing duration after angiography.

Table 1. Mortality data for 229 unoperated male patients based on age at entry into the study and survival after angiography

Age (years)	Alive at start	Exposure years	Deaths observed	Deaths expected[a]	Mortality ratio % (CL)	Extra death rate per 1000	Average AM (%)
28–49	122	829.0	45	4.17	1080 (790–1450)	49	5.4
50–72	107	775.0	43	15.80	272 (200–370)	35	5.5
Interval after angiography (years)							
0–2		425.5	30	3.75	800 (540–1140)	62	7.0
2–5		535.0	25	6.05	413 (270–610)	35	4.7
5		643.5	33	10.17	324 (220–460)	35	5.1
Total [average of total]	229	1604.0	88	19.97	[441 (350–550)]	[42]	[5.5]

[a] According to 1968/1973 Swiss Population Mortality Table (1976)
CL, 95% confidence limits; *AM*, annual mortality

Number of Vessels Involved

The MRs, EDRs, and AMs increased in the presence of two or more diseased coronary vessels and were highest for patients with lesions of the left main coronary artery. Only MRs for single- and triple-vessel involvement were significantly different (see confidence limits Table 2). Among the 75 patients with one-vessel disease the particular vessel involved did not cause a significant change in MR, due to the small number of deaths with isolated right coronary (one of 13) and circumflex artery lesions (two of 12).

Nevertheless, with 11 deaths in 50 patients the incidence of death is higher for patients with lesions of the left anterior descending artery. All of these deaths occurred in patients with 50%–100% stenosis of the proximal third of this artery.

Table 2. Mortality data for 229 unoperated male patients based on number of coronary vessels involved with narrowing of 50% or more

Vessels involved	Alive at start	Mean age	Exposure years	Deaths observed	Deaths expected	Mortality ratio % (CL)	Extra death rate per 1000	Average AM (%)
1	75	48.0	576.0	14	6.58	213 (120–360)	13	2.4
2	76	50.1	568.0	29	7.43	390 (260–560)	38	5.1
3	70	50.1	418.5	39	5.32	733 (520–1000)	80	9.3
LMCA	8	49.4	41.5	6	0.64	938 (350–2050)	129	14.5

CL, 95% confidence limits; *LMCA*, left main coronary artery; *AM*, annual mortality

Left Ventricular Ejection Fraction

The relation between mortality and ejection fraction (EF) was determined in 134 patients. With decreasing EF as a measure of impaired left ventricular function the MRs, EDRs and AMs increased significantly (see confidence limits for MR, Table 3). The mortality data in terms of EF and number of vessels with 50% or more narrowing were analyzed separately. Although no statistical difference in MR could be observed due to the small size of the groups, in patients with EF over 50% there was an apparent trend toward increasing mortality (MR, EDR, and AM) with an increase in the number of vessels involved, the MR being only 119% for one-vessel disease, increasing to 210% and 450% for involvement of two and three vessels, and to 6000% for lesions of the left main coronary artery. With EF of 50% or less the influence of the number of vessels involved was not as evident: MRs were identical for two- and three-vessel disease. EDR and AM were similar for one- and two-vessel involvement.

The mortality for patients with coronary disease and a normal left ventriculogram – MR 95% (95% confidence limits: 30%–220%) – was well within that for the general population and significantly lower than that for patients with one abnormal segment of the left ventricle – MR 392% (240%–600%). The MRs of patients with one abnormal segment were not statistically different (for hypo-

Table 3. Mortality data for 229 unoperated male patients based on ejection fraction and number of coronary vessels with narrowing of 50% or more

EF (%)	Vessels involved	Alive at start	Mean age	Exposure years	Deaths observed	Deaths expected	Mortality ratio % (CL)	Extra death rate per 1000	Average AM (%)
>50		77	49.7	548.5	19	7.86	242 (150–380)	20	3.5
36–50		36	48.8	218.0	19	2.06	922 (550–1440)	78	8.7
≤35		21	49.6	60.0	20	0.55	3636 (2220–5600)	324	33.3
–		95	49.2	777.5	30	9.50	316 (210–450)	26	3.9
>50	1	33	48.7	245.0	4	3.36	119 (30–300)	3	1.6
	2	28	51.9	208.5	7	3.34	210 (80–430)	18	3.4
	3	12	49.6	82.0	5	1.11	450 (140–1050)	47	6.1
	LMCA	4	43.8	13.0	3	0.05	6000	227	23.0
≤50	1	12	50.3	63.5	5	0.56	893 (280–2080)	70	7.9
	2	20	45.1	112.0	12	0.65	1846 (960–3230)	101	10.7
	3	25	51.6	102.5	22	1.40	1571 (990–2370)	201	21.5

EF, ejection fraction; *CL*, 95% confidence limits; *AM*, annual mortality; *LMCA*, left main coronary artery; –, left ventriculogram not performed or calculation of EF not possible

kinesis 394%, for akinesis 419%, and for dyskinesis 352%). With increasing number of abnormally contracting segments MR increased significantly. The MR was 599% (350%–960%) for two and 4118% (2550%–6260%) for three abnormally contracting segments.

Group I – the 61 patients suitable for aortocoronary bypass surgery but not operated on – had an excess mortality of 73% (MR 173%) compared with the general population (Table 4). The MR for the patients not thought to be candidates for coronary surgery (group II) was significantly higher at 736%. Both groups had the same distribution of one-vessel disease (I, 36%; II, 35%). There was more two-vessel involvement (43% versus 29%) and less three-vessel disease in group I (21% versus 36%). Significant differences between the two groups were found on analyzing the impairment of left ventricular function.

Table 4. Mortality data for patients suitable for aortocoronary bypass surgery ($n=229$)

Coronary surgery possible	Alive at start	Mean age	Exposure years	Deaths observed	Deaths expected	Mortality ratio % (CL)	Extra death rate per 1000	Average AM (%)
Yes (group I)	61	50.9	455.0	12	6.93	173 (90–300)	11	2.6
No (group II)	112	48.7	686.0	52	7.07	736 (550–960)	65	7.6
–	56	49.0	463.0	24	5.97	402 (260–600)	39	5.2

CL, 95% confidence limits; –, left ventriculogram not performed; *AM*, annual mortality

Group I had more patients (91%) with EF over 50% and with normal or hypokinetc wall motion (80%). Group II had more patients (61%) with EF of 50% or less and with akinetic or dyskinetic areas in the left ventricle (81%).

History

The 75 patients with one-vessel disease listed in Table 2 (MR 213%, EDR 13) could be divided according to mortality into two groups: one group of 24 patients without myocardial infarction and no deaths, and a second group of 51 patients with a history of myocardial infarction and 14 deaths, having an MR of 408% and an EDR of 29.

In Table 5, the mortality data are analyzed with regard to the patients' history – i.e., presence or absence of angina pectoris and myocardial infarction – and compared with the results of coronary angiography. The MR of group A with angina pectoris only was 116%; of group B with myocardial infarction, 516%; of group C with angina plus myocardial infarction, 727%. The MR of the group with angina pectoris only was significantly lower than those of the other groups (see confidence limits Table 5).

Table 5. Mortality data for 229 unoperated male patients based on history

Groups	Alive at start	Mean age	Exposure years	Deaths observed	Deaths expected	Mortality ratio % (CL)	Extra death rate per 1000	Average AM (%)
A	49	52.3	395.0	8	6.92	116 (50–230)	3	2.0
B	67	47.2	501.5	24	4.65	516 (330–770)	39	4.8
C	106	49.2	655.5	54	7.43	727 (550–950)	71	8.2
O	7	51.0	52.0	2	0.97	206	20	3.8
Total	229	49.3	1604.0	88	19.97	441 (350–550)	42	5.5

A, angina pectoris; *B*, myocardial infarction with ECG evidence of infarction; *C*, A+B; *O*, neither A nor B; *CL*, 95% confidence limits; *AM*, annual mortality

The influence on mortality of the number of vessels involved was clearly detectable only in group A: MR 0% for single-, 87% for double-, and 446% for triple-vessel disease. The MRs in group B were 450%, 460%, and 650%, and in group C 350%, 730%, and 850% respectively.

The mortality for 77 patients with inferior and/or posterior wall infarction (MR 452% [95% confidence limits: 300%–660%], EDR 39 per 1000, AM 5%) was lower than that for 74 patients with anterior and/or lateral infarction (MR 678% [460–950], EDR 57 per 1000, AM 6.7%); this difference was not significant. However, 22 patients with the combination of anterior and inferior wall infarction had a significantly higher MR of 1667% [970–2670] (EDR 164 per 1000, AM 17.4%).

Clinical Follow-up Information on All Patients (n = 250)

At the completion of the study, which was 7–13 years after angiography depending on the individual patient, detailed information was available for 131 of 140 patients still alive. Nine patients were not included in the interview, 95 had died, and contact with 15 had been lost. Of the 131 survivors 46 (35%) were asymptomatic, 58 (44%) had angina pectoris, and 27 (21%) had other main symptoms: shortness of breath, 12; easy fatigability, 11; disabled by stroke, 3; intermittent claudication, 1. There were 105 patients (80%) in functional classes NYHA I and II, 20 (15%) in class III, and 6 (5%) in class IV.

Angina Pectoris

Of the 173 patients with angina pectoris at the time of angiography 68 (39%) had died, 11 were lost to follow-up, and 94 survived. The majority of the surviving patients, 48 (51%), continued to exhibit symptoms of angina pectoris; 23 patients (24%) became asymptomatic and free of pain, 16 developed other symptoms, and seven were not included in the follow-up because of intervening bypass surgery. Ten patients (seven with myocardial infarction) who had had no angina at the time of arteriography became symptomatic. Thirty-eight of the resultant 58 patients with angina pectoris were in NYHA class II, 16 in class III, and four in class IV.

In the group of the 23 patients in whom angina pectoris disappeared between angiography and follow-up at an average of 9.3 years thereafter, 11 presented with one-vessel disease, ten with two-vessel disease, and two with three-vessel disease. The EF could be calculated from the left ventriculogram in 15 patients. In 13 it was over 50%.

Medication

Of the 131 patients interviewed 20 (15%) were not receiving medication. The other 111 patients had been taking drugs regularly during the 3 months preceding the interview. Thirty (23%) were on beta-blocking agents, 70 (53%) on nitrates, 67 (51%) on anticoagulants, 37 (28%) on digitalis, 23 (18%) on diuretics and five on other drugs. Twenty-nine patients received one medicament only and 82 received two or more. The most common combinations were nitrates and anticoagulants for 21 patients and nitrates, anticoagulants, and digitalis for 20 others. All 58 patients with angina pectoris were on long-term medication. Beta-blockers were taken by 25 patients (43%) with angina. Nine of the 23 patients who became asymptomatic during follow-up were not taking any medication, three were taking beta-blocking agents, nine nitrates, nine anticoagulants, two digitalis, two diuretics and one sulfinpyrazone.

Working Status

Fourteen patients were unable to work (six because of angina pectoris), 23 worked part time (17 with angina), 65 worked full time (16 with angina), 22 reached the mandatory retirement age of 65 (14 with angina), and seven retired earlier (four with angina).

"Quality of Life"

To arrive at some meaningful approximation of their "quality of life" we interviewed the 131 patients to ascertain whether they were satisfied with their present situation; 96 (73%) answered affirmatively, 35 (27%) negatively. Angina pectoris accounted for the negative responses in 17 patients. Other complications and diseases were responsible for dissatisfaction in 18: congestive heart failure, four; cerebral vascular accident, four; carcinoma, four; arthritis, one; chronic obstructive lung disease, two; psychiatric disorders, three.

Discussion

Two angiographic parameters are of special importance for predicting the natural history of coronary heart disease: the extent and severity of the disease (number of vessels involved, degree of obstruction) and the degree of left ventricular dysfunction. It was first shown by Friesinger et al. (1970) and amply confirmed by others (Bruschke et al. 1973a; Burggraf and Parker 1975) that the extent of coronary artery atherosclerotic disease, as demonstrated by angiography, is the most important predictor of survival. However, this was subsequently questioned by several authors who concluded that survival is determined only by the degree of left ventricular damage (Hammermeister et al. 1979; Vlietstra et al 1977; Gross et al. 1978). Based on previous and present analyses of our data (Lichtlen and Moccetti 1972; Steinbrunn and Lichtlen 1977), both concepts warrant consideration. On the one hand, our results clearly demonstrate that in patients with impaired left ventricular function mortality is indeed independent of the extent of coronary artery disease, as attested by the group of patients with ejection fractions below 50%. On the other hand, in patients with ejection fractions above 50%, the mortality ratio clearly increased with the number of vessels involved (Table 3).

A similar trend was found in the analysis of patient histories. Mortality among patients manifesting only angina pectoris was low and depended on the number of vessels involved, as had been shown by others (Obermann et al. 1972; Humphries et al. 1974; Webster et al. 1974). In contrast, the high mortality ratio of patients with myocardial infarction depended only to a minor degree on the severity and extent of coronary disease. Hence, we are led to conclude that survival of patients with angina pectoris and normal ejection fractions depends primarily on the extent of coronary artery disease. However, once a myocardial infarction is present and left ventricular function markedly impaired, survival seems to be quite independent of the extent of coronary obstructive disease and is mainly determined by the degree of left ventricular damage. This is supported by the observation that ejection fraction is a strong predictor of survival within this group (Table 3). Furthermore, history is also an indicator of survival, although it was not perceived as such in other studies of coronary disease natural history (Obermann et al. 1972; Bruschke et al. 1973b; Burggraf and Parker 1975; Kannel and Feinleib 1972).

An unexpected finding in this study was the high mortality ratio of patients under the age of 50 (MR 1080% versus 272% for patients above 50 years; Table 1).

This might be explained by the fact that mortality ratio is an index of mortality relative to the general population - one that generally decreases with advancing age. However, the extra death rate for patients below the age of 50 years is also greater than that for patients above 50 years (49 versus 35 per 1000 per year). These figures indicate that our study included a comparatively large proportion of young, high-risk patients. This is most probably due to the indications for coronary angiography at the time of entry into the study, preference having been given to patients under 50 years of age, especially to those with myocardial infarction. This is further reflected in the mean age for patients with only myocardial infarction (47.2 years) versus those with a history of only angina pectoris (52.3 years).

The candidates suitable for bypass surgery, as defined in the present report, also have an excellent prognosis without surgery (Table 4). The selection of this kind of patient for randomized trials with bypass surgery or percutaneous transluminal coronary angioplasty is therefore liable to blur any effect of these interventions on the natural history of coronary disease. A prolongation of life by bypass surgery or transluminal dilatation may be seen only in patients who have a poor prognosis, such as those with infarction, three-vessel disease, lesions of the left main coronary artery, and EF under 50%.

The mortality data for the present study differ considerably from those in previously published reports. It is therefore of special interest to consider them in the light of the MR of the studies performed at the Johns Hopkins Hospital (Friesinger et al. 1970), the University of Alabama Medical Center (Obermann et al. 1972) and the Cleveland Clinic (Bruschke et al. 1973a; Webster et al. 1974), as analyzed by Singer and Levinson (1976) (see Table 6). Direct comparison of these studies is not warranted as there are many variables, known and unknown, among these geographically diverse populations. Furthermore, possible secular changes in fatality rates cannot be excluded. Thus, comparison of these studies with respect to patients with lesions causing 50% or greater narrowing reveals that MRs of our entire group and of our patients with two- and three-vessel involvement were significantly lower (see confidence limits, Table 6). The discrepancy between our results and those from the Johns Hopkins Hospital may be explained by the low average age of 41.5 of the latter group. Their MR of 1060% is in agreement with our data for patients below the age of 50 (MR 1080%; Table 1). The rather short mean follow-up of 21 months for the patients at the University of Alabama might well account for the high MR of 975%, which corresponds to the high MR of the first 2 years of follow-up for our patients (MR 800%, Table 1).

The variance in MR between the data reported by Bruschke et al. (1973a) (740%) and the present data (441%) with narrowing of 50% or more is less clear. There is agreement between the MRs for our patients with severe proximal coronary artery disease and those for patients from the Cleveland Clinic as presented by Webster et al. (1974). It is therefore likely that the study by Bruschke et al. (1973a) was unwillingly biased with respect to selection of an unknown number of good-risk patients for internal mammary artery implantation, with the consequent, relatively high proportion of poor-risk patients remaining in that study group. The percentage of patients who underwent revascularization

Table 6. Relationship between mortality data and number of vessels with obstructive coronary lesions (Singer and Levinson 1976); comparison of findings in four major studies with the present one

	Entry into study	Follow-up (yrs.)	Mean age	A One-vessel disease MR% (CL)	A Two-vessel disease MR% (CL)	A Three-vessel disease MR% (CL)	Total MR% (CL)
John Hopkins (Friesinger et al. 1970) score >4 (≥50% narrowing)	1960–1967	5–12[a]	41.5				1060 (680–1570)
Alabama (Obermann et al. 1972) ≥50% narrowing	1965–1970	1–4	46.8	270	1110 (590–1900)	1300 (730–2150)	975 (650–1390)
Cleveland (Bruschke et al. 1973a) ≥50% narrowing	1963–1965	5–9*	49.7	320 (220–440)	880 (720–1040)	1370 (1050–1740)	740 (640–840)
Zurich ≥50% narrowing	1965–1971	7–13	49.3	213 (120–360)	390 (260–560)	733 (520–1000)	441 (350–550)
Cleveland (Webster et al. 1974) ≥80% narrowing	1960–1965	6–11[a]	49.0	385 (250–560)	865 (670–1100)	1450 (1120–1840)	
Zurich ≥90% narrowing	1965–1971	7–13	49.3	373 (270–510)	767 (510–1110)	1059 (490–2010)	

MR, mortality ratio; *CL*, 95% confidence limits

[a] Data presented only for 0–5 years after angiography

surgery at the time of recruitment is known to be 15% for the study of the University of Alabama Medical Center, 28% for the Johns Hopkins Hospital, and 31% for our own study. The fact remains, however, that the course of the disease in our study appears less severe than that in other investigation; it rather resembles the course described in more recent prospective studies (Harris et al. 1979; Mock et al. 1982) and the prognosis of the medical control groups in the randomized studies of coronary artery bypass surgery (Takaro et al. 1982; European Coronary Surgery Study Group 1982).

This seems to be true as well for the symtoms manifested by the survivors. Despite the inherent limitation of questionnaires for acquiring follow-up data on surviving patients, there are useful observations that can be made. The "quality of life" element is not as discouraging as was supposed by Kannel and Feinleib (1972); most of our patients were only mildly limited in their physical activity. This judgement is sustained by the fact that two-thirds were working and almost three-quarters freely declared that they were satisfied with their situation at the time of the follow-up inquiry. Angina pectoris continued as the principal symptom after 9.3 years (average) following angiography. There was, however, a group of patients in whom remissions of angina occurred, seemingly a group of good-risk patients with one- and two-vessel disease and ejection fractions over 50%, probably reflecting a genuinely benign course of the disease. Their remission was not attributable to drug therapy – most certainly not to beta-blocking agents which were given to only three of these 23 patients. In this connection it is interesting to note that long-term survival and a productive life have also been reported for coronary patients by Gross et al. (1978), even for patients rejected for coronary revascularization surgery.

Acknowledgments. The assistance of Dr. Martin Gander in reviewing some of the cinefilms; the kind cooperation of Manfred Fessel and Lothar Scholl, Life Department, Swiss Reinsurance Company, Zurich; and the help of Dr. Maurice Landy in reviewing the manuscript were very valuable, as were the essential services provided by Erika Lienhard and the late Margret Bücheler.

Summary

In this study 250 patients with obstructions of 50% or more in at least one major coronary artery (left anterior descending, left circumflex, or tight coronary), among them 229 unoperated male patients, were followed up for an average of 7 years after their coronary angiograms. The follow-up for survivors averaged 9.3 (7–13) years. A total of 95 patients (38%) died during this period.

The mortality in this study group was compared with the expected mortality for an age-matched general population by calculating the mortality ratio (MR), which was 441% for the 229 patients. It was lowest for patients over age 50 (272% [95% confidence limits: 200%–370%]), for patients with angina pectoris only (116% [50%–230%]), those with one-vessel disease (231% [120%–360%]), and those with ejection fractions (EF) above 50% (242% [150%–380%]). The MR was significantly higher in patients under 50 years of age (1080% [790%–1450%]), those with myocardial infarction (646% [510%–800%]), those with three-vessel disease (733% [520%–1000%]), those with lesions of the left main coronary artery (938% [350%–2050%]), and with EF below 50% (1494% [1060%–2040%]). Among the surviving patients, 35% were asymptomatic; 80% were in NYHA functional classes I and II; 67% were working (50% full time); and 73% considered their "quality of life" acceptable.

References

Bruschke AVG, Proudfit WL, Sones FM (1973a) Progress study of 590 consecutive nonsurgical cases of coronary disease followed 5–9 years. I. Arteriographic correlations. Circulation 47:1147–1153

Bruschke AVG, Proudfit WL, Sones FM (1973b) Progress study of 590 consecutive nonsurgical cases of coronary disease followed 5–9 years. II. Ventriculographic and other correlations. Circulation 47:1154–1163

Burggraf GW, Parker JO (1975) Prognosis in coronary artery disease. Angiographic, hemodynamic, and clinical factors. Circulation 51:146–156

Dodge HT, Sandler H, Ballew DW, Lord JD (1960) The use of biplane angiocardiography for the measurement of left ventricular volume in man. Am Heart J 60:762–776

European Coronary Surgery Study Group (1982) Prospective randomized study of coronary artery bypass surgery in stable angina pectoris: a progress report on survival. Circulation 65 [Suppl II]:67–71

Friesinger GC, Page EE, Ross RS (1970) Prognostic significance of coronary arteriography. Trans Assoc Am Physicians 83:78–92

Gross H, Vaid AK, Cohen MV (1978) Prognosis in patients rejected for coronary revascularization surgery. Am J Med 64:9–20

Hammermeister KE, DeRouen TA, Dodge HT (1979) Variables predictive of survival in patients with coronary disease. Selection by univariate and multivariate analyses from the clinical, electrocardiographic, exercise, arteriographic, and quantitative angiographic evaluations. Circulation 59:421–430

Harris PJ, Harrel FE, Lee KL, Behar VS, Rosati RA (1979) Survial in medically treated coronary artery disease. Circulation 60:1259–1269.

Humphries JO, Kuller L, Ross RS, Friesinger GC, Page EE (1974) Natural history of ischemic heart disease in relation to arteriographic findings. A twelve-year study of 224 patients. Circulation 49:489–497

Kannel WB, Feinleib M (1972) Natural history of angina pectoris in the Framingham study. Prognosis and survival. Am J Cardiol 29:154–163

Levinson L, Singer RB (1976) Methodology in medical risks. In: Singer RB, Levinson L (eds) Patterns of mortality and survival. Heath, Lexington, pp 9–21

Lew EA, Singer RB (1976) Interpretation of mortality and survival data in medical risks. In: Singer RB, Levinson L (eds) Patterns of mortality and survial. Heath, Lexington, pp 23–32

Lichtlen PR, Moccetti T (1972) Prognostic aspects of coronary angiography (abstract). Circulation 45, 46 [Suppl II]:7

Mock MB, Ringqvist I, Fisher LD, Davis KB, Chaitman BR, Kouchoukos NT, Kaiser GC, Alderman E, Ryan TJ, Russell RO Jr, Mullin S, Fray D, Kilip III T, Participants in the Coronary Artery Surgery Study (1982) Survival of medically treated patients in the coronary artery surgery study (CASS) registry. Circulation 66:562–568

Nelson GR, Cohn PF, Gorlin R (1975) Prognosis in medically treated coronary artery disease. Influence of ejection fraction compared to other parameters. Circulation 52:408–412

Obermann A, Jones WB, Riley CP, Reeves TJ, Sheffield LT, Turner ME (1972) Natural history of coronary artery disease. Bull NY Acad Med 48:1109–1125

Singer RB, Levinson L (1976) Prognostic significance of coronary arteriography in medical risks. In: Singer RB, Levinson L (eds) Patterns of mortality and survival. Heath, Lexington, pp 334–341

Steinbrunn W, Lichtlen PR (1977) Complete 5-year cumulative survival rates in 244 unselected, unoperated coronary patients undergoing angiography (abstract). Circulation 55, 56 [Suppl III]: 174

Swiss Population Mortality Table 1968/1973 (1976) Sterblichkeit nach Todesursachen. Ausscheide- und Überlebensordnungen nach Zivilstand. Statistische Quellenwerke der Schweiz, Vol 577. Eidgenössisches Statistisches Amt, Bern

Takaro T, Hultgren HN, Detre KM, Peduzzi P (1982) The veterans administration cooperative study of stable angina: current status. Circulation 65 [Suppl II]: 60–67

Vlietstra RE, Assad-Morell JL, Frye RL, Elveback LR, Connolly DC, Ritman EL, Pluth JR, Barnhorst DA, Danielson GK, Wallace RB (1977) Survival predictors in coronary artery disease. Medical and surgical comparisons. Mayo Clin Proc 52:85–90

Webster JS, Moberg C, Rincon G (1974) Natural history of severe proximal coronary artery disease as documented by coronary cineangiography. Am J Cardiol 33:195–200

Prognosis of Coronary Heart Disease Patients Evaluated by Data Obtained by Noninvasive Methods

R. A. Bruce
University of Washington, RG-20 Seattle, WA 98195, USA

The study design of the exercise testing unit of a prospective, collaborative community practice experience of many physicians, known as the Seattle Heart Watch, illustrates the prognostic value of the initial clinical examination, and of noninvasive exercise testing (Bruce et al. 1977). The procedures followed are now available, at minimal expense for equipment, to any interested physician, for office or clinic use.

The basic principle is the sampling of different populations of either symptomatic ambulatory cardiac patients or healthy persons, with clinical examination and classification before exercise testing, and then the monitoring of responses to stress (Bruce 1978; Bruce et al. 1974). Follow-up is done by mailing questionnaires periodically to persons included in a computer registry in order to ascertain annual cardiac heart disease (CHD) event rates. These may be either primary or secondary events, although risk factors and exercise predictors are not identical for both types.

The clinical diagnosis of CHD before exercise testing is based on a history of typical angina pectoris, myocardial infarction, and/or prior cardiac "death" with resuscitation by ventricular defibrillation.

It is important to note the a priori predictive value of age and of preliminary clinical classification of the patient. The age-specific probability for secondary events per year ranges from .048 to .08 in men with CHD who are 30–64 years of age (Fig. 1). Mortality is low in such patients under 30 years of age,

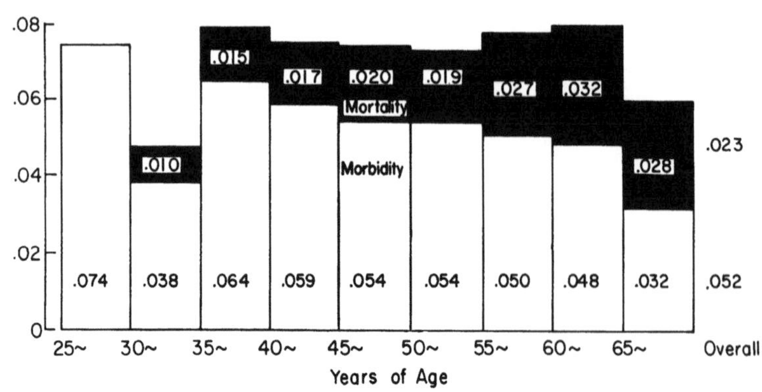

Fig. 1. Age-specific probability of secondary coronary heart disease events in Seattle men with coronary heart disease

while the probability of cardiac death per year reaches 0.32, or 3.2 per 100 man-years, in men 60–64 years old. In contrast, the 1-year probability for secondary CHD events ranges from .055 for men with angina pectoris only to .139 (or 13.9 per 100 man-years) for men with a history of prior cardiac arrest (Fig. 2). Thus, the relative predictive value of a clinical diagnosis ranges from 1.14 to 4.34 times that of age alone. The predictive risk ratio for Secondary CHD relative to primary CHD events in asymptomatic, healthy men, ranges from 15 to 38 : 1.

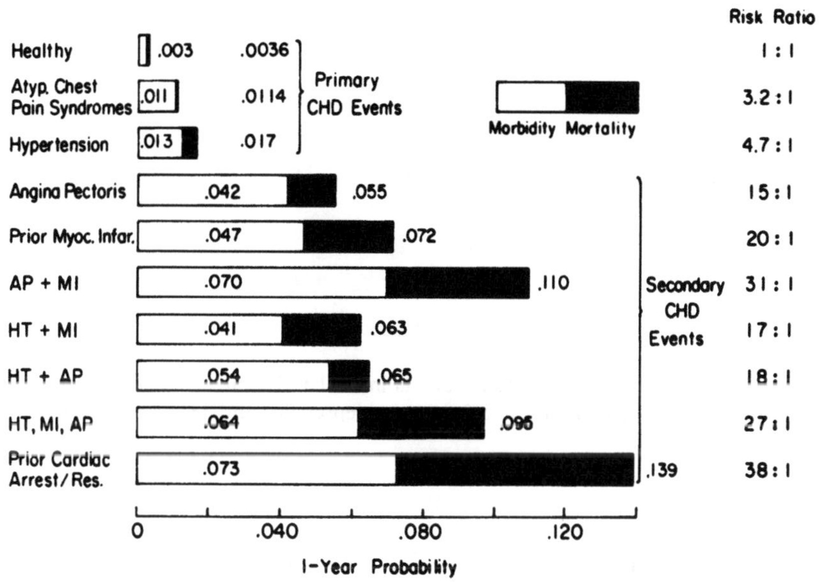

Fig. 2. Risks of CHD morbidity and mortality events, expressed as 1-year probabilities per person, for 5363 men, stratified in relation to preliminary clinical classification before exercise testing. Note the lower probabilities for primary CHD events in men without clinical evidence of coronary disease, versus the higher probabilities for secondary CHD events in patients with coronary disease

The traditional approach to the prognosis of CHD events focuses primarily on the demonstration of ischemic ST segment depression in response to exercise testing. Unfortunately, the incidence of this response in CHD men and women hardly exceeds that observed in either hypertensive or healthy persons; it also increases with age (Bruce 1981).

The predictive value is limited in both non-CHD and CHD patients. Neither of two manifestations of exertional myocardial ischemia – chest pain and ischemic ST segment depression – was observed in 43.5% of men with CHD on exercise testing, yet the subsequent mortality for the group was 21.6 per 1000 man-years. However, the presence of one or both manifestations in the majority of patients was associated with subsequent mortality of 46.1–57.3 per 1000 man-years ($p < .05$).

Stratification of responses to exercise by the number of stages or workloads attained shows an obvious inverse gradient of risk. The range was 15%–20% per year for those patients who were limited to stage I, to 2%–4.5% per year for patients who attained stage IV (Fig. 3). Subdivision of patients into groups according to the presence or absence of ischemic ST segment depression at each stage or workload revealed no significant differences in rates of secondary CHD events.

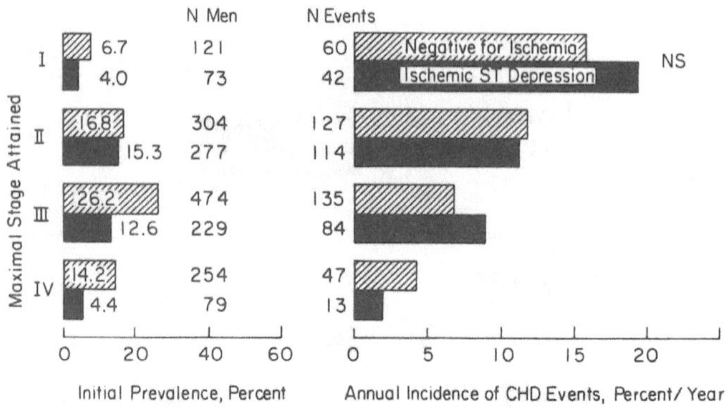

Fig. 3. Variations in secondary CHD events in 1811 CHD men over 4±2 years stratified by absence or presence of ischemic ST segment depression and exercise capacity in terms of highest stage attained

Three important predictors of CHD mortality are parameters of left ventricular dysfunction (Bruce 1977). The first of these is cardiomegaly noted during the physical, or on X-ray examination, before exercise testing. The second is failure to complete 3 min of exercise in stage I (which requires 4–4.5 METs energy expenditure), and the third is failure to raise systolic pressure (as observed by clinical sphygmomanometry) above 130 Torr during exercise. Of 1653 men with CHD tested, 78% exhibited none of these features, and the subsequent CHD mortality for this group was 20 per 1000 man-years of observation. With any one, any two, or all three characteristics present in decreasing numbers of patients tested, mortality increased to 96, 252, and 884 per 1000 man-years of follow-up respectively (Fig. 4).

Because of these disparities in predictive values a stepwise multivariate analysis of 26 clinical and exercise variables was performed (Bruce et al. 1977). In rank order of diminishing statistical significance, the predictive variables were:

1. Number of categorical abnormalities in the resting 12-lead ECG in supine position
2. Cardiomegaly
3. Maximal systolic pressure
4. Arrhythmia severity score
5. Duration of maximal exercise

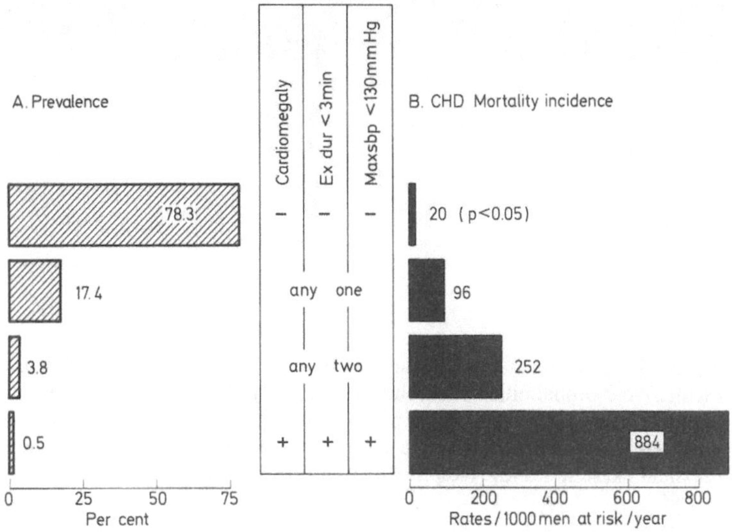

Fig. 4. Comparative prevalence of significant predictors of secondary CHD events in 1653 men with coronary heart disease, and subsequent incidence of cardiac mortality in relation to absence or presence of one or more predictive variables for left ventricular dysfunction. Ex-dur, exercise duration; Maxsbp, maximal systolic blood pressure. (Reprinting from the New England Journal of Medicine, Bruce 1977a)

The corresponding F values were 42.4, 26.7, 16.1, 8.0, and 7.3 respectively. Neither chest pain nor ischemic ST depression, with or following maximal exercise, was significant. These predictive variables were combined with a logistic risk probability estimate for each patient, and survival curves were computed. For the first 85 percentiles of 1852 men with CHD the 2-year survival rate exceeded 96%. For the ramining 15% of patients survival was lower in proportion to predictive variables identified; for the 99th percentile it was only 42% for 2 years.

On the basis of this information, several exertional pathophysiological syndromes for men with CHD have been defined (Bruce et al. 1979). These are (a) neither myocardial ischemia nor left ventricular dysfunction, (b) either of these two syndromes, and (c) the combination of both syndromes. With additional years of observation (average 6) the annual probabilities for CHD morbidity and mortality events have been recalculated for men who remain unoperated. In relation to myocardial ischemia an increase in event rates from .062 to .093 when both chest pain and ST depression occur is barely significant, with a risk ratio of only 1.5:1 ($p<.05$; Fig. 5; Bruce et al. 1981a). In relation to left ventricular dysfunction, however, the increase from .062 to 1.12 per man-year is quite significant ($p<.001$), and the predictive risk ratio is 18:1 (Fig. 6; Bruce et al. 1981).

The amount of prognostic information provided by these pathophysiological syndromes in combination with the preliminary clinical classification has

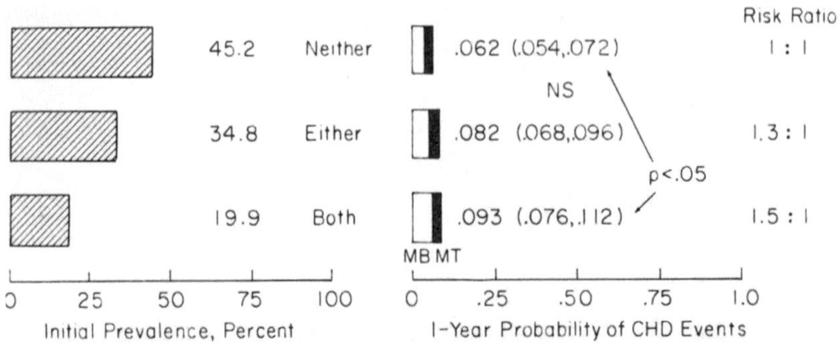

Fig. 5. Revised prevalence of manifestations of exertional myocardial ischemia and subsequent 1-year probabilities of secondary morbidity (*MB*) or mortality (*MT*) events in men with coronary heart disease who remain unoperated (95% confidence intervals are enclosed in *parentheses*). Note limited predictive value of either chest pain or ST segment depression with maximal exercise testing. (Reprinted from Cardiology)

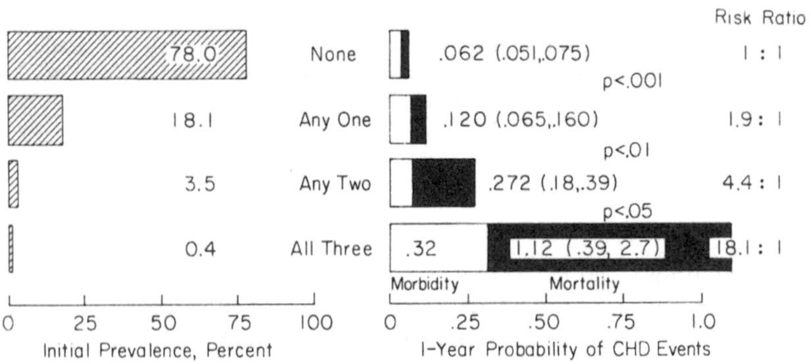

Fig. 6. Revised prevalence of manifestations of left ventricular dysfunction and subsequent incidence of secondary CHD morbidity and mortality in men with coronary heart disease who remain unoperated (95% confidence intervals are enclosed in parentheses). Note the low incidence in 78% of patients. $p > 1.0$ in 0.4% of patients who initially manifested all three criteria (cardiomegaly, exercise duration <3 min, exercise systolic pressure <130 mmHg) because the majority of deaths occurred within 1 year. (Reprinted from Cardiology)

also been determined (Bruce, unpublished observations, 1982). The age-standardized, uncorrected secondary event rates, based on the subsequent spontaneous occurrence of myocardial infarction, sudden cardiac arrest, or cardiac death - sudden or not - have been computed for 1956 men and 369 women with CHD (Fig. 7). The lowest age-standardized annual rates were 30 per 100 man-years and 15.3 per 1000 woman-years in the absence of both pathophysiological syndromes. Myocardial ischemia increased this rate to 46.2 in men, but reduced it to 11.3 in women. The combination of myocardial ischemia and left ventricular dysfunction, as defined by three noninvasive variables, increased the rates to 97.3 and 46.5 respectively in men and women with CHD. The pres-

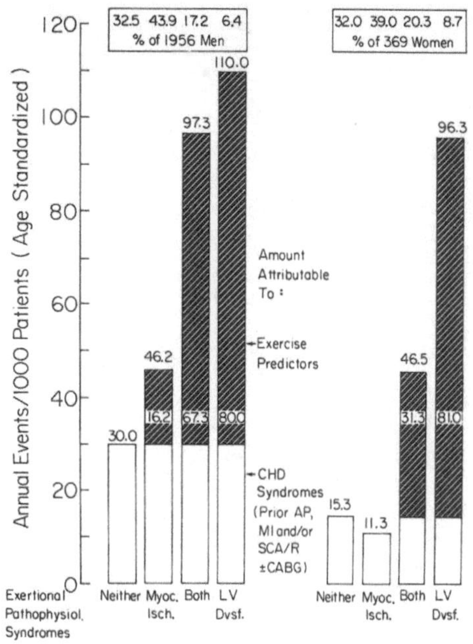

Fig. 7. Comparison of annual secondary event rates per 1000 patients, age standardized, in men and women in relation to absence or presence of either of two exertional pathophysiological syndromes. *MI,* myocardial infarction; *AP,* angina pectoris; *SCA/R* (sudden cardiac arrest/resuscitation); *CABG,* coronary artery bypass graft

ence of left ventricular dysfunction alone, however, was associated with even higher rates of 110 and 96.3 per 1000 person-years for men and women respectively. These risk gradients seem to reflect the natural history of coronary heart disease in men and women.

When these two syndromes were used retrospectively to classify unoperated and operated men with CHD, unexpected results were obtained (Fig. 8; Bruce et al. 1979). The 4-year survival rates of 91% versus 92%, for operated versus unoperated CHD patients with exertional myocardial ischemia, show no significant difference, yet this has been the traditional clinical indication for aortocoronary bypass surgical grafting. Patients with left ventricular dysfunction, whether or not they show exertional myocardial ischemia, manifest a significant difference of in 4-year survival rates of 67% for unoperated as opposed to 94% for operated CHD patients ($p < .01$). In the opinion of the cardiologists who were responsible, all unoperated patients had at least one potentially graftable artery. In retrospect, 34% of operated patients fell into this category, even though in the years of enrollment from 1971 through 1974 left ventricular dysfunction by invasive diagnostic criteria in a patient resting supinely was usually considered a contraindication to bypass surgery.

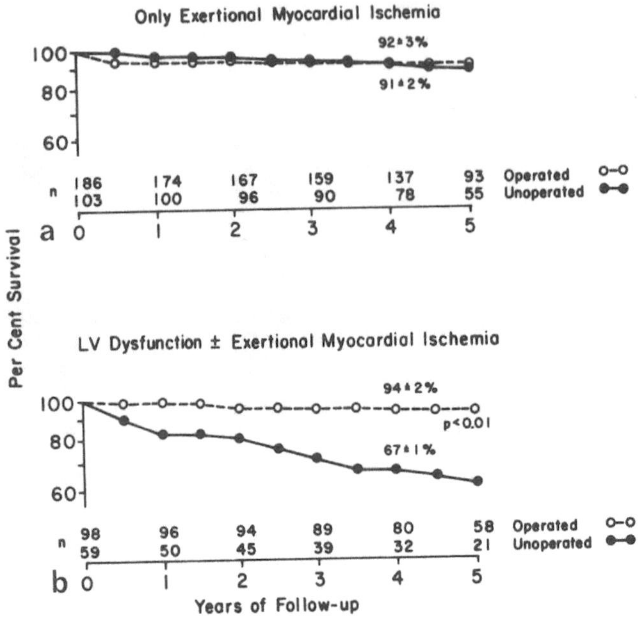

Fig. 8. A Comparison of survival rates in men with coronary heart disease who manifested exertional myocardial ischemia on initial maximal exercise test in relation to subsequent aortocoronary bypass grafting or no surgical treatment. Note similarity of 4-year survival rates. **B** Divergent survival rates in relation to initial manifestation of left ventricular dysfunction, whether or not myocardial ischemia was also manifested, and to subsequent operative or medical (unoperated) treatment. Note significant difference at 4 years ($p < .01$). (Reprinted from Circulation, Bruce et al. 1979)

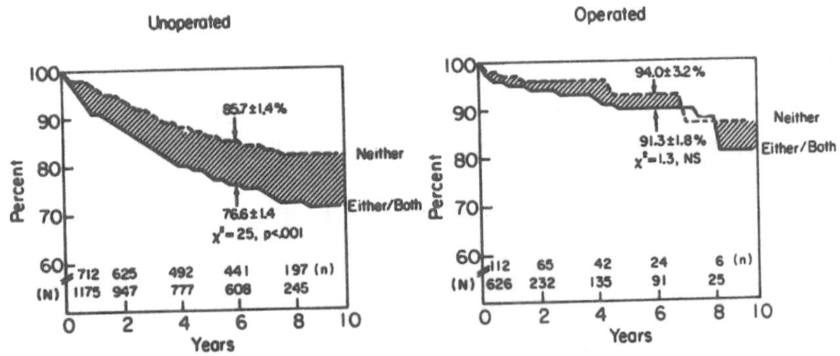

Fig. 9. Comparison of rates of survival without "hard" secondary CHD events in patients with coronary heart disease who remain *unoperated* or who are treated surgically (*operated*). The *shaded zone* indicates the additional predictive information derived from either or both of the two exertional pathophysiological syndromes over that of the original clinical classification of disease. Note the significant contribution of exertional pathophysiological syndromes in unoperated by not in operated patients. The 6-year survival rates are higher in the latter groups. *N*, number of patients observed over subsequent years

The cumulative contribution of exercise testing of operated and unoperated CHD patients shows a significantly lower rate of survival when these secondary CHD events are absent in the patients who, exhibit one or more exertional pathophysiological syndromes at enrollment, and who remain unoperated (Fig. 9).

A network of computer terminals in hospitals clinics and office practices linked by telephone to a central computer provides an immediate summary of preliminary findings, clinical classification, and responses to maximal exercise; the last of these are interpreted in relation to normal standards. Probabilities of CHD events are indicated, and data are stored in a computer register (Bruce, 1981b).

In conclusion, exercise as a noninvasive functional test reproduces and/or reveals symptoms and signs, identifies mechanisms of cardiac impairment, permits appraisal of prognosis in relation to CHD morbidity and mortality, and reveals changes produced by disease and/or therapy.

References

Bruce RA (1977a) Current concepts: exercise testing for evaluation of ventricular function. N Eng J Med 296:671-675

Bruce RA (1978) Exercise testing methods and interpretation. Adv Cardiol 24:6-15

Bruce RA (1981) Human data from Seattle Heart Watch and network registries, 1971-1977. In: Masoro EJ (ed) Handbook of physiology in aging. CRC, Boca Raton

Bruce RA, Gey GO, Cooper MN et al. (1974) Seattle heart watch: initial clinical, circulatory and electrocardiographic responses to maximal exercise. Am J Cardiol 33:459-469

Bruce RA, DeRouen T, Peterson DR., et al. (1977b) Noninvasive predictors of sudden cardiac death in men with coronary heart disease. Predictive value of maximal stress testing. Am J Cardiol 39:833-840

Bruce RA, DeRouen TA, Hammermeister KE (1979) Noninvasive screening criteria for enhanced 4-year survival after aortocornonary bypass surgery. Circulation 60:638

Bruce RA, Hossack KF, DeRouen TA (1981a) Predictive value of symptom-limited exercise for risk assessment for primary and secondary events due to coronary heart disease in men. Cardiology 68 [Suppl 2]: 15-26

Bruce RA, Hossack KF, Belanger L, DeRouen TA, Sobolenski JS, Hofer V, Holzmann T (1981b) A computer terminal program to evaluate cardiovascular functional limits and estimate coronary event risks. West J Med 35:342-350

Prognosis of Coronary Heart Disease Patients Evaluated by Data Obtained by Invasive and Noninvasive Methods

K. Bachmann, W. Niederer, H. Fuchs, and H. Holzberger
Med. Universitäts-Poliklinik, Östliche Stadtmauerstrasse 29, 8520 Erlangen, FRG

The natural course of coronary atherosclerotic heart disease may be considered from various standpoints. No controversy exists about the validity of both noninvasive and invasive methods in the evaluation of long-term prognosis of patients with coronary heart disease (CHD). But, similar to problems in the detection of CHD, indirect markers such as symptoms, electrocardiographic abnormalities and risk factors discriminate only roughly between low-risk and high-risk patients (Sigler 1951; Zukel et al. 1969). They are more likely to affect short-term rather than long-term prognosis (Humphries et al. 1974; Proudfit et al. 1978). There is no close correlation between the severity and extent of coronary artery sclerosis, the number of vessels diseased, and the involvement of the left ventricle which allows the physician to predict accurately the long-term course, especially after the disease has developed (Burggraf and Parker 1975; Humphries et al. 1974). The physician with invasive methods at his disposal focuses primarily on the "X-ray anatomy" of selective coronary angiography (Burggraf and Parker 1975; Bruschke et al. 1973; Hammermeister et al. 1979; Lichtlen 1977, 1977; Proudfit et al. 1978; Taylor et al. 1980).

Patients and Methods

A total of 5281 patients with suspected or already diagnosed CHD were studied angiographically between 1969 and 1976 at Erlangen (Fig. 1). Coronary angiography was performed (a) preoperatively in congenital or acquired heart disease, (b) in arrhythmia, (c) as postoperative follow-up after bypass surgery, and (d) in occlusive arterial disease, where "total angiography" was routine. This may explain the high percentage of noncoronary subjects in the total group; 2983 patients had angiographic evidence of coronary artery disease. Of these, 1596 were graded I and II, with narrowing in lumen diameter of 50% or less, or 51%–75%, which was considered to be hemodynamically insignificant. (This classification differs from the Cleveland follow-up where the borderline between hemodynamically significant and insignificant CHD was at 50% reduction of lumen diameter.) The remaining 1387 patients had CHD which was considered to be hemodynamically effective, with more than 75% stenotic lesions (grade III) or total occlusion (grade IV). Due to a restrictive policy on bypass surgery only 510 patients graded III and IV were regarded as candidates for surgery. Thus, 877 patients remained for medical treatment, who could serve as models for studying the natural course of CHD, which – at least in the symptomatic patient - is never natural. Noncompliance with the advice reduced the group of operative candidates to 351. Of the 159 patients who did not undergo surgery, 24 dropped out during the long-term follow-up; 12 of them underwent delayed surgery. In the nonoperative group there were 28 dropouts, 10 of whom disregarded their classification and underwent surgery elsewhere. Thus, the total group of patients in the study numbered 984, each of them having 75% or more stenosis or occlusion in at least one major coronary artery. There were 912 men aged 28–81 years (mean age, 52.5 years) and 72 women aged 31–76 years (mean age, 52.3 years).

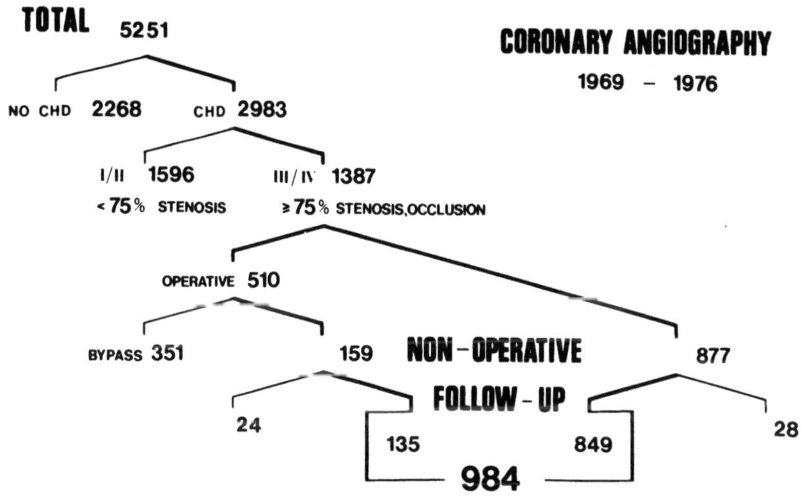

Fig. 1. Distribution of 5251 patients who underwent coronary angiography

All patients had selective cineangiography and ventriculography; a 17-cm image intensifier with a high resolution of 4.2 periods/s (Siemens) was used. The majority were studied by Sones' (Proudfit et al. 1978) method and had additional pharmacodynamic angiography after 10 mg isosorbide dinitrate, given sublingually. The coronary artery lesions were classified according to De Bakey's score and to recommendations of the Grading Committee of the NYHA, taking normal, left dominant, or right dominant circulation into consideration (De Bakey et al. 1968; AHA 1975). According to the coronary score the patients were grouped into classes I (score 1–20), II (score 21–40), and III (score over 40). Diastolic and end-systolic volumes and the ejection fraction (EF) were determined from monoplane left ventricular angiograms taken in the 30° RAO oblique position. The left ventricular pump function was graded I as normal (EF 60% and above), II as moderately depressed (EF 59%–30%), and III as severely reduced (EF below 30%). Statistic analysis was performed according to the actuarial method of Berkson and Gage (1950) with a mean follow-up of 40.1 months, ranging from 12 to 108 months.

Results

Cardiac survival curves for the total group (T), the conservative group (K), and the noncompliant candidates (OP) are shown in Fig. 2a. The cumulative 5-year

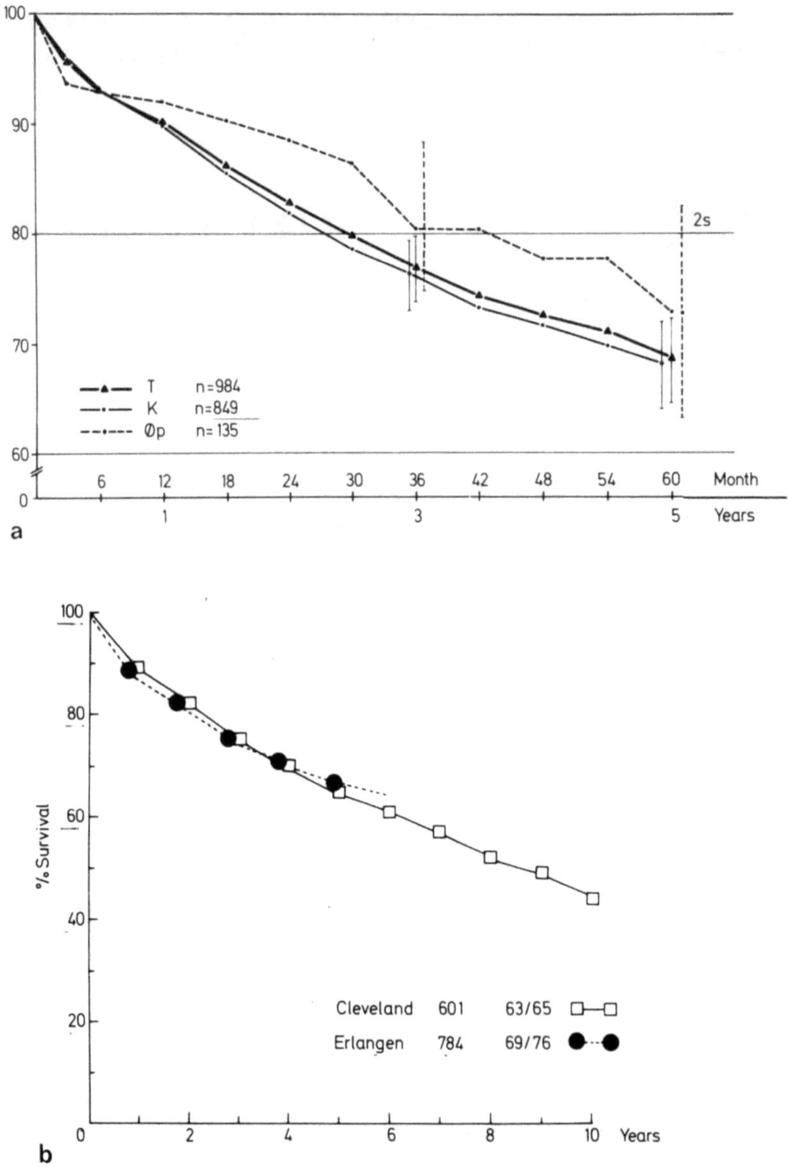

Fig. 2. a The cumulative 5-year survival rate with 95% confidence limits for 984 patients with significant CHD, compared with subgroup K (849 patients who were not considered candidates for coronary bypass surgery) and with subgroup OP (135 candidates for bypass surgery who were not operated on due to misgivings of the patients or the attending physicians. **b** Comparison of the long-term prognosis in the Cleveland Group with our own follow-up

survival rates were 68.5%, 67.9%, and 72.9% respectively. The 5% difference for the 5-year survival rate in both subgroups is not statistically significant. Thus, the following analysis of the influence of sex, age, severity of coronary artery disease, myocardial function, and collaterals can be made with the total group, assuming that the conservative group has the same prognosis as operative candidates who did not undergo bypass surgery.

The overall 5-year mortality in our study is almost identical with the long-term prognosis in the initial 5-year period reported in the Cleveland group, if one compares the cardiac survival of 601 men in the Cleveland group with 784 men aged 60 years or less in our follow-up (Fig. 2b). Because there were different periods of observation as regards medical treatment, we may conclude from these survival curves that changes in medical therapy in the early 1980s, such as the introduction of β-blockers, have not altered long-term prognosis with death as an end point.

In comparing the natural course of CHD according to sex, no statistically significant difference could be demonstrated between the 912 men and 72 women (Fig. 3a). Age did seem to have a statistically significant influence on long-term prognosis, however. The group of patients (K) aged 30–45 and 45–60 years had 5-year survival rates of 85.3% and 70.5% respectively (Fig. 3b). We excluded potential differences of both age-groups due to severity of coronary artery disease and left ventricular pump function by analyzing a more homogeneous group with the coronary score of 20–40 (II) and moderately impaired left ventricular pump function with an EF ranging from 30% to 60% (II). In these selected groups differences in long-term survival could no longer be demonstrated (Fig. 3c). Thus the "coronary factor" and "myocardial factor", and not age per se, are the causes of age-related differences in survival rates as reported by others (Proudfit et al. 1978).

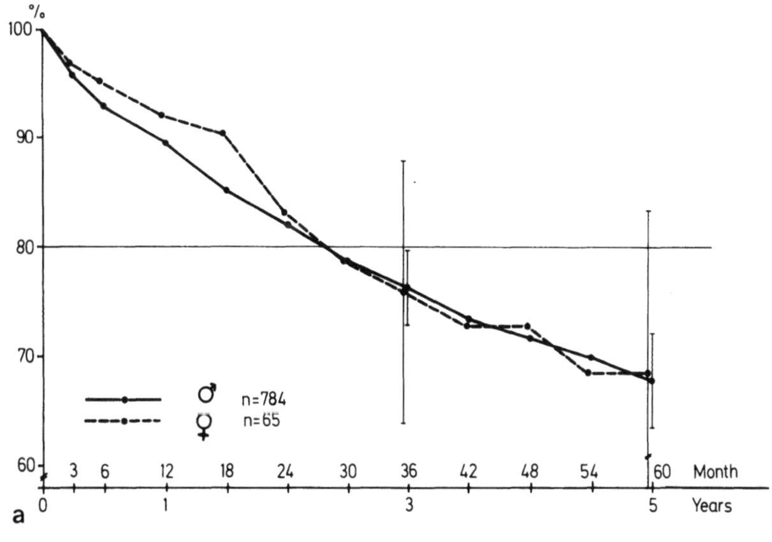

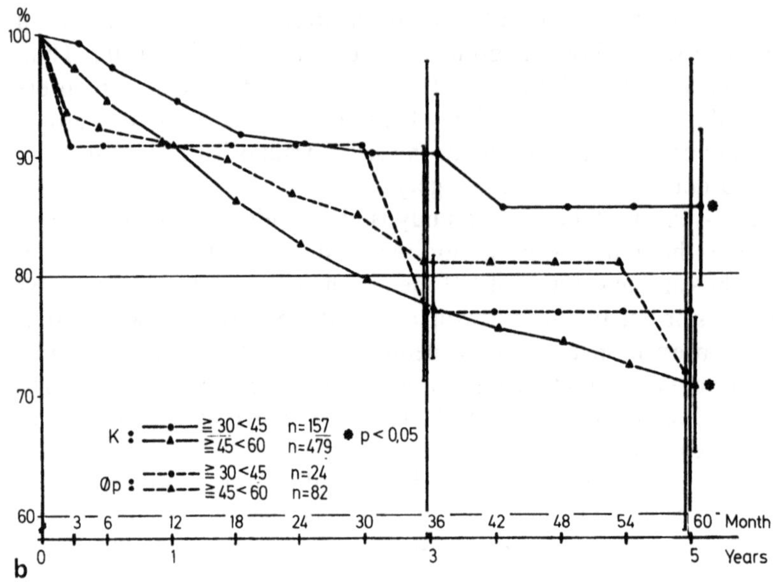

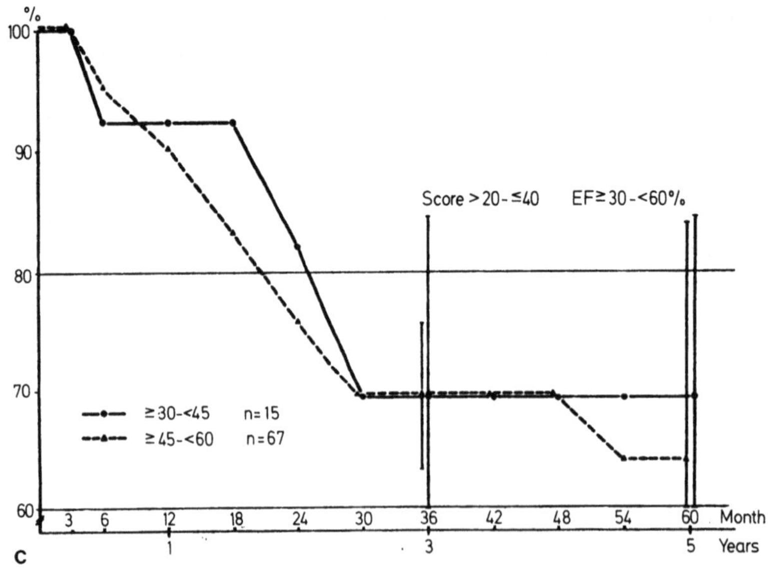

Fig. 3. a Sex-related long-term prognosis in CHD. Age-related 5-year survival, **b** in the groups *K* and *OP*, and **c**, in a homogeneous age-group adjusted for coronary score II and left ventricular ejection fraction II

It is known from the literature that long-term prognosis is markedly influenced by the severity and extent of coronary artery disease and the number of vessels involved (Burggraf and Parker 1975; Hammermeister et al. 1979; Lichtlen 1977, 1979; Steinbrunn and Lichtlen 1977). In our study patients with a maximum coronary score of 20 (I) were linked to a cardiac survival of 89.5%

in the first 5 years. This survival rate declined in the group with a score from 21–40 (II), and above (III), to 67.3% and 44.6% respectively (Fig. 4a). But a score of 35 (II), for example, must not necessarily have such a poor survival of 67.3% at the end of 5 years. The natural course of CHD is influenced in a statistically significant way by the myocardial factor, indicated in our study by left ventricular ejection fraction. Thus, in patients with normal EF (I), EF of 59%–30% (II), and EF of less than 30% (III) the 5-year survival rates are 63.1%, 36.4%, and 11.4% respectively (Fig. 4b). This clearly shows that the coronary

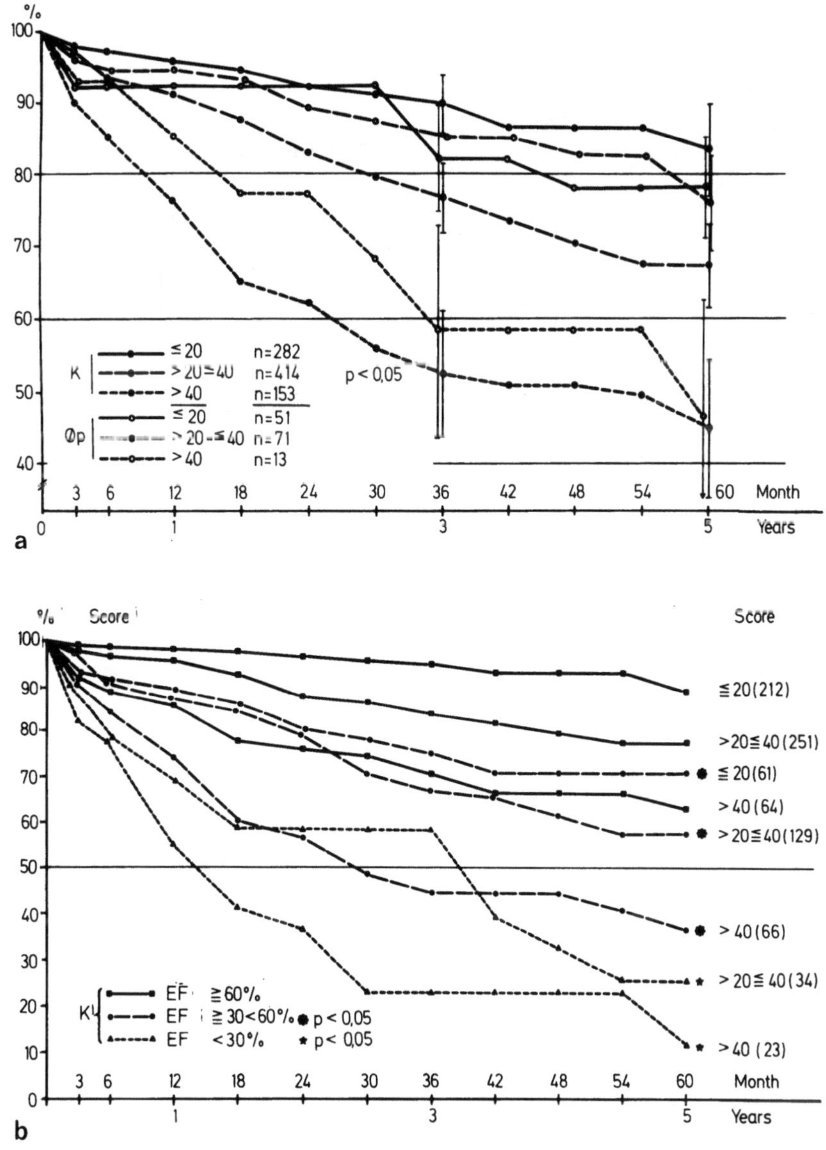

Fig. 4 a–b. Long-term prognosis of CHD **a** in regard to the coronary score and **b** in subgroups adjusted for left ventricular ejection fraction

score does not provide the entire prognostic message. For evaluation of the long-term prognosis one needs additional information about left ventricular pump function and wall abnormalities to decide whether the prognosis is better or worse than indicated by the "X-ray anatomy" of the coronary angiogram alone.

If we look at CHD the other way around, focusing only on left ventricular pump function, there is again a decline in 5-year survival according to the depression of pump function, with rates of 80.1%, 54.6%, and 20.6% respectively in the myocardial groups I, II, and III (Fig. 5a).

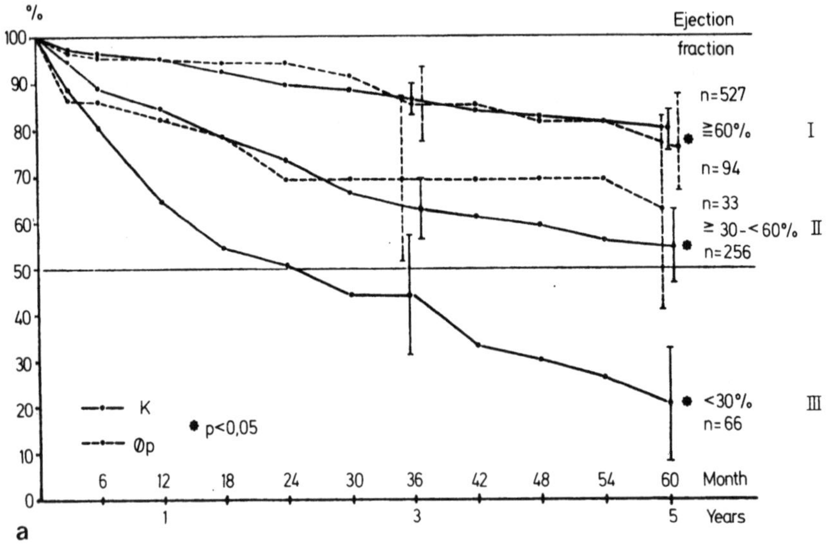

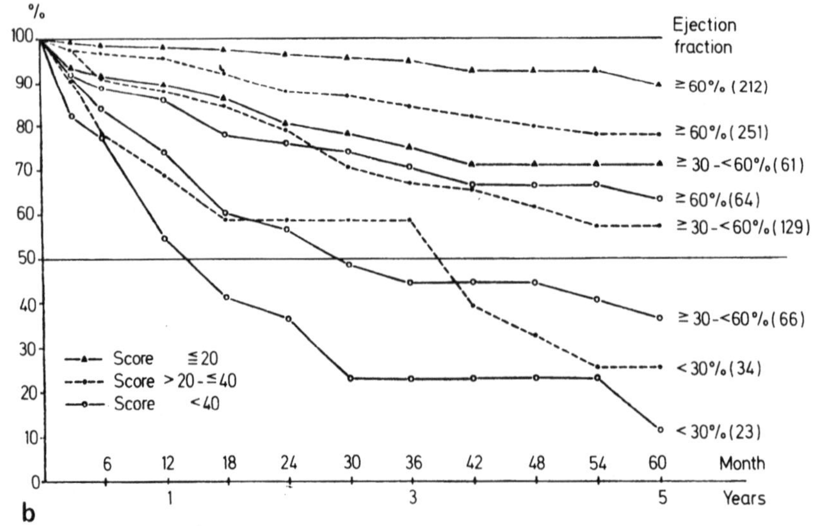

Fig. 5 a–b. Left ventricular ejection fraction, **a** as a predictor of long-term prognosis in CHD and **b** in sub-groups adjusted to the coronary score

Discussion has centered on the influence of collaterals on the natural history of CHD. In a group (K) of 310 patients without collaterals the 5-year survival rate is 70.3%, as compared with 66.4% in 539 patients with collaterals; in The OP subgroup the figures are 79.1% and 64.2% respectively (Fig. 6). These data, in contrast to a reported higher survival rate for coronary patients with collaterals (Webster et al. 1974), should not lead us to the false conclusion that collaterals per se worsen the long-term prognosis. Collateral circulation has to be considered a marker of advanced stages of CHD, and collaterals are therefore linked to a higher mortality than that for patients without angiographic evidence of collateral vessels. This can be documented by a mean coronary score in the "collateral group" of 31.3% as compared with 19.9% in the "noncollateral group."

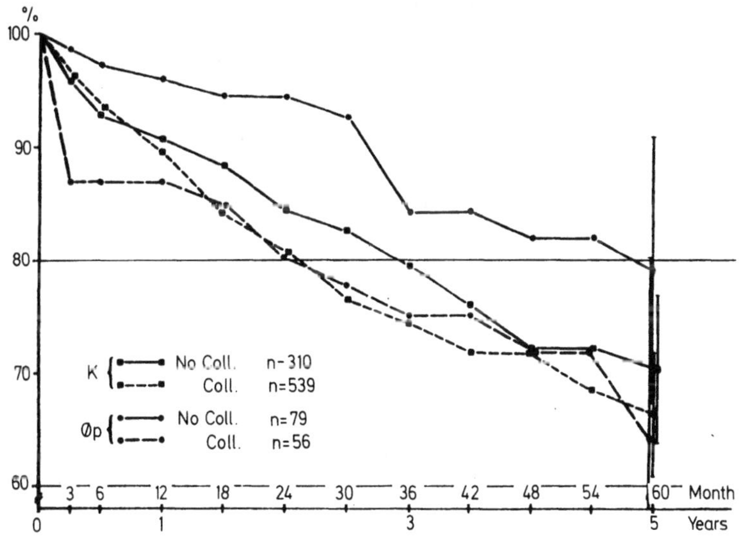

Fig. 6. Survival with CHD and collateral circulation

Returning to the basic influence of the coronary factor and the myocardial factor, the question arises whether we should focus primarily on the coronary score or on the EF. In other words, does the coronary factor dominate over the myocardial factor or vice versa? Or is the combination of both in a prognostic index a more predictive parameter of long-term prognosis? This was the reason for calculating 5-year survival rates for subgroups.

We decided to grade our patients according to a prognosis index which was formed from all potential combinations of the coronary factor (I, II, III) and the myocardial factor (I, II, III). Including normal subjects with coronary factor 0 and myocardial factor I, all possible combinations resulted in ten groups with the prognostic index 1–10 (Fig. 7). In a second step the 5-year survival rate for each index group was calculated and arranged according to the decline in long-term prognosis. When we looked at the 5-year survival rate according to the prognostic index a basic principle was revealed (Fig. 8):

1. For a given coronary score the long-term survival is determined by the left ventricular ejection fraction
2. Patients with an identical myocardial factor are discriminated by the coronary factor
3. In a given prognostic index such as 3, 4 or 5 the myocardial factor dominates over the coronary factor

This demonstrates clearly that long-term survial in coronary heart disease is primarily influenced by left ventricular anatomy and function. This finding is in agreement with reports in the literature that consider EF the most predictive parameter of long-term survival (Hammermeister et al. 1979; Lichtlen 1979).

Thus, the prognostic index of 2, for example, defines the subgroup of coronary patients with a low score of 20 or less and normal left ventricular pump function in whom the 5-year survival rate of 89.2% is close to that of the normal population. There are two indices, numbered 3a and 3b, which differentiate patients with the coronary score of 21–40 from those with 20 or less. Ejection fraction predominates in the long-term prognosis. The patient with more advanced coronary artery disease but still normal pump function (3a) has the better prognosis of 77.7%, as compared with 63.1% for the group with moderately reduced ejection fraction (3b). In the prognostic index of 4, three combinations of the coronary factor and the myocardial factor are possible: III+I, II+II, and I+III. Again, left ventricular pump function is the dominant factor in the determination of 5-year survival rates, declining from 63.1% to 57,3% and 48.5% according to the prognostic indices of 4a, 4b, and 4c.

The prognostic index of 5 includes the two combinations III+II or II+III, and again the long-term prognosis for patients with a coronary score exceeding 40 is better at 36.4%, than 25.4% for patients with less advanced coronary artery

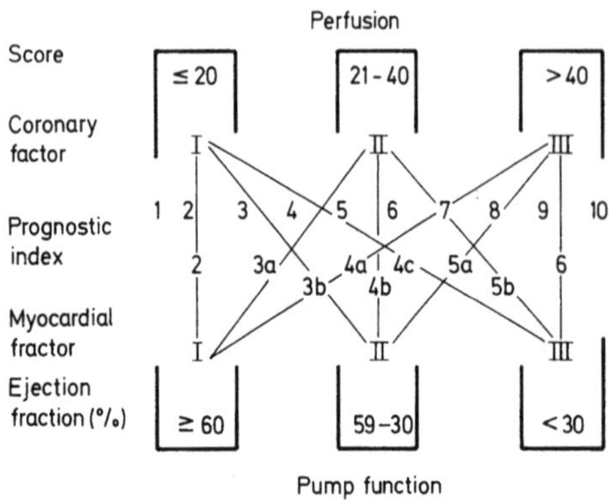

Fig. 7. The prognostic index of CHD as the sum of the *"coronary factor"* and the *"myocardial factor"*

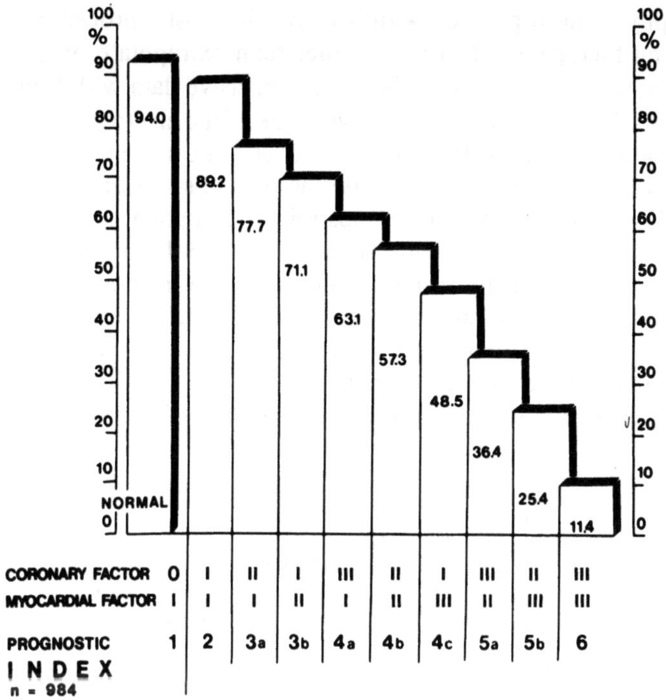

Fig. 8. The prognostic index of CHD as a predictor of 5-year survival in 984 patients with significant coronary artery disease

disease but critically depressed left ventricular pump function marked by an EF of less than 30%.

The coronary index of 6 has only one combination, III + III, which means a coronary score of more than 40 and left ventricular ejection fraction below 30%. Therefore, in this subgroup both the coronary factor and the myocardial factor are at the worst end of the prognostic scale. These high-risk coronary patients have only 11.4% probability of 5-year survival.

The information from the prognostic index is concise and simple. In our experience, the combination of the coronary factor and the myocardial factor in a prognostic index scale of ten different groups seems to be highly predictive in evaluating long-term prognosis. This is why we prefer angiographic data in evaluating the natural history of CHD. It is obvious that symptoms of coronary heart disease, electrocardiographic abnormalities, risk factors, and arrhythmias have some bearing on the natural course of coronary heart disease. But these and other noninvasive parameters correlate poorly with angiographic data. This leads to the conclusion that noninvasive methods are less reliable in predicting longevity. There is no doubt that statistical analysis and constructed survival curves based on angina, ST-segment depression, bundle-branch block, arrhythmias, and risk factors will discriminate to some extent (Kannel and Feinleib 1972; Keys et al. 1971; Sigler 1951; Zukel et al. 1969). But the message of a poor prognosis based on these parameters may motivate both, patient and physician to proceed with invasive diagnostic procedures, especially for making therapeutic decisions, rather than extrapolate on 5- and 10-year survival rates. The poor correlation of noninvasive data with long-term prognosis may be illustrated by the predictive value of the electrocardiogram in postinfarction patients (Fig. 9). In daily routine, electrocardiographic patterns of transmural necrosis are taken to evaluate the patient's short-term and long-term outcome. If we study a group of 123 postinfarction patients with transmural anterior wall infarction and infarction pattern in 1-2, 3-4, and 5-6 precordial leads, only a small, statistically insignificant difference in long-term survival may be seen. The 5-year survival rate in this selected group is 77.4%. But after discrimination by left ventricular pump function the 5-year survival rate will vary, according to the myocardial factor, between 95% and 0%, depending on whether left ventricular pump function is normal, moderately reduced, or critically depressed.

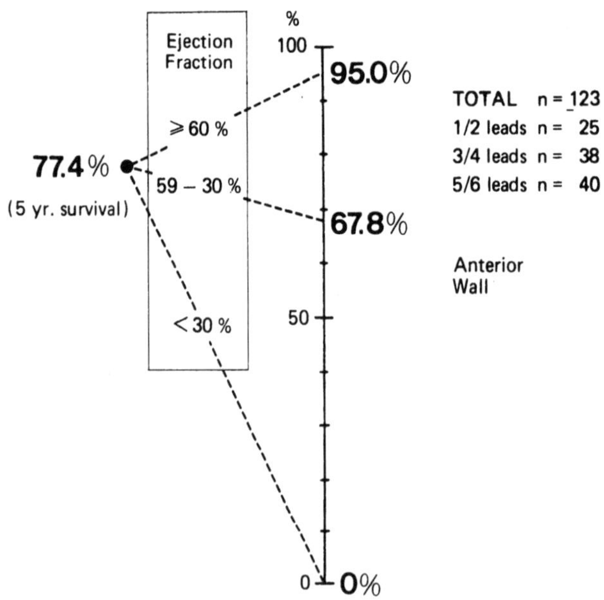

Fig. 9. Five-year survival rate in 123 postmyocardial infarction patients, and in subgroups with identical electrocardiographic patterns of anterior wall infarction but different left ventricular ejection fractions

Conclusion

Evaluation of the natural course of CHD, which is identical with the nonoperative course under medical treatment and usual care, requires information about both the coronary factor and the myocardial factor and, therefore, invasive methods. This does not disqualify noninvasive methods from providing information, especially on short-term prognosis, and thereby evaluating the patient at risk of myocardial infarction. Thus, noninvasive methods are of more help in deciding whether or not coronary angiography should be untertaken. Only the "X-ray anatomy" provides the information needed for precise evaluation of long-term prognosis and therapeutic decisions on medical treatment, bypass surgery, and transluminal dilatation. Angiography is most predictive in the evaluation of the natural course of CHD, and for surpasses all other invasive and noninvasive methods.

References

AHA (1975) Committee for Grading Coronary Artery Disease. Council on Cardiovascular Surgery. A reporting system on patients evaluated for coronary artery disease. Circulation 51:759

Berkson J, Gage, RP (1950) Calculation of survival rates for cancer. Mayo Clin Proc 25:270

Bruschke AVG, Proudfit WL, Sones FM (1973) Clinical course of patients with normal and slightly or moderately abnormal coronary arteriograms. A follow-up study on 500 patients. Circulation 47:936

Burggraf GW, Parker JO (1975) Prognosis in coronary artery disease. Angiographic, hemodynamic and clinical factors. Circulation 57:146

De Bakey ME, Diethrich EB, Liddicoat IE, Garret HE (1968) Poster exhibited at Baylor University Coll Med, Texas Medical Center, Houston

Hammermeister KE, Timothy A, De Rouen TA, Dodge HT (1979) Variables predictive of survival in patients with coronary disease. Circulation: 59:421

Humphries J, O'Neal J, Kuller L, Ross RS, Friesinger GC, Page EE (1974) Natural history of ischemic heart disease in relation to arteriographic findings. A twelve year study of 224 patients. Circulation 49:489

Kannel WB, Feinleib M (1972) Natural history of angina pectoris in the Framingham Study. Prognosis and survival. Am J Cardiol 29:154

Keys A, Tayler HL, Blackburn H, Borgek J, Anderson JT, Simonson E (1971) Mortality and coronary heart disease among men studied for 23 years. Arch Intern Med 128:201

Lichtlen PR (1977) Natural history of coronary artery disease based on coronary angiography, a critical review. In: The first decade of bypass graft surgery for coronary artery disease. Syllabus, Cleveland, p 117

Lichtlen PR (1979) Koronarangiographie und Prognose der koronare Herzkrankheit. In: Lichtlen PR (ed) Koronarangiographie, Perimed, Erlangen

Proudfit WL, Bruschke AVG, Sones F (1978) Natural history of obstructive coronary artery disease. Ten-year study of 601 nonsurgical cases. Prog Cardiovasc Dis 21:53

Sigler LH (1951) Prognosis of angina pectoris and coronary occlusions. Follow-up of 1700 cases. JAMA 146:998

Steinbrunn W, Lichtlen PR (1977) Complete 5-year cumulative survival rates in 244 unselected unoperated coronary patients undergoing angiography. Circulation 55/56 [Suppl III]:174

Taylor GJ, O'Neal J, Humphries J, Mellits ED, Pitt B, Schulze RA, Griffith LSC, Achuff SC (1980) Predictors of clinical course, coronary anatomy and left ventricular function after recovery from acute myocardial infarction. Circulation 62:960

Webster JS, Moberg C, Rincon G (1974) Natural history of servere proximal coronary artery disease as documented by coronary cineangiography. Am J Cardiol 33:195

Zukel WJ, Cohen BM, Mattingly TW, Hrubec Z (1969) Survival following first diagnosis of coronary heart disease. Am Heart J 18:159

Prognosis of Coronary Heart Disease Patients Evaluated by Data Obtained by Angiography and Exercise Testing

R. Balcon, M. Cattell, and K. Wong
London Chest Hospital, Bonner Road, E2, London 9JX, W1, Great Britain

The prognosis in coronary artery disease has been shown, not surprisingly, to be dependent on the severity of the disease as judged by coronary and left ventricular angiography (Oberman et al. 1972; Bruschke et al. 1973; Reeves et al. 1974). The usual system for analysis of the coronary arteriogram has been to describe patients as falling into one-, two-, or three-vessel disease categories. This is a very simple classification which leaves scope for considerable error. Most patients have at least five, and some as many as eight major arteries supplying the left ventricular myocardium. Two patients described as having three-vessel disease could be very different, one with three of eight arteries involved and the other with all eight. Each of these individual vessels is important, and has to be evaluated if the extent of the disease is to be accurately described. The simple approach also takes into account only one major stenosis in each vessel system ignoring other stenoses and the site of the lesions. Importance of site is demonstrated by the well-known poor prognosis in patients with left main coronary lesions (Cohen et al. 1972; Pichard et al. 1973; Webster et al. 1974). The effects of multiple stenoses are probably more than additive, so attention to only the more severe stenoses does not give an adequate representation of the reduction of myocardial blood flow, which is one of the critical factors in determining the symptoms of ischaemic heart disease. A second critical factor is the amount of myocardium prejudiced by a stenosis, which must determine the outcome of sudden events, such as infarction resulting from changes related to that stenosis. Minor lesions cannot be ignored, as they may also be involved in the causation of sudden cardiac events. These factors are, to a variable extent, ameliorated by collateral flow. It is very important, therefore, to take all of them into account when assessing the coronary circulation.

Method

Various systems of scoring coronary angiographic abnormalities have been used in an attempt to overcome some of these difficulties (Friesinger et al. 1970; Gensini 1975). The data presented here combine information obtained by categorising patients according to the number of lesions in the three main coronary trunks with an index of overall severity of coronary disease (Balcon 1980). The index takes into account the site and severity of all lesions in the coronary circulation. It adds weight to lesions that occur in series in any vessel or vessel system and scores vessels that are normal. Each lesion is graded 1–4, 4 being total occlusion; grade 1 is stenosis of less than 50%, 2 of 51%–75%, and 3 of 76%–99%. The coronary circulation is coded for 13 branches, the left main stem and three main trunks, right, anterior descending and circumflex. Eight possible terminal branches are described, three inferior left ventricular branches from the right coronary artery, three circumflex branches, the diagonal and anterior descending beyond the diagonal branch. Not all branches are identified in all patients. The index is mathematically computed by weighting each arterial lesion according to its severity, with weights increasing by 25% for each stenosis grade. Lesions in parallel are added and lesions in series multiplied. The right and left coronary artery systems start with a numerical score of 1 which is then reduced by the lesions present as described. The score for each branch is added and divided by the number of terminal branches identified and the final score (Coronary Index, CI) expressed as a percentage. High scores represent minor disease and low, severe. The left ventricle was scored from the right oblique ventriculogram. The anterior, apical and inferior walls were considered to contract normally, or to be hypokinetic, akinetic or dyskinetic. The average numbers of abnormally contracting segments (LV score) were noted in various subgroups of patients. The angiographic data from which these scores are derived are recorded on computer mark sense cards together with clinical and follow-up data.

Patients

The data bank now consists of information from 4000 patients examined for known or suspected coronary artery disease. The policy determining which patients were investigated and their subsequent management has varied over the years of the study. Initially, all patients suspected of disease underwent angiography, but a more conservative policy has been adopted in the past 3 or 4 years, and some patients with a satisfactory exercise test result have not been catheterised. The surgical policy has also changed and most patients with limiting symptoms are now recommended for surgery even of they have diffuse disease. Some patients with left main stem or severe proximal three-vessel disease have been operated upon mainly for prophylactic reasons. Angiographic and exercise test data are now available from 1512 patients who have been treated medically. A number of them refused surgery. It is a heterogeneous group of patients - some with mild disease, some with diffuse disease thought unsuitable for surgery during the early part of the study, and those who refused operation. Finally, a small group of them were part of a random allocation trial of medical and surgical therapy (Varnauskas et al. 1979).

Results

Accurate survival data depend on full mortality reporting. In this study it is almost 100%, since the patients were identified by the Registrars General of Great Britain. Non-cardiac deaths are excluded if possible but a previous study has shown that there is very little difference in survival curves if all deaths are included (Proudfit et al. 1978). There were 178 deaths (11.8%) in the first 5 years of follow-up. Data are available from 594 bicycle ergometer exercise tests. Patients who achieved a maximum load of 600–750 Kpm/min had a 94% 5-year survival, compared with 76% for those who reached 450 Kpm/min or less ($p<0.02$). There were significant differences ($p<0.05$) between the survival curves of patients divided according to their exercise test end point. Five-year survival for those limited by fatigue was 95%; for those limited by angina or ST segment depression it was 90%, and for those limited by dyspnoea, 87%. Five-year actuarial survival curves were constructed according to the presence of at least 50% stenosis in the left main stem or one, two, or all three main coronary trunks (Fig. 1). Patients with distal disease only are also represented; they have the best survival. The patients with left main stem lesions have the worst, and the curves for three, two, and one main trunk lesion follow, in that order. The difference between the curves is significant ($p<0.01$, Wilcoxon rank sum test). Curves have also been constructed according to coronary index quartiles. These also rank in order of severity of disease, with similar significance levels (Fig. 1). The number of abnormal left ventricular segments increased significantly ($p<0.01$) with increasing severity of coronary disease, except for the left main stem group which was not worse than the three-vessel disease group. The effect of the left ventricular abnormality seems, at least to a certain extent, to be contained in the coronary angiographic data, although an additional independent effect cannot be excluded.

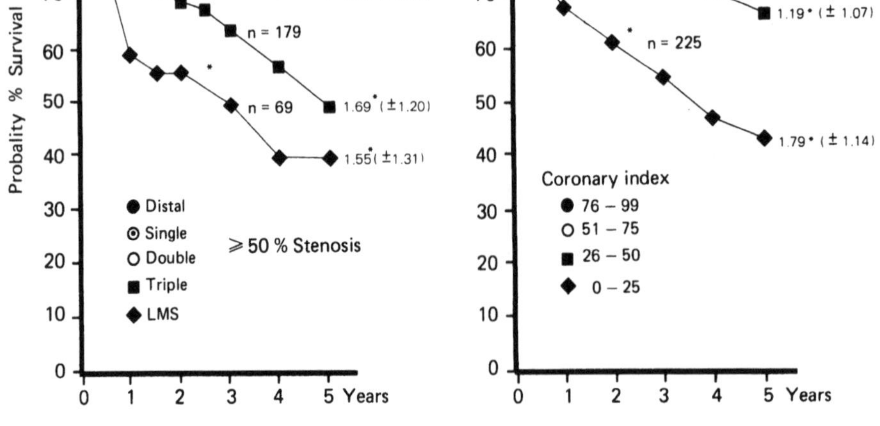

Fig. 1. Curves for 5-year survival constructed according to number of ≥50% main vessel stenoses (*left*) and to Coronary Index (*right*). *Asterisks*, $p<0.01$

These two methods of analysis of the angiographic data provide different information. For example, patients with three main trunk lesions appear in the first three coronary index quartiles (Fig. 2). The data have therefore been combined and survival curves constructed for the appropriate coronary index quartiles within the subgroups with one, two, and three main trunk lesions. Of the patients with three main trunk lesions, 98% had a CI below 50. The 5-year survival was 57% for the whole group, 71% for those with CI 26–50 and 33% for those with CI 0–25. The difference between these and subsequent survival curves is significant at the 1% level unless otherwise stated. The LV score was 1.25 (1.17 SD) for CI group 26–50, and 1.93 ($\pm$1.14 SD) $p<0.001$.

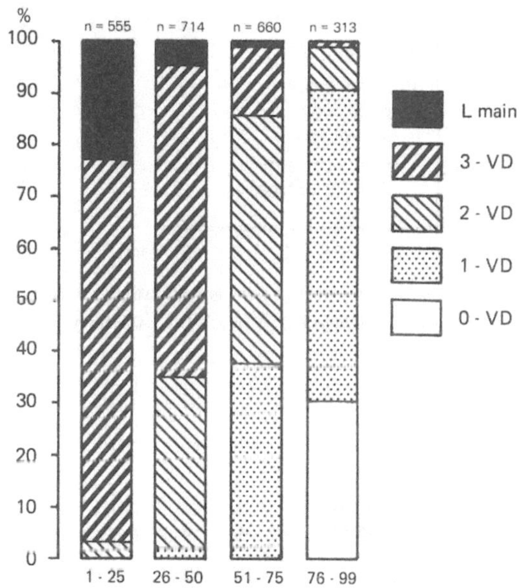

Fig. 2. Correlation of main vessel disease (*VD*) categories [vessel disease $\geq$grade II stenosis (33%–66%)] with Coronary Index quartiles

It is possible that the low-CI group included patients with more severe proximal lesions which completely accounted for the lower score, and the presence of other lesions did not influence the survival pattern. The results are similar, however, if the data are analysed from patients with 75% or more stenosis rather than 50%. The 5-year survival for these patients is similar but at lower levels. It was 35% for the whole group, 66% for the CI 26–50 subgroup, (LV score 1.39$\pm$SD 1.21) and 25% for the CI 0–25 subgroup (LV score 2.13$\pm$SD 1.06). The survival curves for all patients with three main trunk lesions are shown in Fig. 3. The difference between the best and worst is 45%. The patients with one main trunk lesion can be divided into three coronary index subgroups. Five-year survival for CI 26–50 was 93% (LV score 0.53$\pm$SD 0.76), for CI 51–75 was 85% (LV score 0.77$\pm$SD 0.86), and for CI 26–50 was 61% (LV

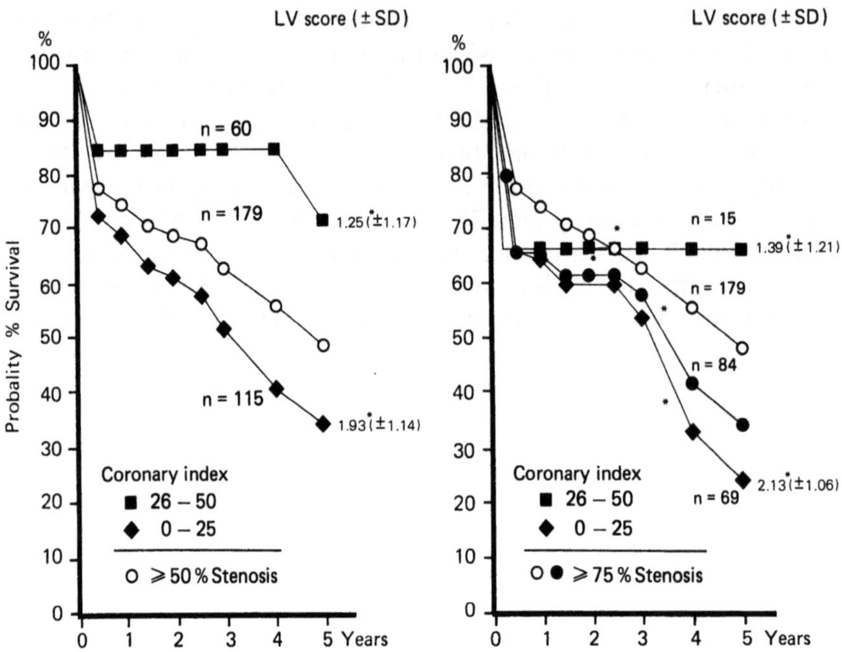

Fig. 3. Five-year survival curves for patients with lesions of three main vessels – *left*, stenoses ≥50%; *right*, stenoses ≥75% – with Coronary Index subgroups. *Asterisks*, $P<0.001$

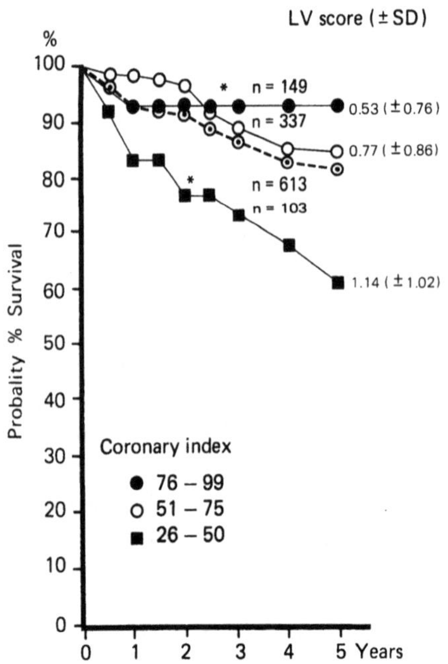

Fig. 4. Five-year survival curves for patients with lesions of one main vessel (≥50% stenosis), with Coronary Index subgroups. *Asterisks*, $p<0.001$

score 1.14±SD 1.02). The figure for the whole group was 81% (Fig. 4). The patients with two main trunk lesions appear to be a more homogeneous group, although the subgroup with CI 63–75 had a 5-year survival of 90% (LV score 0.85±SD 0.95), compared with 71% for the whole group and 70% (LV score 1.20±SD 0.07) for those with CI 0–62.

Discussion

The patients described here were all United Kingdom residents and attended one hospital for cardiological care. In addition to the usual methods of hospital out-patient visits and communication with attending physicians and with patients and their families, indexing of patients with the Registrars General of Great Britain was done. This ensured that mortality reporting was as close to 100% as possible. The addition of registration was in fact the only method that disclosed approximately 30% of the deaths. Caution is therefore needed when judging reports of survival. An early study (Zukel et al. 1969) suggested annual mortality for patients with coronary artery disease of between 3% and 5%, depending upon whether they presented with angina pectoris or myocardial infarction. These patients did not undergo coronary arteriography, so the diagnosis is not confirmed nor is its severity assessed. Later angiographically controlled studies demonstrated that mortality depended on both coronary and left ventricular abnormalities (Oberman et al. 1972, Bruschke et al. 1973, Reeves et al. 1974), was approximately 6% per annum overall, and ranged from approximately 2% for one-vessel disease to 15%–20% for three-vessel disease. The situation was worse for left main stem stenosis. It was also generally worse when the left ventricular angiogram was also abnormal. One group reported a worse prognosis in the first year after investigation (Bruschke et al. 1973).

These patients had a 2.4% annual mortality for the 5-year follow-up period. This is the same as the figure reported by Proudfit et al. (1978) for the first 4 years of a 10-year study of 601 medically treated patients. They did notice, however, that mortality was greater in the subsequent 6 years, at approximately 5% per annum. This and all other studies have found increasing mortality with increasing involvement of main arterial trunks. The effect of disease in the smaller coronary branches and of "noncritical" stenoses has been less well studied. In 1970 Friesinger et al. introduced a scoring system for the coronary arteriogram. Each main vessel was scored 1–5, indicating both severity and diffuseness of the lesions. They demonstrated in a 12-year follow-up that mortality was related to total score (Humphries et al. 1974). Proudfit et al. (1978) also observed an adverse effect of "noncritical" (30%–50%) stenoses of right and circumflex vessels on survival of patients with major lesions of the anterior descending artery. Data reported here show a quite marked effect of distal coronary disease on the survival of patients with involvement of one, two, or three main trunks with, for instance, a 45% difference in 5-year survival within the three-vessel disease group.

The amount of left ventricular damage is clearly also a determinant of survival, but these data suggest that it may not be entirely independent. Hammermeister et al. (1979) found that left ventricular ejection fraction was the most valuable predictor of mortality at 2 years, using a multivariate analysis of 46 variables. They also observed that the addition of information on the coronary lesions did not improve prediction. This was not, in fact, a sufficiently strong predictor in the prior univariate analysis to be included in the multivariate test. The authors, however, intuitively reintroduced it and it was finally selected as one of the four variables most helpful in prediction. The difference in their survival data and those reported is almost certainly related to the shorter follow-up and the use of an indicator of global left ventricular function rather than regional, which represents a more severe abnormality. It is possible - and, in fact, likely - that this affects short-term survival and that in the long term the severity of the coronary disease has a more important effect.

Data derived from exercise tests have been shown to be predictive of future coronary events. The occurrence of chest pain, a low maximum work load, failure to reach 90% of predicted maximal heart rate and "ischaemic" ST-segment depression were predictors both in normal subjects (Bruce et al. 1980) and in patients with coronary disease (Bruce et al. 1977). In this study there was a significant difference in survival between those who achieved 750 Kpm/min or more and the rest of the group. There was a greater difference in the patients with more severe disease (CI 0-50). In this subgroup there was approximately 40% difference in 5-year mortality between those whose maximum was 600 Kpm/min or more and the remainder of the group. The occurrence of chest pain was a predictor of mortality but less so than if the test was terminated by dyspnoea. This is to be expected, since it is a manifestation of global left ventricular ventricular dysfunction which is associated with early mortality.

In summary, mortality in patients with coronary artery disease is dependent on the severity of not only the major stenoses in the main coronary vessels but also the other lesions in both the main and distal vessels. Exercise test results are also predictive of outcome on their own, and add information when the results of angiography are known.

References

Balcon R (1980) Prognostic significance of coronary arteriography. Acta Med Port [Suppl) 1:9

Bruce RA, DeRouen TA, Peterson DR (1977) Noninvasive predictors of sudden cardiac death in men with coronary heart disease. Predictive value of maximal exercise testing. Am J Cardiol 39:833

Bruce RA, DeRouen TA, Hossack KF (1980) Value of maximal exercise tests in risk assessment of primary coronary heart disease events in healthy men. Five years' experience of the Seattle Heart Watch study. Am J Cardol 46:371

Bruschke AVG, Proudfit WL, Sones FM (1973) Progress study of 590 consecutive non-surgical cases of coronary disease followed 5-9 years. Arteriographic correlations. Circulation 47:1147

Cohen MV, Cohn PF, Herman MV, Gorlin R (1972) Diagnosis and prognosis of main left coronary artery obstruction. Circulation 45 [Suppl 1]:57

Friesinger GC, Page EE, Ross RS (1970) Prognostic significance of coronary arteriography. Trans Assoc Am Physicians 83:78

Gensini GC (1975) Coronary arteriography. Futura, New York
Hammermeister KE, DeRouen TA, Dodge HT (1979) Variables predictive of survival in patients with coronary disease. Circulation 59:421
Humphries JO, Kuller L, Ross RS, Friesinger GC, Page EE (1974) Natural history of ischemic heart disease in relation to arteriographic findings. Circulation 49:489–497
Oberman A, Jones WB, Riley CP (1972) Natural history of coronary artery disease. Bull NY Acad Med 48:1109–1125
Pichard AD, Sheldon WC, Shinji K, Effler DB, Sones FM, (Jnr) (1973) Severe arteriosclerotic obstruction of the left main coronary artery: follow-up results in 176 patients. Circulation 48 [Suppl 4]:53
Proudfit WL, Bruschke AV, Sones FM (1978) Natural history of obstructive coronary artery disease: ten year study of 601 non-surgical cases. Prog Cardiovasc Dis 21:2, 53
Reeves TJ, Oberman A, Jones WB, Sheffield LT (1974) Natural history of angina pectoris. Am J Cardol 33:423
Varnauskas E (1979) European coronary surgery study group. Lancet 1:889
Webster JS, Moberg C, Rincon G (1974) Natural history of severe proximed coronary artery disease as documented by coronary cineangiography. Am J Cardiol 33:195–200
Zukel WL, Cohen BM, Mattingly TW, Hrubec Z (1969) Survival following first diagnosis of coronary heart disease. Am Heart J 78:159

Prognostic Relevance of Findings from Invasive and Noninvasive Investigations in Coronary Heart Disease Patients

M. Kaltenbach and W.-D. Bussmann

Klinikum der Johann Wolfgang Goethe-Universität, Zentrum der Inneren Medizin, Abteilung für Kardiologie, Theodor-Stern-Kai 7, 6000 Frankfurt/Main 70, FRG

More than 200 years ago Heberden noticed that among patients with disorders of the chest, the group with typical angina pectoris had a much worse prognosis as compared with patients with atypical, i.e., non-stress-related chest pain. Many years later it became clear that typical angina pectoris is the consequence of coronary artery obstruction. The term coronary heart disease refers to coronary atherosclerosis, the most common cause of coronary artery narrowing, and to its clinical manifestations such as angina pectoris and myocardial infarction.

Patients with diagnosed coronary heart disease can be subdivided according to prognosis. The two main prognostic indicators are the degree of coronary artery obstruction and the degree of left ventricular dysfunction (Friesinger et al. 1970, Bruschke et al. 1973). Despite the fact that myocardial infarction is the consequence of coronary obstruction the two parameters are not necessarily closely related in any given patient. In some patients - particularly younger ones - we may observe very severe myocardial damage despite involvement of only one major coronary artery, while in others we may be faced with normal left ventricular function in spite of severe obstruction of all major coronary arteries. Figures 1 and 2 show typical examples.

In 1973 Bruschke et al. published the prognostic implications of coronary angiographic findings based on the extensive experience of the Cleveland Clinic. Many investigators have confirmed these findings, which showed a close correlation between the degree of coronary artery narrowing and the long-term prognosis. Bruschke found that involvement of one, two, or three vessels or of the left main coronary artery had a significant influence on 7-year survival. One-, two-, and three-vessel disease was defined as vessel narrowing of 50% or more seen on coronary arteriography. Bruschke has noted, however, that obstructions of less than 50% are also of importance. If patients with single-vessel disease have additional involvement of the other vessels to a lesser degree than 50% the prognosis is markedly worse than that for patients with single-vessel disease without any involvement of other branches (Fig. 3).

More quantitative information from the coronary arteriogram can be derived if a scoring system is used, taking into account the degree of narrowing, the localization and extension of coronary obstructions, and predominance of the right or left coronary artery (Kaltenbach 1975; Figs. 4 and 5). Using such a score we found very good correlation to 7-year survival in patients catheterized in the years 1970–1973 and followed up over the next 7 years. Subgroups formed according to this score represent patient groups with 7-year survival rates ranging from more than 95% to 40% (Fig. 6).

To evaluate the influence of left ventricular impairment on prognosis Bruschke subdivided his patients according to normal left ventricular function, local dysfunction, and diffuse scar formation. He found a marked correlation to prognosis.

A more quantitative evaluation of the left ventriculogram can be based on a scoring system with values between 0 and 12. If patients are grouped according to this score the significant discrimination of long-term survival is apparent. Patients with very severe ventricular dysfunction apparently have a particularly bad prognosis (Fig. 7).

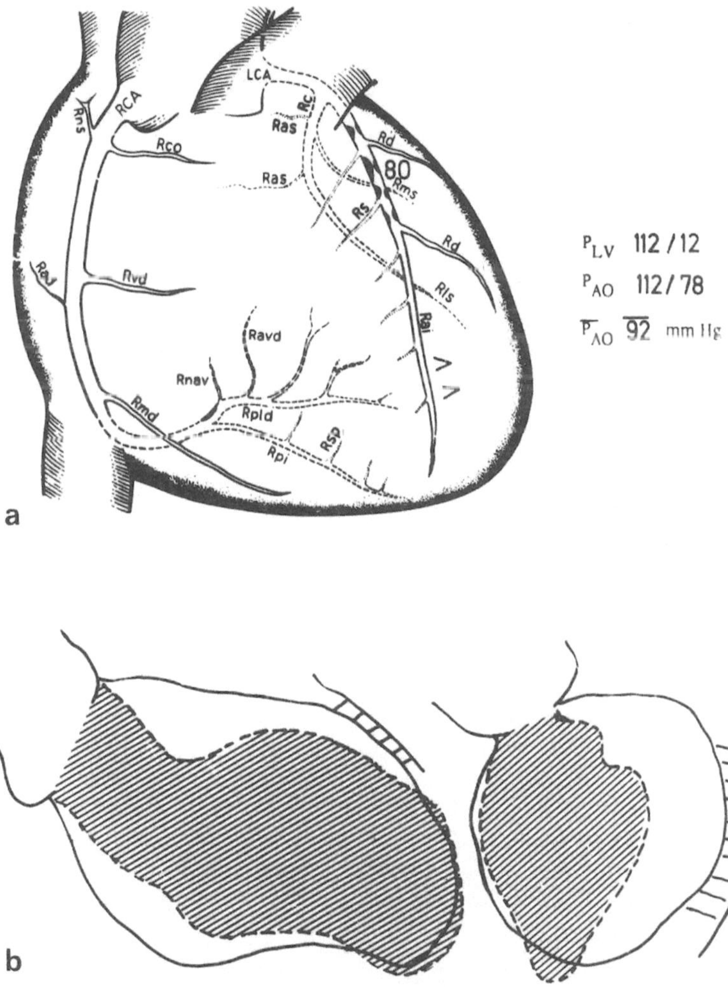

Fig. 1. a Eighty percent stenosis of left anterior descending artery in a 43-year-old man, with right predominance; despite only single-vessel involvement there is severe left ventricular dysfunction. **b** Ventriculograms of end diastole and end systole; RAO (*left*), LAO (*right*). There is extensive akinesia of the septum and anterior wall

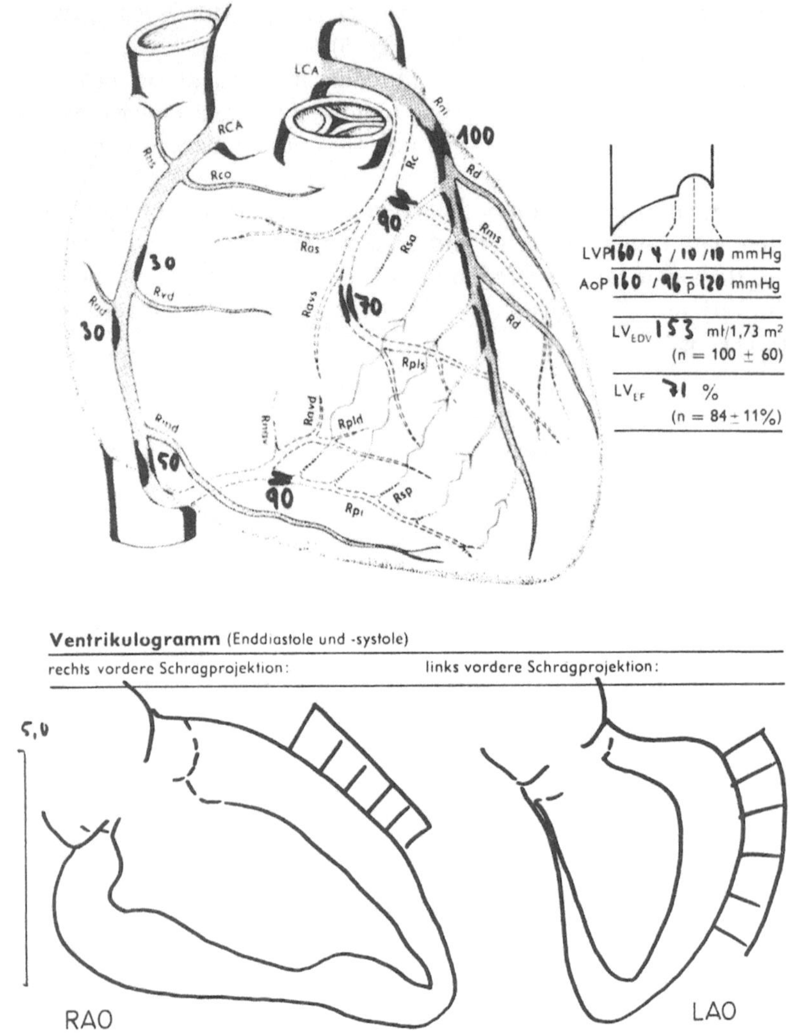
LCA
RCA
Rco
100
90
70
30
30
50
90
Ras
Rsa
Ravs
Rvd
Rpls
Rpld
Rsp
Rpi
Rd
Rms
Rc
LVP 160 / 4 / 10 / 10 mmHg
AoP 160 / 96 p̄ 120 mmHg
LV EDV 153 ml/1,73 m²
(n = 100 ± 60)
LV EF 71 %
(n = 84 ± 11%)
Ventrikulogramm (Enddiastole und -systole)
rechts vordere Schragprojektion:
links vordere Schragprojektion:
5,0
RAO
LAO

a

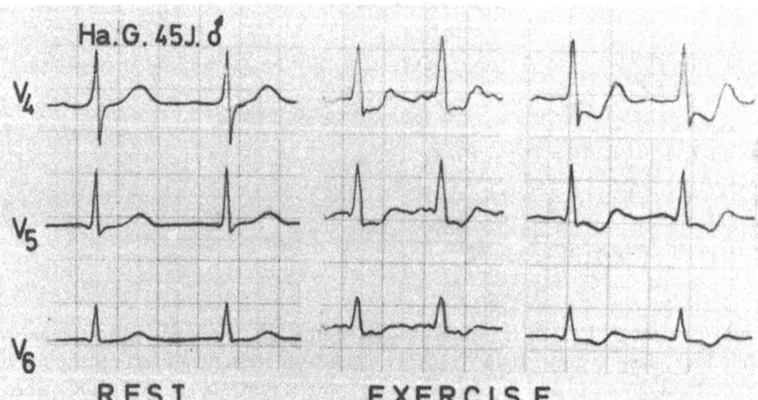
Ha.G. 45J. ♂
V4
V5
V6
REST
EXERCISE

b

◀ **Fig. 2. a** Triple-vessel disease in a 45-year-old man. There is obstruction of the left anterior descending artery (*Ria*) and subtotal stenosis of the right coronary artery (*RCA*) and the circumflex artery (*Rms* and *Rpls*). Despite severe coronary artery involvement left ventricular function remains normal. *Numbers* on diagram refer to percentage of stenosis: 10%–20%, wall irregularity; 30%–90%, stenosis; 100%, occlusion. Ventriculograms of end diastole and end systole. *n*, normal values
b ECG from same patient at rest, and showing ischemic ST depression during (*middle*) and after (*right*) exercise

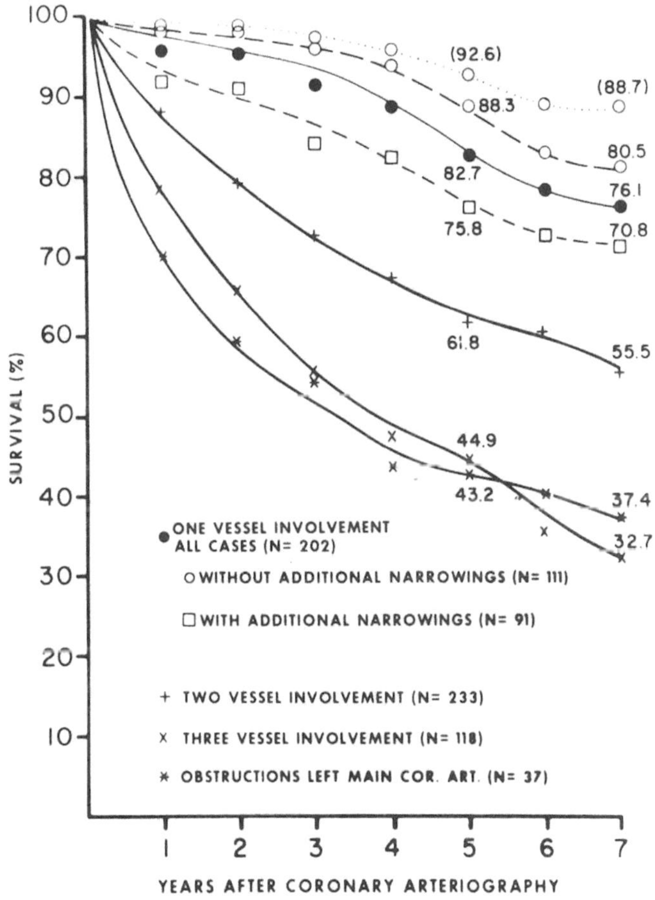

Fig. 3. Seven-year survival according to severity of coronary artery involvement. One-, two-, and three-vessel, and left main involvement are clearly correlated to prognosis. *Dotted line* represents cardiac mortality alone for the group with only single-vessel disease; in the other groups cardiac mortality and total mortality were similar. (Bruschke et al. 1973a)

If the degree of coronary artery obstruction and the degree of left ventricular impairment are correlated, it becomes evident that in patients with very severe left ventricular dysfunction prognosis is extremely poor, regardless of whether one, two, or three vessels are involved (Fig. 8).

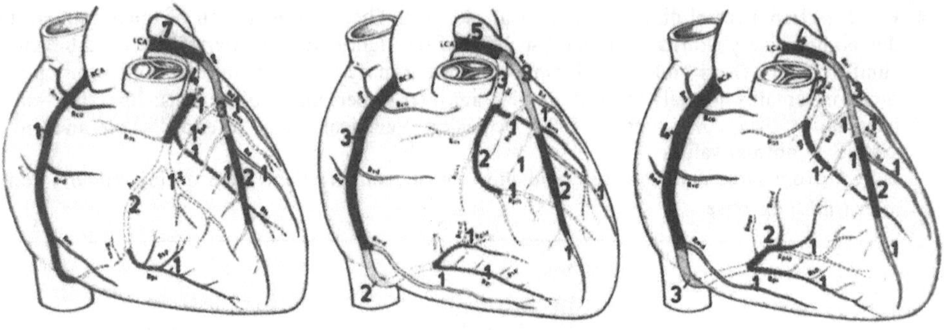

Left predominance Balanced perfusion Right predominance

Stenosis %	1-39	40-59	60-79	80-99	100
Factor	1	2	3	4	5

a

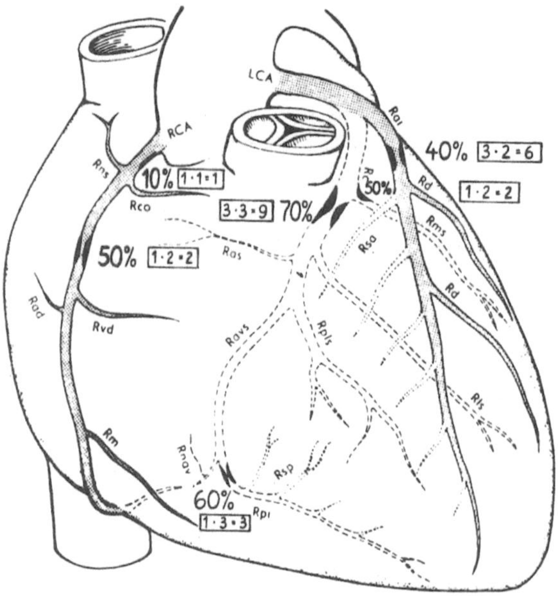

b Score = 2 + 1 + 3 + 9 + 2 + 6 = 23

Fig. 4. a Coronary scoring system. Each segment has a number according to hemodynamic importance in respect to perfusion type. If stenosis is present, the number of the involved segment is multiplied by a factor, according to the degree of narrowing (*table*). The sum of the values obtained for each stenosis represents the severity of coronary artery involvement
b Example of scoring, in which the sum of the values of six different stenoses is 23

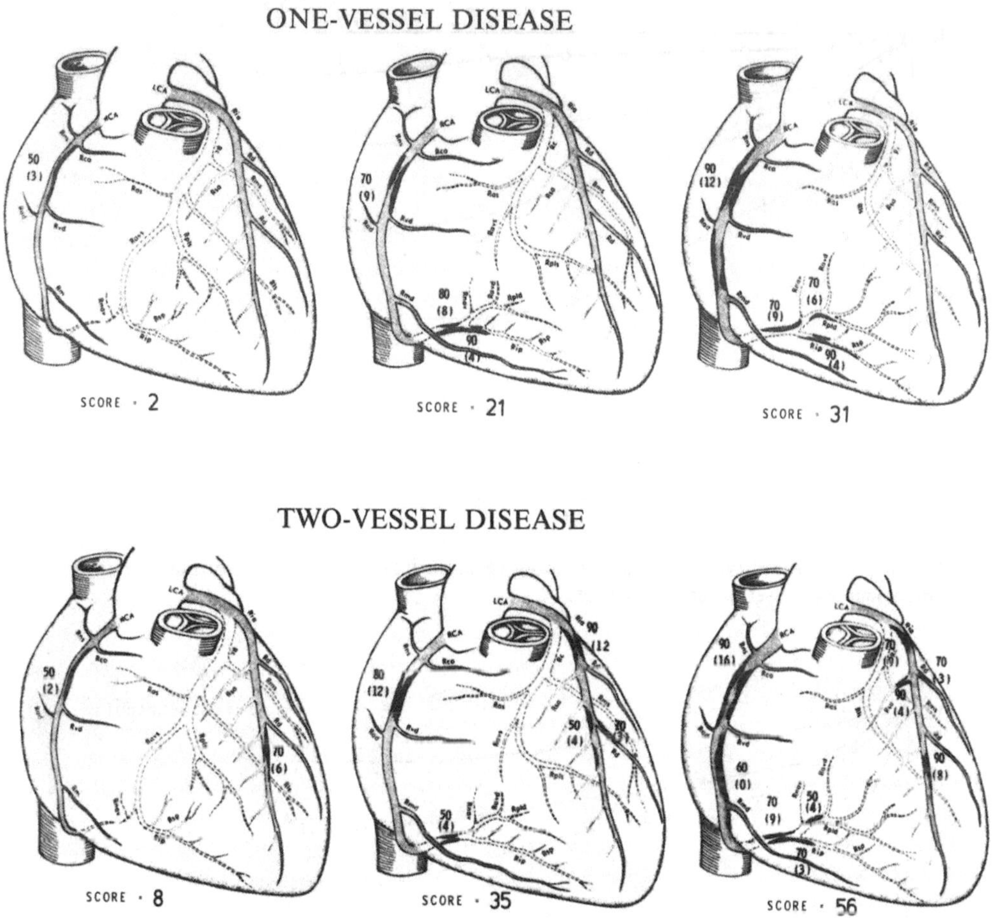

Fig. 5. Three examples each of one- and two-vessel disease. In one-vessel disease the coronary score ranges from 2 to 31, and in two-vessel disease from 8 to 56, illustrating the wide overlap of coronary artery involvement in the two types of disease

It is therefore of practical importance to investigate what noninvasive parameters are available which represent left ventricular function in patients with coronary heart disease. Apart from echocardiography and nuclear ventriculography, heart volume is an easily obtainable noninvasive parameter. In coronary heart disease, impaired left ventricular function results in reduced ejection fraction with increased systolic and end-diastolic volume. The reduced ventricular compliance is the reason for elevated end-diastolic left ventricular pressure, which results in pulmonary artery hypertension with left atrial and right heart enlargement.

Heart volume measurements from teleroentgenograms of the chest, taken with the patient in supine position, can provide a useful parameter of myocardial function, discriminating between patients with different prognoses. 7-year survival rates according to left ventricular score derived from the cineangio-

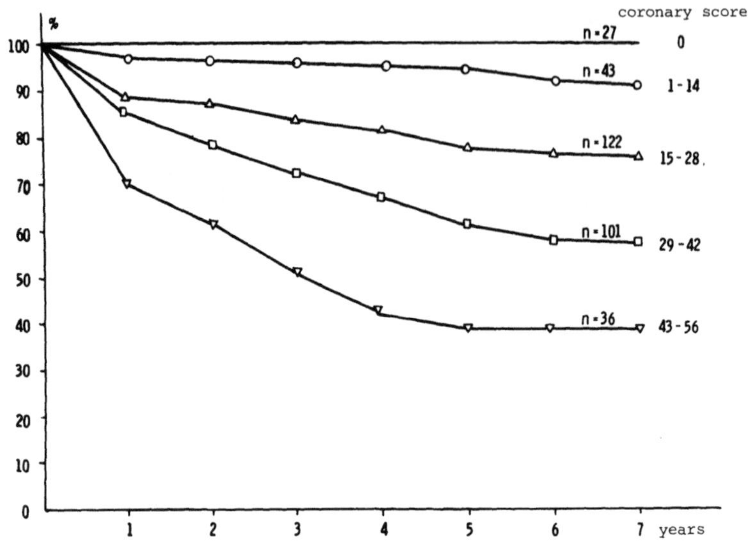

Fig. 6. Seven-year survival for patients grouped according to severity of coronary artery involvement, expressed as coronary score

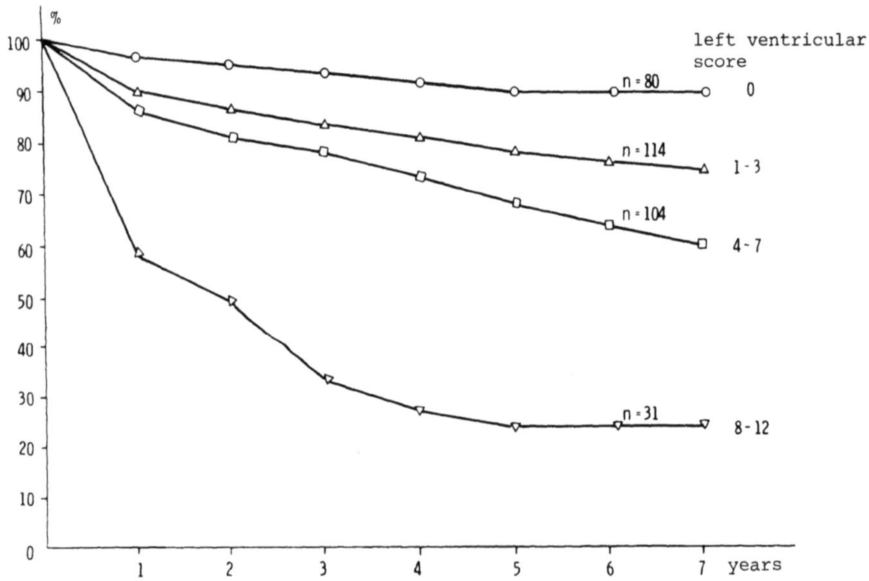

Fig. 7. Seven-year survival for patients grouped according to severity of left ventricular impairment, expressed as a score of 0–12

gram and from heart-volume determination (Fig. 9) shows very similar patterns.

For noninvasive evaluation of myocardial ischemia the exercise electrocardiogram is the method most often used. It has been known for many years that

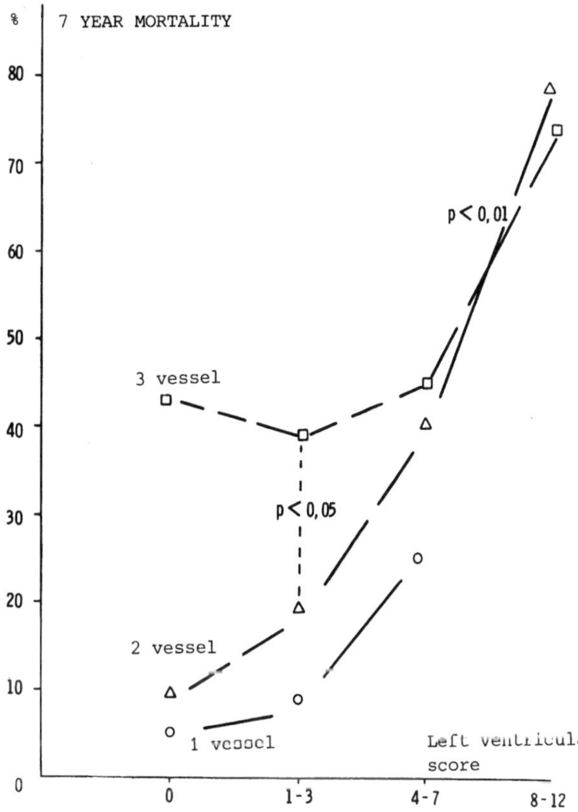

Fig. 8. Seven-year mortality in relation to involvement of one, two, or three vessels, and to severity of left ventricular impairment

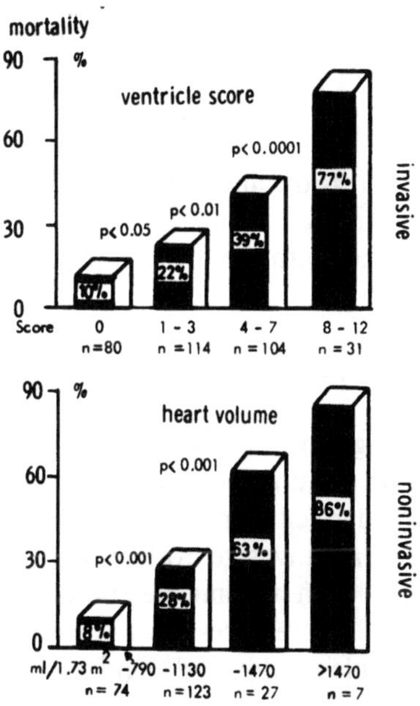

Fig. 9. Seven-year mortality in relation to left ventricular impairment, as derived from ventriculograms (*invasive*) and from heart volume determined from teleroentgenograms of the chest (*noninvasive*) taken with the patient in a supine position

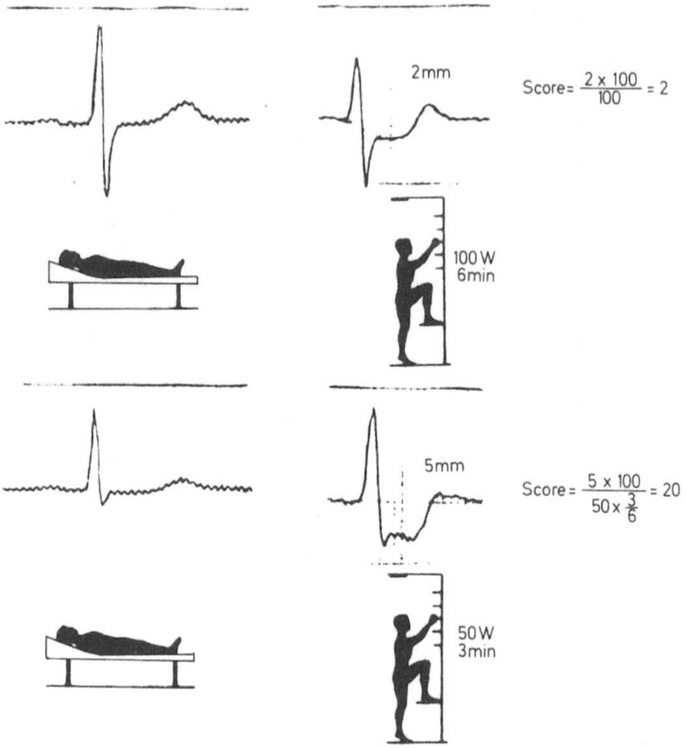

Fig. 10. Quantitative evaluation of an exercise ECG. The score is a quotient, with ST depression in millimeters times 100 as numerator, and workload in watts as denominator. If the workload is tolerated for less than 6 min, the value in watt has to be moderated by a factor according to the number of minutes, e.g., 3 min = *3/6*

prognosis is related to the result of exercise testing (Kaltenbach et al. 1967); in recent years a quantitative relationship between the result of exercise testing and the survival rate has been established. Quantitative evaluation of the exercise electrocardiogram can be achieved by taking into account the degree of ST depression and the workload tolerated (Fig. 10). With this quantification a clear relationship to prognosis can be seen. Figure 11 shows this parameter, together with the three others, in realtion to 7-year mortality.

Summary

Prognosis in coronary heart disease is related to coronary artery involvement and to functional impairment of the left ventricle. Prognostic parameters can be derived from invasive and noninvasive findings. Of particular importance is the noninvasive evaluation of left ventricular function.

Heart volume determination has proven to be extremely useful. Further studies are necessary to determine the value of echocardiography, nuclear ventriculography, and digitized contrast angiography.

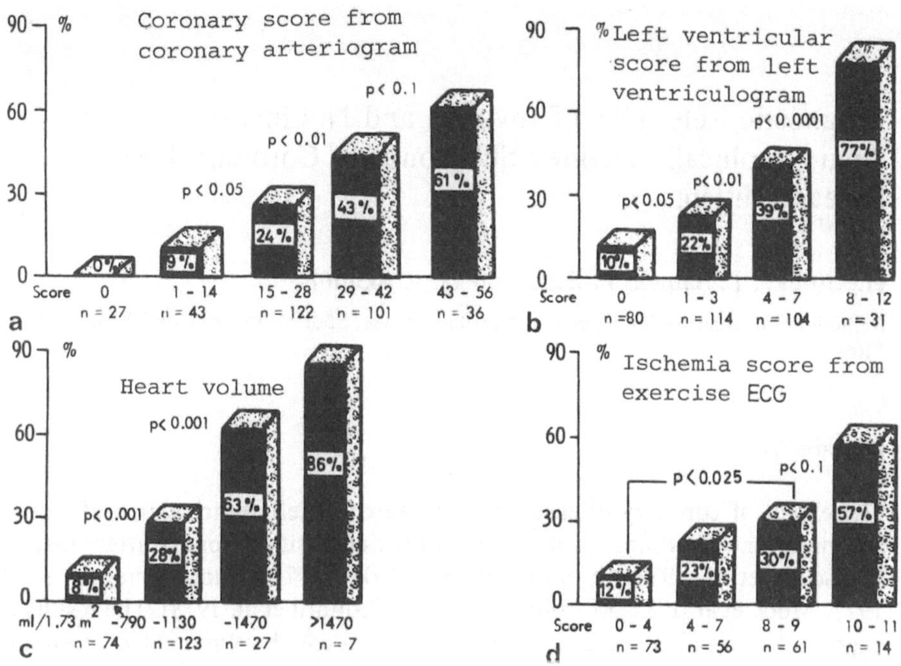

Fig. 11. a–d Seven-year mortality in relation to prognostic parameters, derived from invasive (**a** and **b**) and noninvasive (**c** and **d**) studies

For office-based practical evaluation, the patient's history remains the essenital tool. Presence or absence of angina pectoris, of sustained myocardial infarction and heart failure is most important. Risk factors such as cigarette smoking, diabetes, and hypertension are of additional value. Beside the electrocardiogram at rest and during exercise, evaluation of heart size by teleroentgenography of the chest is most valuable if heart volume determinations are performed.

References

Bruschke AVG, Proudfit WL, Sones FM Jr (1973a) Progress study of 590 consecutive nonsurgical cases of coronary disease followed 5–9 years. I. Arterographic correlations; II. Ventriculographic and other correlations. Circulation 47:1147

Friesinger GC, Page EE, Ross RS (1970) Prognostic significance of coronary arteriography. Trans Assoc Am Physicians 83:78

Kaltenbach M (1975) Quantitative Bewertung koronarographischer Befunde mit Hilfe eines Punktsystems (Score). Z Kardiol 64:597–606

Kaltenbach M, Schäfer R, Klepzig H (1967) Die prognostische Bedeutung des Belastungs-Elektrokardiogramms. Med Klin 62:710–713

Prognostic Relevance of Invasive and Noninvasive Data in Angiographically Defined Subgroups of Coronary Heart Disease Patients

H. Gohlke, L. Samek, P. Betz, and H. Roskamm

Rehabilitationszentrum für Herz- und Kreislaufkranke, Südring 15, 7812 Bad Krozingen, FRG

Introduction

The extent of coronary disease and the degree of left ventricular dysfunction are important determinants of survival in patients with coronary artery disease (Bruschke et al. 1973a, b; Burggraf and Parker 1975; Hammermeister et al. 1977; Mock et al. 1982; Murphy et al. 1977; Proudfit et al. 1978). The results of exercise testing also correlate with the subsequent development of coronary events in a normal population (McDonald 1979) and in different groups of patients with coronary disease (Cole and Ellestadt 1978; Samek et al. 1975; Starling et al. 1980; Payne et al. 1978; Weiner et al. 1978; Tubau et al. 1980). This correlation has been related to the fact that exercise tests are more often positive in patients with multi-vessel disease (Starling et al. 1980) and patients with multi-vessel disease are more likely to have a poor prognosis.

The objectives of the present study were to analyze whether exercise testing can give additional prognostic information in patients whose degree of left ventricular function and extent of coronary artery disease are angiographically determined.

Materials and Methods

Patient Selection

Between 1975 and 1978, 2883 patients underwent coronary angiography for suspected coronary artery disease or for preoperative evaluation. Of these patients, 757 underwent bypass surgery within 6 months after angiography. In 1772 of the remaining 2126 cases both a coronary angiogram and an exercise test were available for review. These patients were followed up for a mean of 4.5 years (Table 1).

Patients included in this study were not part of a randomized or controlled study; patients with significant coronary disease were chosen for medical management because their anginal symptoms were adequately controlled with antianginal medication and/or modification of life style, or because coronary anatomy did not appear suitable for bypass surgery.

Table 1. Selection and characteristics of 1772 medically treated patients

Selection	No. of patients
Angiography for suspected coronary artery disease or for preoperative evaluation between 1975 and 1978	2883
Bypass surgery within 6 months after angiography	757
Exercise test not available	414
Patients treated medically, exercise test and angiography available	1772
Characteristics	
Male/Female	1595/177
Mean age at angiography (years ± SD)	49.9 ± 6
Mean follow-up after angiography in years (range)	4.5 (3–7)

Coronary Angiography

Coronary angiography was performed using Sones' technique in the majority of patients (90%) and Judkins' technique in the remainder. Sublingual nitroglycerine was usually given before angiography. The right and left coronary systems were visualized in sufficient projections to delineate the morphology of the entire coronary system. Angled caudocranial views were used routinely.

Lesions in the coronary arteries were analyzed by measuring the reduction in luminal diameter with an optical gauge in reference to the size of the artery just proximal to the obstruction. A luminal diameter reduction of more than 50% was considered significant.

Left Ventricular Angiography

Left ventricular angiography was performed in the RAO projection (30°) at 50 frames per second in all patients. The left ventricle was divided into five segments according to the AHA recommendations (AHA Committee Report 1975).

The left ventricle was considered to be normal if there was only mild hypokinesia in one segment. Mild impairment of left ventricular function was considered to be present when there was akinesia of one segment and mild hypokinesia in a second segment; moderate impairment of left ventricular function was considered to be present if there were two akinetic segments; severe impairment of left ventricular function was considered to be present if there was severe hypokinesia or akinesia in almost all segments of the left ventricle.

Exercise ECG and Hemodynamics

Exercise tests were performed with an electrically braked bicycle ergometer (Siemens Elema) with the patient in the supine position. A 5-F Swan-Ganz catheter was inserted percutaneously into an antecubital vein and advanced to the pulmonary artery. Pulmonary artery and pulmonary capillary wedge pressure were measured at rest. A nine-lead ECG (I, II, III, aVR, aVL, aVF, V2, V4, V5) was recorded before and immediately after exercise. During exercise, leads V2, V4, and V5 were recorded at the end of each minute at 50 mm/s. Exercise was started at 25 or 50 watts and increased by 25 or 50 watts every 6 min until fatigue, severe angina pectoris, or more than .3 mV ST-segment depression occurred, or 80% of the age-predicted maximal heart rate was reached. Pulmonary artery pressure was recorded throughout exercise, and pulmonary capillary wedge pressure was measured after 4–5 min on each exercise level. The oxygen saturation in the central pulmonary artery was determined at rest and after 6 min on each exercise level. Arterial oxygen saturation was determined from the hyperemic earlobe. Cardiac output at rest and during maximal exercise was determined according to Fick's principle, using the assumed O_2 consumption taken from a table for the corresponding exercise level, corrected for age and sex (Reindell et al. 1967). The following features were analyzed:

1. Maximal exercise tolerance in watts
2. Angina-free exercise tolerance in watts
3. Maximal heart rate during exercise
4. The peak heart rate blood pressure product
5. Occurrence of angina pectoris
6. Pulmonary capillary wedge pressure at rest and during maximal exercise
7. Cardiac output at rest and during maximal exercise.

Follow-Up

Follow-up was done with questionnaires sent out in September 1982, or by means of repeat visits in our outpatient clinic. Follow-up was 98% complete in patients with significant coronary artery disease, regardless of the number of vessels involved. It was less complete in patients without significant coronary artery disease. End point for follow-up was death of the patient. In case of bypass surgery after 6 months of follow-up the patient was withdrawn from the study at the time of surgery.

Statistical Analysis

Survival curves were computed according to Cutler and Ederer (1958). Following a recommendation of Collins et al. (1980), the comparison of survival between different groups was tested according to Mantle and Haenszel (1959). A probability level of less than .05 was considered significant.

The correlation between the exercise parameters and subsequent death was determined using multivariate analysis of the parameters with Cox' model of proportional hazards regression (1972). Calculations were performed on a PDP 11/45 computer.

Results

The results of coronary angiography in the 1772 patients are shown in Table 2. There were 403 patients with either normal coronary arteries or ≤50% luminal diameter narrowing in a major coronary artery. The number of patients with single-, double-, or triple-vessel disease was 495, 413, and 461 respectively. The mean age increased slightly with severity of coronary artery disease. During a mean follow-up of 4.5 years 182 patients died.

The gross survival rates for up to 6 years after angiography in these patients are shown in Fig. 1 and they illustrate the typical trend for less favorable survival with increasing number of diseased vessels ($p<0.0001$).

Table 2. Angiographic findings in 1772 medically treated patients

No. of diseased vessels	No. of patients	Mean age (years ± SD)
Stenosis <50%, or normal coronary arteries	403	47.3±7.7
One	495	49.6±6.6
Two	413	50.0±5.8
Three	461	52.3±5.9

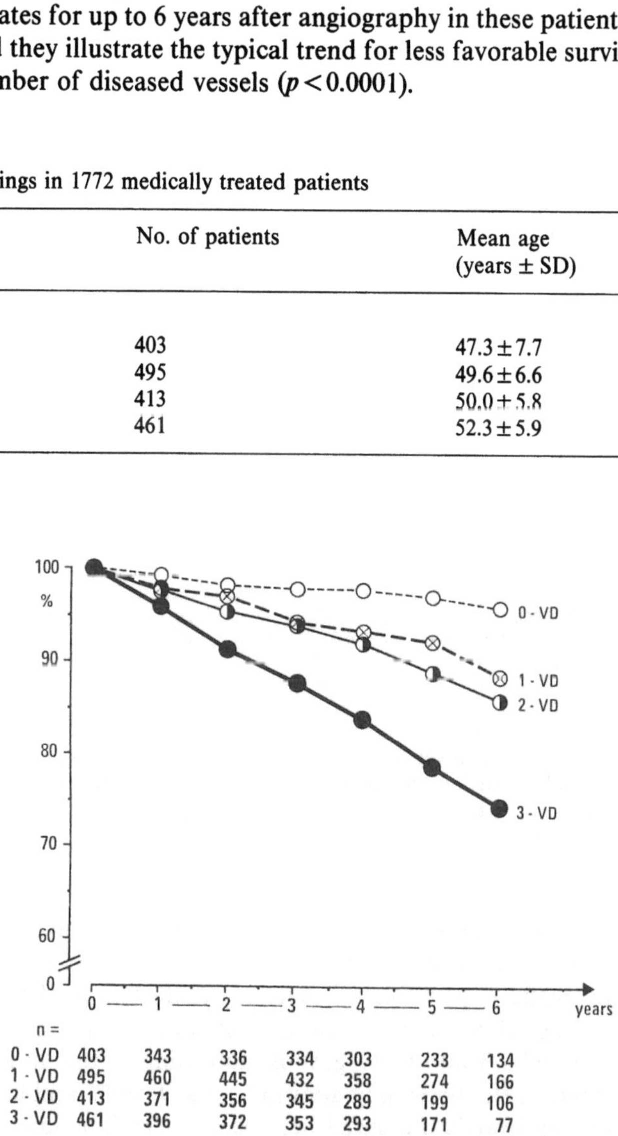

Fig. 1. Survival curves of patients with zero-, one-, two-, and three-vessel disease, independent of left ventricular function ($p<0.0001$, global testing for differences in survival). *Numbers* indicate number of patients in each group at the beginning of the indicated year of follow-up.

If the patients are grouped according to the degree of left ventricular dysfunction (Fig. 2) the difference in survival between those with normal left ventricular function and those with severe left ventricular dysfunction becomes greater than the difference in survival between patients with no vessel involvement and those with triple-vessel disease; however, the number of patients with severe left ventricular dysfunction is small ($p < 0.001$).

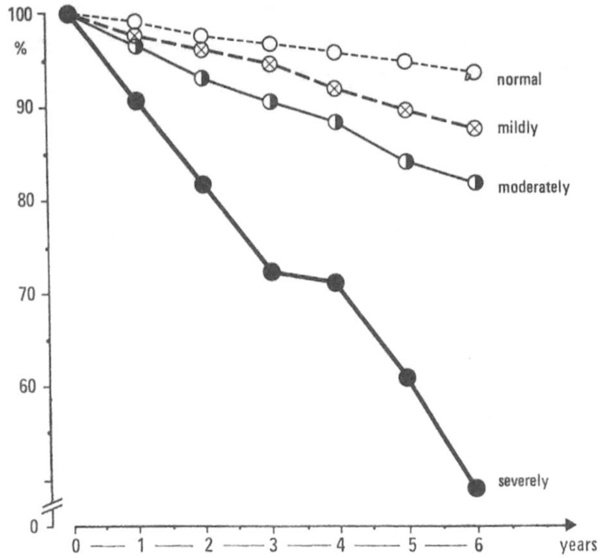

LV - function							
normal	605	531	513	506	458	383	235
mildly	817	729	704	682	554	332	171
moderately	287	258	245	235	194	134	62
severely	59	48	43	38	34	25	12

Fig. 2. Survival curves of patients with normal, mildly, moderately, or severely impaired left ventricular function, independent of the number of vessels diseased ($n = 1772$; $p < 0.0001$). *Numbers* indicate number of patients in each group at the beginning of the indicated year of follow-up.

Because patients with poor left ventricular function as determined by angiography are known to have a poor prognosis, we confined our analysis of the prognostic importance of exercise parameters to the following subgroups of patients: Those with normal or only mildly impaired left ventricular function were divided into three groups, according to the number of diseased vessels (groups I, II, and III). In addition, patients with double- or triple-vessel disease and moderately impaired left ventricular function were grouped together (group IV) because of the smaller number of patients available for analysis (Table 3). Thus, patients with angiographically severe left ventricular dysfunction and those with single vessel disease and moderately impaired left ventricular function are not considered in this analysis.

Table 3. Definition of groups I–IV based on angiographic assessment[a]

Group	No. of vessels diseased	Left ventricular function	No. of patients
I	One	Normal or mildly impaired	410
II	Two	Normal or mildly impaired	316
III	Three	Normal or mildly impaired	308
IV	Two or three	Moderately impaired	204

[a] Patients with single-vessel disease and moderately or severely impaired LV function, and those with two- or three-vessel disease and severely impaired LV function are not included

The medical treatment used in these four groups is summarized in Table 4; the majority of patients received more than one drug; between 8% and 14% of patients took no medication.

Table 4. Medical treatment in groups I–IV

	Group (% of patients)			
Treatment	I	II	III	IV
β-Blockers	44	50	53	54
Nitrates	63	74	75	76
Ca^{++} antagonists	22	26	21	28
Antihypertensives	14	17	14	10.3
Diuretics	4.0	4.4	6.1	6.4
Digitalis	25	25	24	37
No medication	14	8	12.6	8.4

The survival curves in the four groups analyzed are shown in Fig. 3. The previously seen trend to less favorable survival of patients with more severe disease is seen again here, but the difference between patients with single- and triple-vessel disease (groups I and III) is slightly less after patients with severe left ventricular dysfunction have been excluded. The difference in survival between the four groups remains highly significant ($p < 0.0001$).

We examined the prognostic importance of the noninvasive and the invasive exercise parameters in the four groups. According to the distribution of each exercise variable, the patients in groups I, II, and III were divided into three approximately equal sized groups. Thus, in group I the third of patients with the highest exercise tolerance was grouped together (the highest tercile) and compared with the third of patients with the lowest exercise tolerance (the lowest tercile). The survival curves of these terciles were computed according to Cutler and Ederer (1958). The survival curves of the middle terciles were between those of the highest and the lowest tercile for all variables. Patients in group IV were divided into two halves based on the exercise variables because of the smaller number of patients available. The *p* value refers to global differences in the survival curves of the three terciles or of both halves of the corresponding variable; only the 5-year survival rates of the highest and lowest tercile (halves) are given in Table 5.

Using the noninvasive exercise variables, such as maximal exercise tolerance, angina-free exercise tolerance, and maximal heart rate achieved, there was a trend to better survival in the highest tercile in all subgroups. This trend, based on noninvasive parameters reached statistical significance only for patients in group II.

Survival was significantly better for patients in group II with higher exercise tolerance and higher angina-free exercise tolerance, and in those achieving a higher maximal heart rate. The magnitude of this difference in 5-year survival between the highest and the lowest tercile in patients with double-vessel disease is comparable to the difference in survival between patients which single- and triple-vessel disease, i.e., approximately 15%.

In patients with single-vessel disease, the overall mortality was lower and the trend for better survival in the highest terciles did not reach statistical significance. In patients with triple-vessel disease, mortality was high even in the highest tercile of the exercise parameters. Here again, the difference in mortality did not reach statistical significance (Table 5).

Analysis of maximal cardiac output and pulmonary capillary wedge pressure, the invasive exercise parameters obtained during maximal exercise test-

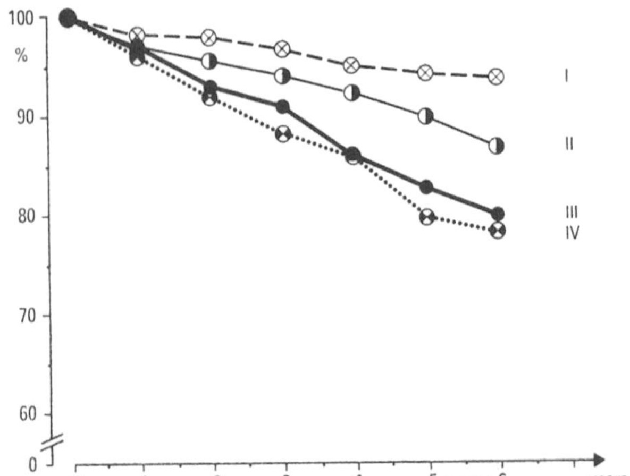

I	410	381	370	359	296	226	144
II	316	283	273	264	225	151	83
III	308	264	249	242	199	113	52
IV	204	180	170	160	130	85	40

Fig. 3. Survival curves in four angiographically defined groups (I, II, III, IV) of patients with significant coronary artery disease ($n = 1238$). For definitions of groups see Table 3; $p \ll 0.0001$. *Numbers* indicate number of patients in each group at the beginning of the indicated year of follow-up.

Table 5. Five-year survival rates for highest and lowest terciles (groups I–III) and halves (group IV) based on noninvasive exercise parameters and maximal cardiac output

Group	*n*	Tercile	Maximal exercise tolerance			Angina-free exercise tolerance			Maximal heart rate			Maximal cardiac output		
			Cutpoints (watts)	Survival (%)		Cutpoints (watts)	Survival (%)		Cutpoints (Beats/min)	Survival (%)		Cutpoints (Liters/min)	Survival (%)	
I	410	Highest	>110	97±2	n.s.	>90	95±2	n.s.	>140	97±2	n.s.	>15	96±2	a
		Lowest	<90	92±3		<60	93±2		<110	93±2		<12	87±4	
II	316	Highest	>110	95±2	b	>70	96±2	b	>125	95±2	a	>14	96±2	a
		Lowest	<90	81±5		<40	78±5		<110	82±4		<10	80±6	
III	308	Highest	>90	86±4	n.s.	>70	88±4	n.s.	>110	88±3	n.s.	>13	92±3	b
		Lowest	<60	79±4		<40	82±3		<100	82±4		<10	73±5	
IV	204	Upper half	>60	88±4	a	>40	80±5	n.s.	>105	83±4	n.s.	>11	90±3	b
		Lower half	<60	72±5		<40	78±5		<105	75±5		<11	68±5	

[a] $p<0.05$ [b] $p<0.005$

ing, revealed a significant difference in survival in all three subgroups between the lowest and the highest tercile of maximal cardiac output and in the higher and lower half in subgroup IV (Table 5). The difference in 5-year survival between the highest and lowest tercile was 9% ($p<0.05$), 16% ($p<0.05$), and 19% ($p<0.005$) in groups I, II, and III respectively. Among patients in group IV, the difference in survival between the higher and the lower half was 22% ($p<0.005$).

Table 6. Univariate analysis of variables correlating with subsequent death in four subgroups

	Group (p value)[a]			
Noninvasive variables	I	II	III	IV
Age	0.0018		0.07	
Maximal exercise tolerance	0.03	0.017	0.08	0.048
Angina-free exercise tolerance		0.019		
Maximal heart rate	0.0147	0.033		
ST↓ during exercise ≥0.1			0.033	
Invasive variables				
Maximal cardiac output	0.0017	0.0034	0.0086	0.0021
Maximal pulmonary capillary wedge pressure during exercise				0.0053

[a] Only p values of <0.1 are listed

Univariate analysis (Table 6) of noninvasive exercise parameters with the proportional hazards regression model of Cox (1972) showed that in patients with single-vessel disease (group I) age correlated best with subsequent death, and the maximal heart rate was only second, followed by maximal exercise tolerance. In patients with double-vessel disease (group II) univariate analysis with this model shows that age is no longer important, and the parameters of exercise testing become determinants of survival; maximal exercise tolerance is the most significant factor. In patients with triple-vessel disease (group III) the occurrence of ST-segment depression correlates with subsequent death. In patients with double or triple vessel disease and moderately impaired left ventricular function (group IV), exercise tolerance is the most important noninvasive variable for the prediction of subsequent death.

If maximal cardiac output and maximal pulmonary capillary wedge pressure are included in the uni- or multivariate analysis, maximal cardiac output is the most important variable correlating with subsequent cardiac death in all four groups (Table 6). However, age in group I and exercise-induced ST-segment depression in group III remain of independent importance. In group IV the maximal cardiac output and the maximal pulmonary capillary wedge pressure are independent prognostic factors. Thus, using noninvasive parameters in patients with double-vessel disease and normal or mildly impaired left ventricular function, exercise testing is able to differentiate those at low risk for death during a 5-year follow-up period from those at substantially higher risk for death during the same period.

Using cardiac output as an invasive parameter obtained during exercise testing a significant difference in survival becomes evident in all four groups between the lowest and the highest tercile (groups I, II, III) or half (group IV).

Discussion

The classification of patients with coronary artery disease into subgroups according to the number of diseased vessels (Bruschke et al. 1973a) has gained wide acceptance, but it has also been criticized (Selzer 1982). Several authors have developed a scoring system that can give a more precise picture of the extent of coronary artery disease (Friesinger et al. 1970; Gensini 1975; Kaltenbach 1975) in a given patient or in groups of patients.

Despite the theoretical advantage of a more precise classification with one of these scoring systems, the simple original classification of patients into groups with single-, double-, and triple-vessel disease has been used in most of the major studies, such as the VA-study (Murphy et al. 1977), the European Coronary Surgery Study (1980), and the CASS-Study (Mock et al. 1982). If left ventricular function is taken into consideration the prognosis of such patients is further delineated.

The 5-year survival rates for our subgroups I, II, and III are similar to those reported in the CASS-Study for patients with comparable left ventricular function; the 5-year survival rates of groups II and III are also similar to those of medically treated patients with double- and triple-vessel disease in the European Coronary Surgery Study, in which only patients with ejection fractions above 50% were randomized. Thus, the 5-year survival rate of patients with good left ventricular function is related to the number of vessels diseased, and is similar in the United States and Europe.

Previous studies have correlated the results of exercise testing with subsequent cardiac events or subsequent death in a normal population (McDonald 1979), in patients in the chronic phase of myocardial infarction (Samek et al. 1975), and in patients soon after myocardial infarction (Starling et al. 1980; Koppes et al. 1980; Theroux et al. 1980). The results of exercise testing allow a classification of high-risk subgroups in each category of individuals or patients.

The prediction of a future event is enhanced if a normal exercise test becomes abnormal on repeat examination (McDonald 1979). The correlation of the results of exercise testing has been related to the fact that exercise tests are more likely positive in patients with multivessel disease or with severe left ventricular dysfunction (Starling et al. 1980), and these patients, in turn, are more likely to have a poor prognosis (Bruschke et al. 1973b). We excluded patients with severely impaired left ventricular function as determined by angiography, because these patients are known to have a poor prognosis. Thus, exercise testing was able to delineate high and low risk subgroups in angiographically homogeneous groups of patients.

In the group of patients with double-vessel disease and good left ventricular function, noninvasive exercise parameters appear particularly useful for separating those with a good prognosis (5-year-survival, 96%) from those with a markedly reduced prognosis (5-year-survival, 81%). The difference in survival between the highest and lowest terciles in group II is similar to, or even greater than, the difference in survival between patients with single- and triple-vessel disease. Among patients with triple-vessel disease, the prognosis for those with better exercise capacity or higher angina threshold, or for those achieving higher heart rates, is slightly but not significantly better than the prognosis for those in the lower terciles. Patients in our group IV with a higher exercise tolerance had a significantly better prognosis than patients with a lower exercise tolerance, but the differences using the other noninvasive exercise parameters are not significant.

Using the invasively obtained exercise parameters, maximal cardiac output and maximal pulmonary capillary wedge pressure, a significant difference in survival is evident in all four subgroups of patients between the lowest and the highest tercile or half of cardiac output. In patients in group IV the maximal pulmonary capillary wedge pressure is of independent prognostic importance in multivariate stepwise regression analysis, and probably reflects the degree of left ventricular dysfunction during exercise.

Surprisingly, the maximal pulmonary capillary wedge pressure during exercise in patients with good resting function of the left ventricle does not correlate with subsequent death. This finding must be interpreted with caution because a large number of patients with high pulmonary capillary wedge pressures underwent bypass surgery, the decision to operate having been based partly on this variable.

The magnitude of the difference in survival between the lowest and the highest tercile of cardiac output increases with the extent of coronary disease. The difference in survival between the lowest and the highest tercile was significant even in patients with single vessel disease (group I). In patients in group II noninvasive parameters reached a similar differentiation of high- and low-risk subgroups. In patients in groups III and IV, maximal cardiac output was able to identify patients with a markedly impaired prognosis. The difference in survival between the high- and low-risk groups was almost twice as large as that between patients with single- and triple-vessel disease.

Based on these results, exercise testing appears to provide independent prognostic information, once left ventricular function and the extent of coronary artery disease has been determined by angiography. Exercise testing is not only a means of quantitating the limitation of exercise capacity; in conjunction with the angiographic findings it provides additional prognostic information. The power of exercise testing to differentiate between high- and low-risk subgroups is similar to that of coronary angiography.

Both tests, coronary angiography and exercise testing, provide complementary information, and exercise testing should not be considered redundant even if performed after coronary angiography.

References

AHA Committee Report (1975) A reporting system on patients evaluated for coronary artery disease. Circulation 51 (April): 5

Bruschke AVG, Proudfit WL, Sones FM Jr (1973a) Progress study of 590 consecutive non-surgical cases of coronary disease followed 5-9 years. I. Arteriographic correlations. Circulation 47: 1147

Bruschke AVG, Proudfit WL, Sones FM Jr (1973b) Progress study of 590 consecutive non-surgical cases of coronary disease followed 5-9 years. II. Ventriculographic and other correlations. Circulation 47: 1154

Burggraf WL, Parker JO (1975) Prognosis in coronary artery disease. Angiographic, hemodynamic and clinical factors. Circulation 51: 146

Cole JP, Ellestad M (1978) Significance of chest pain during treadmill exercise: Correlation with coronary events. Am J Cardiol 41: 227

Collins D, Peduzzi P, Detre K (1980) A computer program for comparing survival experience of two groups after adjustment for relevant covariates. Comp Programs Biomed 11: 119

Cutler S, Ederer F (1958) Maximum utilization of the life table method in analyzing survival. J Chronic Dis 8: 699

Cox DR (1972) Regression models and life tables. J Roy Statist Soc 34: 187

European Coronary Surgery Study Group (1980) Prospective randomized study of coronary artery bypass surgery in stable angina pectoris. Second interim report. Lancet II: 491

Friesinger GC, Page EE, Ross RS (1970) Prognostic significance of coronary arteriography. Trans Assoc Am Physicians 83: 78

Gensini GE (1975) Coronary arteriography. Futura, New York, p 271

Hammermeister KE, DeRouen TA, Murray JA, Dodge HT (1977) Effect of coronary saphenous vein bypass grafting on death and sudden death. Am J Cardiol 39: 925

Kaltenbach M (1975) Quantitative Bewertung koronarangiographischer Befunde mit Hilfe eines Punktesystems (Score). Z Kardiol 64: 597

Koppes GM, Kruyer W, Beckmann CH, Jones FG (1980) Response to exercise early after uncomplicated acute myocardial infarction in patients receiving no medication: Long-term follow-up. Am J Cardiol 46: 764

Mantel N, Haenszel W (1959) Statistical aspects of the analysis of data from retrospective studies of disease. JNCI 22: 719

McDonald L (1979) Very early recognition of coronary heart disease. In: Yu P, Goodwin J (eds) Progress in cardiology, vol 8. Lea and Febiger, Philadelphia, p 147

Mock MB, participants of the Coronary Artery Surgery Study (1982) Survival of medically treated patients in the Coronary Artery Surgery Study (CASS) registry. Circulation 66: 562

Murphy ML, Hultgren HN, Detre K, Thomsen J, Takaro T (1977) Treatment of chronic stable angina. A preliminary report of survival data of the randomized Veterans Administration Cooperative Study. Engl J Med 297: 621

Paine TD, Dye LE, Roitman DI, Sheffield LT, Rackley CE, Russel RO, Rogers WJ (1978) Relation of graded exercise test findings after myocardial infarction to extent of coronary artery disease and left ventricular dysfunction. Am J Cardiol 42: 716

Proudfit WL, Bruschke AVG, Sones FM Jr (1978) Natural history of obstructive coronary artery disease: Ten years' study of 601 nonsurgical cases. Prog Cardiovasc Dis 21: 53

Reindell H, König K, Roskamm H (1967) Funktionsdiagnostik des gesunden und kranken Herzens. Thieme, Stuttgart, pp 248–249

Samek L, Roskamm H, Rentrop P, Kaiser P, Stürzenhofecker P, Schober B, Görnandt L, Velden R (1975) Belastungsprüfungen und Koronarangiogramm im chronischen Infarktstadium. Z Kardiol 64: 809

Selzer A (1982) On the limitation of therapeutic intervention trials in ischemic heart disease: A clinican's viewpoint. Am J Cardiol 49: 252

Starling MR, Crawford MH, Kennedy GT, O'Rourke RA (1980) Exercise testing early after myocardial infarction: Predictive value for subsequent unstable angina and death. Am J Cardiol 46: 909

Theroux P, Waters DD, Halpen C, Debaisieux J, Mizgala HF (1980) Prognostic value of exercise testing after myocardial infarction. N Engl J Med 301:341
Tubau JF, Chaitman BR, Bourassa MG, Waters DD (1980) Detection of multivessel coronary disease after myocardial infarction using exercise stress testing and multiple ECG lead systems. Circulation 61:44
Weiner DA, McCabe C, Klein MD, Ryan TJ (1978) ST segment changes post-infarction: predictive value for multivessel coronary disease and left ventricular aneurysm. Circulation 58:887

Angiographic Findings and Prognosis in Asymptomatic Men with Rest and Exercise Electrocardiographic Abnormalities*

V. F. Froelicher

Department of Medicine, Cardiology Division, University of California, San Diego, CA 92103, USA

Introduction

Mortality due to coronary heart disease (CHD) has begun to decline, perhaps owing to changing life-style patterns. However, morbidity rates probably have not been altered and CHD remains the leading cause of death in most developed countries. Since it will be some time before its primary prevention is a reality, it is advisable to evaluente screening methods for detecting latent CHD while methods for primary prevention evolve. Screening can be defined as the presumptive identification of unrecognized disease by the utilization of tests, examinations, and other procedures which can be applied rapidly (Froom et al. 1979). The relative value of techniques for identifying individuals who have asymptomatic CHD should be assessed in order to optimally and cost-effectively direct secondary preventive efforts towards those with disease. Resting electrocardiographic assessment, risk factor screening, exercise testing, and other newer techniques will be discussed here.

Eight criteria have been proposed for the selection of a screening procedure (Breslow and Sommers 1977); (a) the procedure is acceptable and appropriate; (b) the quantity and/or quality of life can be favorably altered; (c) the results of intervention outweigh any adverse effects; (d) the target disease has an asymptomatic period during which detection and treatment can reduce morbidity and/or mortality; (e) acceptable treatments are available; (f) the prevalence and seriousness of the disease or condition justify the cost of intervention; (g) the procedure is relatively easy and inexpensive; and, (h) resources are available for diagnostic or therapeutic intervention.

In order to evaluate the value of any screening test, sensitivity, specificity, predicative value, and relative risk must be calculated (Froelicher 1983). Sensitivity is the percentage of times a test produces an abnormal response when those with disease are tested. Specificity is the percentage of times a test gives a normal response when those without disease are tested – a definition quite different from the conventional use of word "specific." These two values are inversely related and are determined by the discriminant value chosen for the test result that separates positives from negatives. The predictive value of an abnormal test is the percentage of individuals with an abnormal test who have disease. The relative risk of an abnormal test response is the relative chance of

* Supported by the Ischemic Heart Disease Specialized Center of Research (SCOR) HL 17682 awarded by the National Heart, Lung, and Blood Institute to Dr. John Ross

having disease if the test is abnormal compared to having disease if the test is normal. The values for these last two terms are dependent upon the prevalence of disease in the population being tested.

A basic step in applying any testing procedure for the separation of normal subjects from patients with a disease is to determine a value measured by the test that best separates the two groups. One problem is that there is usually a considerable overlap of measurement values of a test in the groups with and without disease. Consider two bell-shaped normal distribution curves, one representing a normal population and the other representing a population with disease, with a certain amount of overlap of the two curves (see Fig. 1). Along the vertical axis is the number of patients and along the horizontal axis could be the value for such measurements as Q-wave size, exercise-induced ST-segment depression, or CPK. The optimal test would be able to achieve the most marked separation of these two bell-shaped curves and minimize the overlap. Unfortunately, most of the tests currently used for the diagnosis of coronary artery disease, including the exercise test, have a considerable overlap of the range of measurements for the normal population and for those with heart disease. Therefore, problems arise when a certain value is used to separate these two groups (e.g., 1-mm ST-segment depression, a 10-mm Hg drop in systolic blood pressure, less than 5 METS of functional capacity, three beats of ventricular tachycardia). If the value is set far to the right (e.g., 2 mm of ST-segment depression) in order to identify nearly all the normal subjects as being free of disease, the test will have a high specificity. However, a substantial number of those with disease will be called normal. If a value is chosen far to the left (e.g., 0.5 mm ST-segment depression), which identifies nearly all those with disease as being abnormal and gives the test a high sensitivity, then many normal subjects are identified as abnormal. If a value is chosen that equally mislabels the normal subjects and those with disease, the test will have its highest predictive accuracy. However, there may be reasons for wanting to adjust a test to have a relatively higher sensitivity or relatively higher specificity than possible when

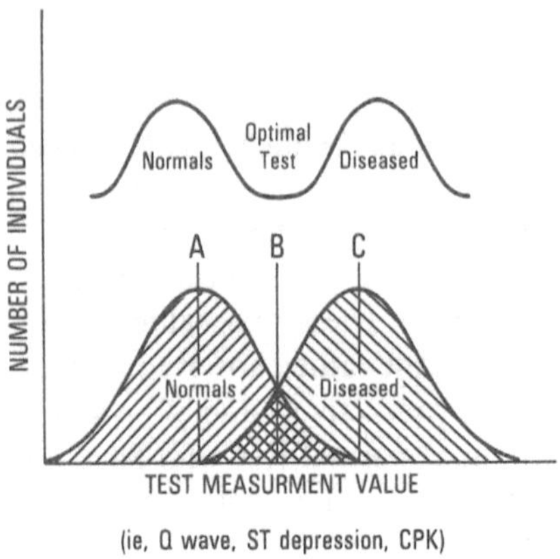

Fig. 1. Example of how a discriminant value determines sensitivity and specificity

predictive accuracy is optimal. But it must be kept in mind that sensitivity and specificity are inversely related; that is, when sensitivity is the highest specificity is the lowest, and vice versa. Any test has a range of inversely related sensitivities and specificities that can be chosen by selecting a certain discriminant or diagnostic value.

The Resting Electrocardiogramm as a Screening Technique

As part of the Copenhagen City Heart Study, nearly 20000 men and women, 20 years of age or older, each had a resting 12-lead electrocardiogramm (Ostor et al. 1981). The Minnesota Code was used to classify the electrocardiograms. The prevalence of all electrocardiographic findings, with the exception of axis deviation, high-amplitude R waves, minor Q-wave abnormalities, and prolonged or short PR interval, was very low, below the age of 40 in men and 50 in women. Rates for Q-wave abnormalities, left-axis deviation, ST depression, premature beats, and atrial fibrillation increased with age, and were higher for men than for women. A strong association between total mortality and major ST depression and T-wave abnormalities, Q-wave patterns, and left bundle branch block existed. During a period from 1976 to 1980, 489 subjects died, but there were only a few deaths in those under the age of 50. Due to this and because the prevalence of electrocardiographic abnormalities was low in the young, relative risk was only significant in those 50 or older. Over 50% of the deaths were noncardiovascular. The relative risk of ST-segment depression was up to five and of some Q-wave abnormalities, three.

Rose and colleagues (1978) performed electrocardiograms (limb leads only) on 8403 male civil servants aged 40–64 and coded them using the Minnesota Code. Coronary heart disease mortality rates were established over the ensuing 5 years (657 men died). Q waves, left-axis deviation, ST depression, T-wave changes, ventricular conduction defects, and atrial fibrillation were related to mortality. However, there was little significance to increased R-wave amplitude, QT interval, premature beats, or heart rate extremes. Among the 6% of men with patterns suggesting ischemia, the subsequent coronary heart disease mortality was little more than 1% per year and even lower in those who were asymptomatic but an approximately five fold risk ratio was found.

As part of the Busselton City Study in Australia, 2119 randomly selected subjects each had a 12-lead electrocardiogram and these were coded according to the Minnesota Code (Cullen et al. 1982). In addition, all subjects completed the Rose chest-pain questionnaire. Subjects were between the ages of 40 and 79 and included both men and women. Between 1967 and 1979 mortality in this group was determined, and the 13-year rate from cardiovascular disease was significantly higher in those with an initial electrocardiogram that showed Q wave and QS patterns, left-axis deviation, ST-segment depression and T-wave abnormalities, atrial fibrillation, or premature ventricular beats. In subjects free of angina and other electrocardiographic abnormalities, ventricular extra systoles were associated with a significantly higher mortality from cardiovascular disease compared with controls. Q-wave patterns had the highest risk ratio (3.7 ×), whereas the other abnormalities had about a 2 × risk ratio.

As part of the Manitoba Study, a cohort of 3983 men with a mean age of 30 years at entry were followed up with annual examinations, including electrocardiograms, from 1948 on (Rabkin et al. 1982). During the 30-year observation period, 70 cases of sudden death occurred in men without previous clinical manifestations of heart disease. The prevalence of electrocardiographic abnormalities before sudden death was 71%. The frequencies of these abnormalities were 31% for major ST- and T-wave abnormalities, 16% for ventricular extra beats, 13% for left ventricular hypertrophy, 7% for left bundle branch block. Left bundle branch block had a 14 times higher risk for sudden death, while ST- and T-wave abnormalities, increased R wave, and premature beats had relative risks as high as five. It must be remembered that this was a serial electrocardiographic study with electrocardiograms usually obtained each year, and specificity was not determined.

In 2000 Framingham Study participants, the 12-lead electrocardiogram failed to correctly classify over half of the persons with clinically definite heart disease (Dawber et al. 1952). The sensitivity was about 50% and specificity 90%. The utility of the electrocardiogram for assessing prior infarction can be evaluated by comparing results with postmortem findings or by comparing results with those from survivors of previously documented infarctions. Levine and Phillips (1951) found that only 20% of old infarcts found at autopsy were correctly identified by the antemortem electrocardiogramm. Electrocardiographic abnormalities may not persist in patients with a previously documented myocardial infarction (Wasserman et al. 1982). In the Framingham Study, 18% of infarction patients had no electrocardiographic abnormalities on subsequent examination. However, the electrocardiogram has a much greater prognostic value in survivors of a coronary heart disease event than in apparently healthy populations.

Angiographic Findings in Asymptomatic Men with Resting Electrocardiographic Abnormalities

Cardiac catheterization was used to evaluate 298 asymptomatic, apparently healthy aircrew men with electrocardiographic abnormalities (Froelicher et al. 1977). These men were identified from annual electrocardiograms and exercise tests used to screen them for latent heart disease. Data from 27 additional symptomatic aircrew men who underwent cardiac catheterization because of mild angina pectoris were also included. The men were grouped according to the major reason for cardiac catheterization. The order of groups by increasing prevalence of coronary artery disease was as follows: abnormal treadmill (labile lead), supraventricular tachycardia, right bundle branch block, left bundle branch block, abnormal treadmill, ventricular irritability, probable infarct, and angina. In Table 1 the specific findings among these groups are presented. Table 2 presents the risk factors and funktional values from treadmill testing

Table 1. Angiographic findings and risk-factor data in 325 aircrew men grouped by major reason for cardiac catheterization[a]

Group	Age (yr)[b]	No. (% of group) with significant CAD	No. (% of group) with no CAD	Serum cholesterol (mg/100 ml)[b]	Serum triglycerides (mg/100 ml)[b]	Blood pressure (mm Hg)[b]	Positive smoking history (% of group)	Positive family history for CAD (% of group)
RBBB ($n=41$)	41±7	8 (20)	29 (7)	224±40	140± 45	125±11 / 81±7	54	27
LBBB ($n=34$)	42±5	8 (24)	23 (68)	223±29	124± 39	129±13 / 82±10	65	29
Labile lead abnormal treadmill test ($n=27$)	38±7	1 (4)	22 (82)	233±38	150± 72	131±11 / 86±8	44	42
Abnormal treadmill test ($n=111$)	43±7	34 (31)	60 (54)	245±47	157± 85	133±15 / 85±10	52	38
Supraventricular tachycardia ($n=36$)	38±7	5 (14)	29 (81)	2[illegible]7±29	116± 41	127±11 / 83±8	44	36
Ventricular irritability ($n=24$)	45±6	9 (38)	12 (50)	2[illegible]0±28	153± 58	132±12 / 85±10	54	21
Probable infarction ($n=25$)	41±8	14 (56)	8 (32)	269±61	152± 55	132±15 / 86±9	80	64
Angina ($n=27$)	44±8	19 (70)	7 (26)	245±34	182±118	130±10 / 84±8	67	74
All ($n=325$)	42±7	98 (30)	190 (58)	237±43	148± 73	130±13 / 84±9	56	39

CAD, coronary artery disease; *significant CAD*, 50% or more luminal occlusion; ***LBBB***, left bundle branch block; ***RBBB***, right bundle branch block

[a] Minimal angiographic coronary artery disease was found in the men not included in the column for either significant or no coronary artery disease. The percent of men with significant coronary artery disease in each group is the predictive value of that group classification

[b] Values expressed as mean ± standard deviation

Table 2. Risk factors and maximal treadmill functional data in 325 aircrew men grouped by angiographic findings

Angiographic CAD	No. (%) of men	Age (yr)[a]	Serum cholesterol (mg/100 ml)[a]	Serum triglycerides (mg/100 ml)[a]	Blood pressure (mm Hg)[a]	Positive smoking history (% of group)	Positive family history for CAD (% of group)	VO_2 (cc O_2/kg/min)[a]	Double product[a,b]	Maximal heart rate (beats/min)[a]
None	190 (58.5)	40±7	224±35	130±53	$\frac{129\pm12}{83\pm9}$	46	34	37.0±5.7	36.7±4.7	184±11
Minimal	37 (11.4)	42±6	249±40	168±67	$\frac{129\pm11}{82\pm9}$	76	41	35.4±4.5	36.4±4.8	183±11
Significant	98 (30.2)	45±6	256±50	172±97	$\frac{134\pm15}{86\pm10}$	67	50	34.8±5.6	34.4±5.3	175±13

CAD, coronary artery disease; VO_2, oxygen consumption
[a] Values expressed as mean ± standard deviation
[b] (Maximal systolic blood pressure × maximal heart rate)/10^3

by the presence of angiographic coronary disease; Table 3 is the same data by vessel score in the 98 men with significant disease. Approximately 60% of men were completely free of angiographic coronary artery disease. The electrocardiographic abnormalities studied have a poorer predictive value for coronary artery disease in asymptomatic, apparently healthy men than they do in a hospital or clinical population. This has been confirmed by follow-up studies in this population as well as in others.

Exercise Testing as a Screening Procedure

Hartley and colleagues (1979) reported an exercise electrocardiographic testing program designed to examine large numbers of people effectively, conveniently, and inexpensively. This study was designed to evaluate the possible future application of exercise testing as a routine tool. A bicycle ergometer was used and multi-lead testing performed. More than 1800 people were examined in 3 years with as many as 55 tests performed per day at a cost of U.S.$60 - 70 each. The program was considered successful for rendering screening conveniently, at low cost, and with accuracy.

Table 4 summarizes six follow-up studies that utilized maximal or near-maximal exercise electrocardiographic testing to screen asymptomatic individuals for latent CHD, and one that evaluated men and women with atypical chest pain. The populations in these studies were tested, and followed up for the CHD end points of angina, acute myocardial infarction, and sudden death. Angiographic findings were not used as end points in these studies.

Bruce and McDonough (1969) studied 221 clinically normal men in Seattle, aged 35–82 years. A CB5 bipolar lead was used and 0.1 mV or more of ST-segment depression was the criterion for an abnormal response, which occurred with 10%. They were followed up for 5 years. The sensitivity was 60%; i.e., 60% of those who had had an abnormal treadmill test when they entered the study developed CHD over the follow-up period. The specificity was 91%, i.e., 91% of those who had had a normal treadmill test did not develop CHD. The probability of developing CHD with an abnormal treadmill test (the predictive value of an abnormal response) was 13.6%; that is 13.6% of those who had had an abnormal electrocardiographic response developed CHD. The relative risk of developing CHD over the follow-up period was 13.6 times greater for those who had an abnormal ST-segment response to treadmill testing than for those who had a normal response.

Aronow and colleagues (1975) tested 100 normal men in Los Angeles, aged 38–64 years, and followed them up for 5 years. Risk-factor analysis was not performed, but all subjects were normotensive. A V5 lead was used and 0.1 mV or more of ST-segment depression was the criterion for an abnormal response.

Cumming and colleagues (1975) reported their 3-year follow-up for CHD end points in 510 asymptomatic men, 40–65 years of age. Maximal or near-maximal effort was exerted and a CM5 lead was monitored. The criterion for abnormal was 0.2 mV or more of ST-segment depression.

Table 3. Risk factors and maximal treadmil functional data in 98 aircrew men with significant coronary artery disease, grouped by number of vessels involved

Vessels with significant CAD	No. (%) of men	Age (yr)[a]	Serum cholesterol (mg/100 ml)[a]	Serum tri-glycerides (mg/100 ml)[a]	Blood pressure (mm Hg)[a]	Positive smoking history (% of group)	Positive family history for CAD (% of group)	VO_2 (cc O_2/kg/min)[a]	Double product[a]	Maximal heart plate (beats/min)[a]
One	45 (45.9)	44±6	243±35	157± 72	132±12 / 85±9	64	44	35.7±5.4	33.7±4.8	175±13
Two	40 (40.8)	46±6	266±62	194±128	137±18 / 88±11	70	53	33.7±5.4	36.3±5.6	178±13
Three	13 (13.3)	46±7	273±43	154±37	135±16 / 85±9	69	62	34.1±6.7	30.6±3.7	164±10

CAD, coronary artery disease; VO_2, oxygen consumption
[a] Values expressed as mean ± standard deviation

Table 4. Results of ECG testing, in six prospective studies screening asymptomatic men for latent coronary artery disease and one evaluating men and women with atypical chest pain, using only ST-segment depression as criterion for abnormal

Investigators	No.	Incidence CAD (%)	Follow-up (years)	Abnormal exercise test (%)	Sensitivity (%)[a]	Specificity (%)[b]	Predictive value (%)[c]	Relative risk
Bruce and McDonough (1969)	221	2.3	5.0	11	60	91	14	14×
Aronow and Cassidy (1975)	100	9.0	5.0	16	67	92	46	14×
Cumming et al. (1975)	510	4.7	3.0	13	58	90	25	10×
Froelicher et al. (1975)	1390	3.3	6.3	10	61	92	20	14×
Allen et al. (1980)	356 (men >40 yrs)	9.6	5.0	23	41	79	17	2.4×
Bruce et al. (1980a)	2365	2.0	6.0	11	30	91	5	3.5×
Manca et al. (1978)	947 (men)	5.0	5.2	18	67	84	18	10×
	508 (women)	1.6	5.2	28	88	73	5	15×
Average (men only)	–	–	–	15	55	88	21	10×

[a] Subjects with CAD who have an abnormal ECG response to exercise
[b] Normals who have a normal ECG response
[c] Abnormal ECG responders who have CAD

At the United States School of Aerospace Medicine, 1390 asymptomatic men, 20–54 years of age, who did not have any of the known causes for false-positive treadmill tests were screened for latent CHD by maximal treadmill testing and followed up for a mean of 6.3 years (Froelicher et al. 1975). The main lead used was CC5, but additional leads were obtained with the subjects in the supine position, post exercise. The criterion for abnormal was 0.1 mV or more horizontal or down-sloping ST-segment depression.

In Italy, Manca and colleagues (1978) studied 974 mean and 508 women who were referred for exercise testing because of atypical chest pain. Those with typical symptoms of angina pectoris, valvular disease, hypertension, bundle branch block, arrhythmias, Wolff-Parkinson-White syndrome, left ventricular hypertrophy with strain, significant resting repolarization abnormalities, and previous myocardial infarction were excluded. No patient received drugs such as digitalis, beta-blockers, antiarrhythmics, or diuretics in the 2 weeks preceding exercise testing. Exercise was done after routine hyperventilation, using a supine bicycle, until at least 85% of the predicted maximal heart rate was reached. The conventional 12 electrocardiogram leads were recorded during and after the exercise test. Criterion for an abnormal response was 0.1 mV or more of horizontal or down-sloping ST-segment depression; response was abnormal for 18% of the men and 28% of the women. The end points for CHD were myocardial infarction or sudden death, and there was a mean follow-up of 5.2 years. The overall incidence of CHD was 5% in the men and 1.6% in the women. The sensitivity was 67% in the men versus 88% in the women. The specificity of the test in the men was 84% versus 73% in the women. The predictive value of a positive test was 18% in men, but only 5% in women. Men with positive tests had a relative risk of 10 for developing clinical manifestations of CHD; the relative risk for women with positive tests was 15. This study clearly shows how predictive value is influenced by the prevalence of CHD in the population under study, and that the specificity of the exercise test is lower in women. The latter finding has recently been confirmed again by the Gotesburg group (Bengtsson et al. 1981).

Allen and colleagues (1980) recently reported a 5-year follow-up of 888 asymptomatic men and women without known CHD who had initially undergone maximal treadmill testing. When tested, none of the subjects were on medications that would affect the electrocardiogram, nor did they have bundle branch block, a strain pattern, or pathologic Q waves. None had clinical evidence of pulmonary disease or vascular disease. No subject developed serious arrhytmias, conduction abnormalities, or chest pain in conjunction with the exercise test. Maximal treadmill testing was performed following the Ellestad protocol, and leads CM5 and V1, and a bipolar vertical lead were recorded. Subjects were exercised until they reached 100% of predicted maximal heart rate, fatigue, or marked dyspnea. Flat ST-segment depression of 0.1 mV or greater and down-sloping of the ST segment were considered positive responses. Subjects with major ST-segment changes at rest were excluded. If there were minor changes in the ST-segment before exercise, an additional .15 mV of depression at 80 ms from the J point were required to indicate an abnormal exercise test. R-wave amplitude was measured for an average of six beats during a control period and immediately after exercise, and an increase or no change in the R wave immediately after exercise compared with control was defined as an abnormal response. A decrease in R-wave amplitude was defined as a normal response.

The original population included 1077 subjects, and 888 (82.5%) were contacted for follow-up. Of the 113 subjects who had initally had abnormal exercise tests, 105 were located (92.9%). There was a 1.1% incidence of coronary heart disease per year. End points for CHD were angina pectoris, myocardial infarction, or sudden cardiac death. Only two of 221 men aged 40 years or less developed end points, and none of these had ST-segment abnormalities, an abnormal R-wave response, or an exercise duration of 5 min or less. Hence, in this study, abnormal maximal treadmill test results did not correlate with subsequent CHD in asymptomatic men 40 years of age or younger. This contrasts with a similar study that had 563 men 30–39 years of age and a 1.4% incidence of CHD (Manca et al. 1978). The exercise electrocardiogram was found to have 50% sensitivity, 95% specificity, 13% predictive value, and a relative risk of 17; thus, it still had value in this age range (see Table 5).

Table 5. Performance of the exercise ECG in asymptomatic men less than 40 years of age

Investigators	No.	Age range	Incidence of CHD (%)	Follow-up (years)	Abnormal exercise test (%)	Sensitivity (%)	Specificity (%)	Predictive value (%)	Relative risk
Froelicher et al. (1975)	563	30–39	1.4	6.3	5.5	50	95	13	17×
Allen et al. (1980)	221	<40	0.9	5.0	3.6	0	96	0	0

Allen and colleagues (1980) concluded that the exercise test was only of value in men older than 40 years, for whom subsequent CHD within 5 years was predicted by an abnormal ST-segment response, an increase or no change in R-wave, and an exercise duration of 5 min or less. The ST segment, R wave, and exercise duration criteria had sensitivities of 41%, 47%, and 26% respectively. The sensitivity of a test which was interpreted as positive when either ST or R-wave criteria were present was 65%. Adding exercise duration of 5 min or less as a third alternative criterion for a positive test did not change sensitivity. The performance of the exercise test responses is summarized in Table 6. When all three criteria were present a sensitivity of 29% with a specificity of 100% was achieved. In men older than 40 years the ST-segment criteria had a sensitivity of 41%, specificity of 79%, predictive value of 17%, and relative risk of 2.4. With the exception of predictive value, these values are strinkingly lower than those found in earlier studies (see Table 4).

Table 6. The performance of the abnormal exercise test responses in men greater than 40 years of age in the study of Allen et al. (1980)

Abnormal response	Sensitivity (%)	Specificity (%)	Predictive value (%)	Risk ratio
ST depression	41	79	17	2×
Rw→↑	47	78	19	3×
Duration	27	96	43	6×
ST and Rw	40	86	27	5×
ST and duration	24	99	71	11×
Rw and duration	33	99	82	12×
All three	29	100	100	17×

Rw, R-wave

Of the 311 women followed up by Allen and his co-workers, ten developed CHD end points. The authors found that ST depression and R-wave response did not correlate with subsequent development of CHD. However, exercise duration of 3 min or less proved to be a significant predictor of CHD. Four of 13 women with limited exercise tolerance developed CHD. When used as a criterion for abnormal, exercise duration of 3 min or less in asymptomatic women had a sensitivity of 40%, specificity of 97%, predictive value of 31%, and relative risk of 15.

Contrary to the conclusions of Allen et al., we feel, in view of these findings, that maximal exercise tests may prove to be of value in screening asymptomatic women and younger men for CHD. Limited follow-up of 80% of the original population and the low incidence of CHD end points in all the women and in men less than 40 years of age are limitations of this study.

Bruce and colleagues (1980a) recently reported the 6-year follow-up of 2365 clinically healthy men (mean age, 45 years) who were exercise-tested as part of the Seattle Heart Watch. They underwent symptom-limited maximal treadmill testing using neither ST depression nor target heart rates as end points of maximal exercise. The Bruce protocol was used, and a bipolar CB5 lead was monitored. Conventional risk factors were assessed at the time of the initial examination in a subset of the population. Follow-up was done by questionnaire, with morbidity defined as hospital admission. Forty-seven men (2%) experienced coronary heart disease morbidity or mortality. Univariate analysis of the individual conventional risk factors (positive family history, hypertension, smoking, hypercholesterolemia) did not show a statistically significant increase in the 5-year probability of primary CHD events. Only when the sum of risk factors in an individual was assessed did conventional risk factors become statistically significant in relation to the event rate. Four variables from treadmill testing were predictive, including (a) exercise duration of less than 6 min (which requires 6–7 METS, or multiples of resting oxygen consumption); (b) 0.1 mV ST depression during recovery; (c) greater than 10% heart rate impairment (defined as the percent reduction of age-adjusted maximal heart rate); and (d) chest pain during maximal exertion. The ST-segment criteria had a sensitivity of 30%, specificity of 89%, predictive value of 5.3%, and a risk ratio of 3.3. Angina and exercise duration each had sensitivities of about 6%. Heart rate impairment had a sensitivity of 19%, and was comparable to ST-segment depression for the other parameters.

Table 7 summarizes the performance of the exercise test predictors. The presence of two or more of the exercise test predictors identified men in all age-groups who were at increased risk. Furthermore, it was found that, in the presence of one or more conventional risk factors, as the prevalence of exertional risk predictors rose from none to any three the relative risk rose from 1 to 30. The group that had one or more conventional risk factors and two or more exertional risk predictors was found to have the highest 5-year probability of CHD. However, in the absence of conventional risk factors, exercise testing failed to provide additional prognostic information in normal men.

Table 7. Performance of the abnormal exercise test results in the Seattle Heart Watch

Abnormality	Sensitivity (%)	Specificity (%)	Predictive value (%)	Relative risk
ST↓	30	91	5	3.5×
Angina	6	99	15	8×
Duration	6	99	19	10×
HRI	19	93	7	4×

HRI, heart rate impairment

Coronary Angiography in Asymptomatic Men with Abnormal Treadmill Tests

Froelicher et al. (1977) performed coronary angiography on 111 asymptomatic men with an abnormal electrocardiographic response to treadmill testing. Only one-third of the subjects had at least one lesion 50% or greater in a major coronary artery. Barnard and colleagues (1975) used near-maximal treadmill testing to screen randomly selected Los Angeles firefighters. Ten percent showed an abnormal exercise-induced elektrocardiographic response despite low risk factors for CHD. Six men with an abnormal exercise test elected to undergo cardiac catheterization (Barnard et al. 1976). One had severe three-vessel disease, and another had a 50% obstruction of the left circumflex coronary artery. The other four men had normal studies. Borer and colleagues (1975) reported their angiographic findings in 11 asymptomatic individuals with hyperlipidemia and an abnormal exercise electrocardiographic test. Only 37% of these individuals were found to have angiographic CHD. Erikssen et al. (1976) reported their angiograhic findings in 105 men aged 40–59 from a working population with one or more of the following criteria: (a) a positive questionnaire for angina pectoris; (b) typical angina during a near-maximal bicycle test; (c) an abnormal exercise electrocardiogram. The exercise test had a predictive value of 84% if a slowly ascending ST segment was included. The higher predictive value in this study might be due to the more advanced age of their population and to the inclusion of men with angina. These angiographic studies confirm the low predictive value of an abnormal exercise test response also found in the epidemiological studies of populations with a low prevalence of CHD.

The Predictive Model

More false-positive responses are found when a testing procedure is used in a population with a low prevalence of disease than in a population with a high prevalence of disease. This explains the greater number of false positive found when using a test as a screening procedure in an asymptomatic population as compared with using it as a diagnostic procedure in patients with symptoms consistent with CHD. No matter what techniques are used, there is a reciprocal relationship between sensitivity and specificity. The more specific a test is (i.e., the more able it is to determine who is disease free), the less sensitive it is. The values for sensitivity and specificity can be altered by adjusting the criterion for abnormal. For instance, when the criterion for an abnormal exercise-induced ST-segment response is altered to 0.2 mV depression to make it more specific for coronary artery disease, the sensitivity of the test can be cut in half. For unknown reasons, the specificity of the ST response is decreased when the test is used in patients with vasoregulatory abnormality, left ventricular hypertrophy, mitral valve prolapse, or ST depression at rest, or when it is used in women. Various computerized electrocardiographic criteria for ischemia have been proposed (Bhargava et al. 1981). However, the most promising techniques recommended to increase the senitivity and specificity of screening are the following:

1. Thallium perfusion imaging
2. Radionuclide ventriculography during bicycle exercise and post treadmill exercise
3. Cardiac fluoroscopy for coronary artery calcification
4. Cardiokymography
5. Total cholesterol/HDL ratio, conventional risk factors
6. ECG-gated chest X-ray per and post exercise
7. Computerized multifactorial risk prediction using Bayesion statistics (CANDENZA marketed by Cardiokinetcs)
8. Systolic time intervals during and after exercise

Thallium-201 Exercise Testing

Caralis and colleagues (1979) performed thallium-201 exercise testing and coronary angiography to evaluate asymptomatic individuals with abnormal ST-segment responses to exercise testing. In 3496 consecutive treadmill tests, 22 individuals developed 0.2 mV or more of asymptomatic horizontal ST-segment depression; 15 agreed to be evaluated further with thallium scintigraphy and coronary angiography. Of the 15 individuals with an abnormal exercise test, five had normal scans with exercise, whereas ten developed new defects. The thallium exercise scans classified 13 of 15 patients properly, with one false negative and one false positive. This was not a valid epidemiological study since it was performed selectively and coronary angiography was the end point.

Nolewajka and colleagues (1981) performed thallium treadmill tests on 58 asymptomatic men as part of a screening study. The risk for coronary heart disease was determined using the Framingham risk equation. The risk calculation was greater in those with abnormal exercise studies than in those who had normal studies. Six had abnormal thallium scans (five consistent with ischemia, one with scar). Three of the subjects with abnormal thallium studies underwent coronary angiography, and all had normal coronary arteries. Surprisingly, two of these had left bundle branch block (one with exercise only, the other at rest) which may account for the false-positive scans. The disappointment in these results was compounded by the psychological stress to the individuals who were told they had "abnormal" results.

Uhl and colleagues (1981a) performed single-dose exercise and delayed thallium scintigrams on 191 aircrew men prior to undergoing coronary angiography because of abnormal exercise electrocardiograms. Of these, 41 men had significant angiographic disease, for a predictive value of the electrocardiogram of 21% versus 74% for scintigraphy. The specificity of the computer-processed scans was 90%. There were mixed results in the 15 men with minimal disease (less than 50% occlusion); ten had abnormal scans, and five had normal. The high sensitivity and specificity of these computer-enhanced thallium scintigrams in this population of apparently healthy men is a strong support for its use as a second-line screening procedure. If both an abnormal exercise electrocardiogram and abnormal perfusion scintigram had been required before angiography was performed, 136 of those free of coronary disease would not have needed to undergo angiography.

Studies from many centers have shown that gated blood-pool ejection fractions are accurate and reproducible at both rest and exercise, but the determination of wall motion abnormalities is much less reliable. This is disappointing, since segmental dysfunction precedes global dysfunction during exercise and should be more specific for coronary disease, which is usually a regional disease.

The only reported application of exercise radionuclide angiograms to detect coronary artery disease in asymptomatic men compared global ejection fraction changes with visual evaluation of segmental wall motion and the visual interpretation of thallium perfusion scintigraphy in 32 men (Uhl et al. 1982). The thallium study had a better sensitivity (92%) than did global (85%) or regional (62%) abnormalities by radionuclide angiograms without loss of specificity (95% versus 85% and 95% respectively).

The results of resting and exercise electrocardiograms, thallium myocardial perfusion imaging, and equilibrium radionuclide angiography were analyzed in 71 consecutive patients referred to our laboratory for diagnosis or evaluation of CHD (Pfisterer et al. 1980). The overall sensitivity for the resting and exercise electrocardiogram was 66%, for the thallium-201 scan 74%, for both combined 79%, and for the ejection fraction response to exercise 97%. The specificity was lowest with supine bicycle radionuclide angiography, but all patients with false-positive results had cardiomyopathies. Thus, supine bicycle radionuclide angiography is highly specific for left ventricular dysfunction, rather than for CHD. The following approach to evaluating patients with symptoms suggestive of CHD was proposed. The resting and exercise electrocardiogram remain the first step. The next step should be radionuclide angiography at rest and during exercise to assess left ventricular function. If normal, radionuclide angiography almost absolutely excludes left ventricular dysfunction and hemodynamically significant CHD. If abnormal, the workup should then proceed to cardiac catheterization if this is clinically indicated.

At the University of California in San Diego we have presented an approach using radionuclide angiography to increase the sensitivity and specificity of treadmill testing (Battler et al. 1980). Labeled technetium was administered intravenously in order to perform sequential left ventricular ventriculography in ten CHD patients and eight normal subjects. All 18 subjects underwent maximal treadmill testing. Ejection fractions were measured from 2 to 4, 4 to 6, and 8 to 10 min of recovery. At 8 to 10 min of recovery all of the normals, but none of the CHD patients, had higher ejection fractions than the resting ejection fraction. The addition of regional wall-motion analysis post-treadmill testing could add further discriminant value. Post-treadmill analysis could be more sensitive than the supine bicycle technique because of the higher work loads achieved, and an increase in specificity could possibly be obtained over standard ST-segment analysis by detecting regional wall-motion abnormalities.

As yet, there has not been adequate research application of the radionuclide exercise techniques to the asymptomatic population. However, both procedures seem to have great promise, since they have been reported to have greater sensitivity when compared with the exercise electrocardiogram in symptomatic populations. Specificity in the asymptomatic population, where it is best determined, has yet to be demonstrated. However, Foster and colleagues (1981) have shown that the exercise ejection fraction can drop in normal individuals. Several studies have demonstrated a specificity as low as 60% with exercise radionuclide ventriculography, which makes it as bad as flipping a coin to identify normals.

Cardiokymography

The cardiokymograph (CKG) is an electronic device that produces a representation of regional left ventricular wall motion noninvasively. It generates an electromagnetic field, and motion within the field causes a change in the frequency of an oscillator. A change in frequency is converted into a change in voltage proportional to the motion. The CKG produced a recording similar to the apexcardiogram (ACG) and the kinetocardiogram (KCG). The advantage of the CKG is that it records absolute cardiac motion without chest motion, thus eliminating the problem of distortion inherent in both the ACG and the KCG. There is considerable tissue penetration, so the CKG responds to deeper cardiac motion as well as to precordial surface movement. CKG recordings have been shown to be predictive of ventriculographic wall-motion abnormalities.

Silverberg and colleagues (1980) reported their use of the post-exercise CKG in 157 patients, including 27 apparently healthy volunteers and 130 patients with suspected CHD who underwent coronary angiography. The subjects performed a progressive symptom-limited maximal treadmill test. The CKG was recorded within 2 min of termination of exercise, and every minute thereafter for 10 min. Two sets of empirical criteria for an abnormal CKG pattern were defined in relation to known effects of ischemia on regional wall motion. The first abnormality was defined as paradoxical systolic outward motion. The second abnormality was defined as development of total absence of inward motion, a resultant holosystolic outward motion, or systolic outward motion occurring for less than the entire period of ejection, but not preceded by inward motion. For detecting CHD in atypical chest pain patients, the CKG had a higher sensitivity, specificity, and predictive value than the electrocardiogram. However, no statistical difference existed between the electrocardiogram and the CKG in asymptomatic patients. This may be explained by the distribution of disease in this study: patients with atypical chest pain had a 30% prevalence of disease, while asymptomatic patients had a 64% prevalence of angiographic coronary artery disease. Exercise-induced CKG abnormalities persisted longer during recovery than did electrocardiographic changes. Although the CKG had higher sensitivity and specificity than the electrocardiogram for the detection of coronary disease in patients with atypical chest pain, the results could have been due to the population sample selected for this study. This device is now commercially available, and Weiner and colleagues have duplicated these results (Weiner et al. 1983).

Coronary Artery Calcification on Fluoroscopy

Kelly et al. (1978) reported the use of cardiac fluoroscopy as a prescreening tool before exercise-testing asymptomatic men. In one study, 129 healthy men (average age 49) were evaluated with cardiac fluoroscopy to detect coronary artery calcification, followed by a submaximal exercise test. Of the 108 subjects who completed the exercise test, 37, or 34%, had at least one fluoroscopically detected calcified coronary artery. Of this group of subjects with positive fluoroscopy, 13, or 35%, had an abnormal ST-segment response to the exercise test. Of the 68 subjects with normal fluoroscopy, only 3, or 4%, had an abnormal exercise response. Consequently, those with calcification of at least one coronary artery had a ninefold increased risk of having an abnormal exercise electrocardiographic test. Of the 16 subjects with an abnormal exercise test, 81% had calcification of at least one coronary artery. The location of the calcific deposit conferred greater risk for exercise-induced ischemic changes than did multi-vessel involvement. Forty-seven percent of men with calcification in the left anterior descending coronary artery had an abnormal exercise electrocardiogram, versus 33% and 16% of persons with left circumflex and right coronary artery calcifications respectively.

In a second study, the 13 men who had both coronary artery calcification and an abnormal exercise test underwent coronary angiography (Langou et al. 1981). They had a mean age of 44, none had any symptoms or signs of CHD, and all had a normal resting electrocardiogram. Coronary artery calcification was first detected by fluoroscopy in one artery in ten men, in two arteries in two men, and in three arteries in one man. On angiography, CHD was considered clinically significant if there was greater than 50% narrowing in any major coronary branch. Coronary arteriography revealed 12 men with clinically significant CHD: single-vessel in four, double in five, and triple in three men. One man had only a minor lesion. There was a 3-year follow-up of these 13 patients; three developed typical angina, and one developed a transmural myocardial infarction. The results of this study suggest that the combination of coronary artery calcification and an abnormal exercise test is highly predictive of CHD. However, the sensitivity and specificity of the combination of these procedures remain to be clarified. Questions that remain are: Did the three subjects with an abnormal exercise test and no fluroscopically detected coronary artery calcification have angiographic disease, and what of the 24 individuals with coronary artery calcification and a normal exercise electrocardiogram? This is certainly a usual population, since even the exercise test alone had a very high predictive value, higher than expected in asymptomatic subjects.

Lipid Screening in Conjunction with Exercise Testing

Total cholesterol high-density lipoprotein cholesterol (TC/HDL) ratios have been shown to be directly correlated with CHD risk. In a study by Williams and colleagues (1979) of 2568 asymptomatic men, a TC/HDL ratio of 4 correlated with a very low CHD conventional risk-factor rating, and a TC/HDL ratio of 8 was correlated with very high risk for CHD. Uhl and colleagues (1981b) measured fasting TC and HDL in 572 asymptomatic aircrew men. Of these, 132 had an abnormal treadmill test and underwent coronary angiography. Coronary disease defined as a 50% or greater lesion was found in 16, with the rest having minimal ($n=14$) or no CHD ($n=102$). The 14 men with minimal CHD had TC/HDL values that differed from the normals ($p<.001$). Two of the 16 with angiographic coronary artery disease had TC/HDL ratios of less than 6, while four of the 102 angiographic normals had a ratio of greater than 6. Only 42 of 440 (9.5%) with a normal treadmill had a TC/HDL ratio greater than 6: 87% of those with CHD had TC/HDL ratios greater than 6. A limitation of this study is that true sensitivity cannot be determined, since only those with an abnormal treadmill test underwent coronary angiography.

Electrocardiographic-Gated Chest X-Rays

Dinsmore and colleagues (1979) reported the use of electrocardiographic-triggered chest X-rays to diagnose CHD. A bicycle ergometer was pedaled directly in front of an X-ray film cassette, and chest X-rays were taken at rest and at peak exercise. Wall motion abnormalities, volume change, or pulmonary hypertension were criteria for ischemia. They suggest that this procedure is suitable for screening the apparently healthy population, but no data are yet available.

Computerized Probability Estimates

Diamond and Forrester (1979) have reviewed the literature to estimate pretest likelihood of disease by age, sex, symptoms, and the Framingham risk equation (based on blood pressure, smoking, glucose intolerance, resting electrocardiogram, and cholesterol). In addition, they have considered the sensitivity and specificity of four diagnostic tests (the exercise test, cardiokymography, thallium, and cardiac fluoroscopy) and applied Bayes' Theorem. This has been assimilated in a computer program written in Apple Basic that can be used to determine probabilities of coronary disease for a given individual after entry of any of the above data. CADENZA is the acronym for this program, which is commercially available (Cardiokinetics, Seattle, Washington).

Hlatky and colleagues (1982) have attempted to validate CADENZA and another method of probability calculation by comparing diagnostic accuracy with that of 91 cardiologists who evaluated the clinical summaries of eight randomly selected patients. For each patient, the cardiologist assessed the probability of coronary heart disease after reviewing the clinical history, physical examination, and laboratory data, including an exercise test. The probability of coronary disease was also obtained for each patient using identical information from a published table of data based on age, sex, symptoms, and degree of ST-segment change during exercise, and from a computer program using the age, sex, risk factors, resting electrocardiogram, and multiple exercise measurements. With the coronary angiogram as the standard, the average diagnostic accuracy was best for the computer program. One wonders if the computer program would be helpful for internists or family practitioners, and what the findings would have been if more than just eight patients had been included.

Systolic Intervals

Sugiura et al. (1981) have reported that systolic intervals measured using ear densitography during exercise appear to improve the sensitivity and specificity of the exercise test. These workers recorded ear densitograms using a photoelectric ear piece attached to the pinna of the ear enabling measurements of the pre-ejection period and left ventricular ejection time. Ten patients with coronary heart disease were compared with 17 normal men. Despite nearly identical heart rate and blood pressure responses, men with coronary heart disease had a significantly greater reduction of pre-ejection period at 1 min and 4 min during exercise, as well as a greater decrease in the PEP/LVET ratio. They felt that the early fall in the PEP/LVET ratio represented limited functional reserve and that the subsequent increase was consistent with functional deterioration. Louis and colleagues (1977) noted prolongation of left ventricular ejection time post exercise and suggested that this enhanced the diagnostic power of the exercise test. These approaches need further evaluation to determine if they have additional value as compared with standard exercise measurement.

Prognosis for Asymptomatic Individuals with Angiographic Coronary Disease

Hickman and co-workers (1980) at the United States Air Force School of Aerospace Medicine followed up 90 asymptomatic men, aged 45–54 years, with angiographic coronary disease without previous infarction, for a mean of 57 ± 25 months; 16 patients developed angina at a mean of 31 ± 5 months, four had myocardial infarctions, and two died suddenly. The events occurred at similar rates in those with one-, two-, or three-vessel disease. Nineteen remained asymptomatic at 45 ± 9 months. Five developed angina, one died suddenly and three underwent coronary bypass surgery while still asymptomatic. Ten of 21 men with events (45%) had three or more risk factors, while only seven of the 64 who remained asymptomatic had at least three risk factors. Thus, the presence of several risk factors predicted angina, infarction, or sudden death better than the angiographic severity of disease did. The 5-year prognosis was good even in those with high-risk lesions and the event rate was only 6% per year. Asymptomatic coronary artery disease has a better prognosis for the same vessel scores than when the disease is asymptomatic. Perhaps this is explained by differences both in the severity of the lesions within diseased vessels and in ventricular function.

Kent et al. (1982) have reported 147 asymptomatic or mildly symptomatic patients with coronary heart disease who were followed prospectively for an average of 2 years. They had ejection fractions greater than 20% and none had significant left main disease. Twenty-eight percent had significant one-vessel, 31% had two-vessel, and 41% had three-vessel coronary disease. Ejection fraction was 55% or greater in 70% of the patients. Thirty-five percent of the patients had a normal electrocardiogram, while 30% had evidence of a previous myocardial infarction. During the follow-up period there were eight deaths. There was an annual mortality of 3% for the entire group, 1.5% for patients with single- and double-vessel disease, and 6% for those with triple-vessel disease. In those with triple-vessel disease, exercise testing enabled better identification of high- and a low-risk groups. In spite of a history of mild symptoms, 25% of the patients with triple-vessel disease exhibited poor exercise tolerance; of these, 40% either died (for an annual mortality of 9%), or had progressive symptoms requiring an operation. In those with good exercise capacity, only 22% died or had progressive symptoms, giving an annual mortality of 4%. The prognosis is excellent in patients with no or mild symptoms with one- or two-vessel disease. In those with three-vessel disease and with good exercise capacity, there was an annual mortality of 4%, versus 9% in those with three-vessel disease and poor exercise capacity.

Conclusions

Risk-factor screening directs attention to a relatively small number of individuals who will develop coronary disease, while the majority of those with events are in the moderate risk group. Again, sensitivity and specificity are limited even with the optimal setting of discriminant values.

The resting electrocardiogram lacks sensitivity and specificity for detecting silent coronary disease, however, it is an inexpensive and readily available technique (Barrett et al. 1981). There are probable health care benefits from obtaining a baseline electrocardiogram in most individuals because of the wide range of normal variation and the possibility of finding serial changes.

The exercise test is usually more sensitive than other approaches since it brings out abnormalities not present at rest. Since an abnormal exercise electrocardiogram is neither 100% sensitive nor specific, an abnormal test does not absolutely predict the presence of CHD or its future development, nor does a normal test rule out disease or the future occurrence of coronary events. Some of those who are going to develop coronary disease will change from a normal to an abnormal response when retested, so, possibly, serial testing will increase sensitivity. However, McHenry et al. (1981) have reported that a change from a negative to a positive test is no more predictive than an initially abnormal test and an individual has been reported who changed from a normal to an abnormal test, but was free of angiographically significant disease (Thompson et al. 1975).

Exercise testing may prove to have another value for asymptomatic populations in addition to its screening capabilities. Bruce et al. (1980b) examined the motivational effects of maximal exercise testing for modifying risk factors and health habits. A questionnaire was sent to nearly 3000 men, 35–65 years of age, who had undergone symptom-limited treadmill testing at least 1 year earlier. Individuals were asked if the treadmill test had motivated them to stop smoking (if a smoker), increase daily exercise, purposely lose weight, reduce the amount of dietary fat, or take medication for hypertension. There was a 69% response to this questionnaire, and 63% of the responders indicated that they had modified one or more risk factors and health habits, and that they attributed this change to the exercise test. In fact, a greater percentage of patients with abnormal function aerobic impairment than of normal subjects reported changing risk factors or health habits.

Of particular interest is the fact that exercise-induced wall-motion abnormalities can precede, and occur, without electrocardiographic changes, as shown by both animal (Theroux et al. 1974) and human studies (Upton et al. 1980). Development of a technique that accurately and reproducibly detects exercise-induced regional wall-motion abnormalities could revolutionize identification of latent CHD.

Newer procedures, including cardiokymography, thallium, radionuclide ventriculography, computerized probability analysis, cardiac fluoroscopy, and systolic intervals need further study in asymptomatic populations before they are routinely used for screening purposes or as a secondary line of testing. But screening for coronary disease has little general application unless risk-factor intervention is effective (The MRFIT Research Group 1982; Hjerman et al. 1981).

References

Allen WH, Aronow WS, Goodman P, Stinson P (1980) Five-year follow-up of maximal treadmill stress test in asymptomatic men and women. Circulation 62:522

Aronow WS, Cassidy JK (1975) Five-year follow-up of double Master's test, maximal treadmill stress test, and resting and postexercise apexcardiogram in asymptomatic persons. Circulation 52:616

Barnard RJ, Gardner GW, Diaco NV, Kattus AA (1975) Near-maximal ECG stress testing and coronary artery disease risk-factor analysis in Los Angeles City fire fighters. J Occup 17:693

Barnard RJ, Gardner GW, Diaco NV (1976) "Ischemic" heart disease in fire fighters with normal coronary arteries. Occup Med 18:818

Barrett PA, Peter CT, Swan HJC, Singh BN, Mandel WJ (1981) The frequency and prognostic significance of electrocardiographic abnormalities in clinically normal individuals. Prog Cardiovasc Dis 23:299

Battler A, Slutsky R, Pfisterer M et al. (1980) Left ventricular ejection fraction changes during recovery from treadmill exercise: A preliminary report of a new method for detecting coronary artery disease. Clin Cardiol 3:14

Bengtsson C, Grimby G, Lindquist O, Noppa H, Sigurdsson JA, Vedin JA (1981) Prognosis of women with exercise-induced ECG changes - results from a longitudinal population study. Cardiology 68:9

Bhargava V, Watanabe K, Froelicher V (1981) Progress in computer analysis of the exercise ECG. Am J Cardiol 47:1143

Borer JS, Brensike JF, Redwood DR et al. (1975) Limitations of the electrocardiographic response to exercise in predicting coronary artery disease. N Eng J Med 193:367

Breslow L, Sommers AR (1977) The lifetime health monitoring program: practical approach to preventive medicine. N Engl J Med 296:601

Bruce RA, McDonough JR (1969) Stress testing in screening for cardiovascular disease. Bull NY Acad Med 45:1299

Bruce RA, DeRouen TA, Hossack KF (1980a) Value of maximal exercise tests in risk assessment of primary coronary heart disease events in healthy men. Am J Cardiol 46:371

Bruce RA, DeRouen TA, Hossack KF (1980b) Pilot study examining the motivational effects of maximal exercise testing to modify risk factors and health habits. Cardiology 66:111

Caralis DG, Bailey I, Kennedy HL, Pitt B (1979) Thallium-201 myocardial imaging in evaluation of asymptomatic individuals with ischaemic ST segment depression on exercise electrocardiogram. Br Heart J 42:562

Cullen K, Stenhouse NS, Wearne KL, Cumpston GN (1982) Electrocardiograms and 13 year cardiovascular mortality in Busselton study. Br Heart J 47:209

Cumming GR, Samm J, Borysyk L et al. (1975) Electrocardiographic changes during exercise in asymptomatic men: 3-year follow-up. Can Med Assoc J 112:578

Dawber TR, Kannel WB, Love DE, Streeper RB (1952) The Framingham study. Circulation 5:559

Diamond GA, Forrester JS (1979) Analysis of probability as an aid in the clinical diagnosis of coronary artery disease. N Engl J Med 300:1350

Dinsmore RE, Wernikoff RE, Miller SW, Pohost GM, Block PC, Potsaid MS (1979) Evaluation of left ventricular free wall asynergy due to coronary artery disease: use of an interlaced ECG-gated radiography system. AJR 132: 909
Erikssen J, Enge I, Forfang K, Storstein O (1976) False-positive diagnostic tests and coronary angiographic findings in 105 presumably healthy males. Circulation 54:371
Foster C, Anholm JD, Hellmann CK, Carpenter J, Pollack ML, Schmidt DH (1981) Left ventricular function during sudden strenuous exercise. Circulation 63:592–596
Froelicher, VF (1983) Exercise testing and training. Le Jacq, New York
Froelicher VF, Thomas M, Pillow C et al. (1975) An epidemiological study of asymptomatic men screened with exercise testing for latent coronary heart disease. Am J Cardiol 34:770
Froelicher VF, Thompson AJ, Wolthuis R, Fuchs R, Balusek R, Longo MR, Triebwasser JH, Lancaster MC (1977) Angiographic findings in asymptomatic aircrewmen with electrocardiographic abnormalities. Am J Cardiol 39:32
Froom J, Boisseau V, Sherman A (1979) Selective screening for lead poisoning in an urban teaching practice. J Fam Pract 65:9
Hartley LH, Herd JA, Day WC, Abusamra J, Howes B (1979) An exercise testing program for large populations. JAMA 241:269
Hickmann JR, Uhl GS, Cook RL, Engel PJ, Hopkifk JAC (1980) A natural history study of asymptomatic coronary disease. Am J Cardiol 45:422
Hjermann I, Holme I, VelveByre K, Leren P (1981) Effect of diet and smoking intervention on the incidence of coronary heart disease. Lancet 2:1305
Hlatky M, Bovinick E, Brundage B (1982) Diagnostic accuracy of cardiologists compared with probability calculations using Bayes' rule. Am J Cardiol 49:1927
Kelley MJ, Huang EK, Langou RA (1978) Correlation of fluoroscopically detected coronary artery calcification with exercise stress testing in asymptomatic men. Radiology 129:1
Kent KM, Rosing DR, Ewels CJ, Lipson L, Bonow R, Epstein SE (1982) Prognosis of asymptomatic or mildly symptomatic patients with coronary artery disease. Am J Cardiol 49:1823
Langou RA, Huang EK, Kelley MJ et al. (1981) Predictive accuracy of coronary artery calcification and abnormal exercise test for coronary artery disease in asymptomatic man. Circulation 62:1196
Levine HD, Phillips E (1951) The electrocardiogram and myocardial infarction. N Engl J Med 245:833
Louis RP, Marsh DG, Sherman JA, Forester WF, Schaal SF (1977) Enhanced diagnostic power of exercise testing for myocardial ischemia by addition of post-exercise left ventricular ejection time. Am J Cardiol 39:767
Manca C, Cas LD, Albertini D, Baldi G, Visioli O (1978) Different prognostic value of exercise electrocardiogram in men and women. Cardiology 63:312
McHenry PL, Richmond HW, Weisenberger BL, Rodway JS, Perry GF, Jordan JW (1981) Evaluation of abnormal exercise electrocardiogram in appenrently healthy subjects: Labile repolarization (ST-T) abnormalities as a cause of false-positive responses. Am J Cardiol 47:1152
The MRFIT Research Group (1982) Risk factor changes and mortality. JAMA 248:1465
Nolewajka AJ, Kostuk WJ, Howard J, Rechnitzer PA, Cunningham DA (1981) 201 Thallium stress myocardial imaging: An evaluation of fifty-eight asymptomatic males. Clin Cardiol 4:134
Ostor E, Schnohr, Jensen G, Nyboe J, Hansen AT (1981) Electrocardiographic findings and their association with mortality in the Copenhagen City Heart Study. Eur Heart J 2:317
Pfisterer ME, Williams RJ, Gordon DG et al. (1980) Comparison of rest/exercise ECG, thallium-201 scans and radionuclide angiography in patients with suspected coronary artery disease. Cardiology 66:45
Rabkin SW, Mathewson FAL, Tate RB (1982) The electrocardiogram in apparently healthy men and the risk of sudden death. Br Heart J 47:546
Rose G, Baxter PJ, Reid DD, McCartney P (1978) Prevalence and prognosis of electrocardiographic findings in middle-aged men. Br Heart J 40:636

Silverberg RA, Diamond GA, Vas R et al. (1980) Noninvasive diagnosis of coronary artery disease: The cardiokymographic stress test. Circulation 61:5579

Sugiura T, Doi Y, Haffty B, Moreau K, Bishop R, Singh J, Spodick D (1981) Noninvasive assessment of left ventricular performance in patients with ischemic heart disease: ear densitographic study during uninterrupted treadmill exercise. Am J Cardiol 48:101

Therox P, Franklin D, Ross J Jr et al. (1974) Regional myocardial function during acute coronary artery occlusion and its modifications by pharmacologic agents in the dog. Circ Res 35:986

Thompson AJ, Froelicher VF, Longo MR, Triebwasser JH (1975) Normal coronary angiography in an aircrewman with serial exercise test changes. Aviat Space Environ Med 46:69

Uhl GS, Kay TN, Hickman JR (1981a) Computer-enhanced thallium scintigrams in asymptomatic men with abnormal exercise tests. Am J Cardiol 48:1037

Uhl GS, Troxler RG, Hickman JR, Clark D (1981b) Angiographic correlation of coronary artery disease with high-density lipoprotein cholesterol in asymptomatic men. Am J Cardiol 48:903

Uhl GS, Kay TN, Hickman JR (1982) Comparison of exercise radionuclide angiography and thallium perfusion imaging in detecting coronary disease in asymptomatic men. J. Cardiac Rehab 2:118

Upton MT, Rerych SK, Newman GE et al. (1980) Detecting abnormalities in left ventricular function during exercise before angina and ST-segment depression. Circulation 62:341

Wasserman AG, Bren GB, Ross AM, Richardson DW, Hutchinson RG, Rios JC (1982) Prognostic implications of diagnostic Q waves after myocardial infarction. Circulation 65:1451

Weiner D, McCabe C, Dagostino G, Cutler S, Ryan T (1983) Cardiokymography during exercise testing Amerdour Card 51:1307–1311.

Williams P, Robinson D, Bailey A (1979) High-density lipoprotein and coronary risk factors in normal men. Lancet I:72

Prognostication in the Patient with Coronary Artery Disease: Preliminary Results of Radionuclide Cineangiographic Studies*

J. S. Borer**, J. Wallis***, J. Holmes, H. L. Goldberg, J. W. Moses, and J. Fisher

The New York Hospital, Cornell Medical Center, Department of Medicine, Division of Cardiology, 525 East 68th Street, New York, NY 10021, USA

Radionuclide cineangiography during exercise has frequently been demonstrated to be of value in the diagnosis of coronary artery disease (Borer et al. 1977, 1979, 1980). However, the quantitative nature of the technique lends itself readily not only to the detection of disease, but also – by permitting determination of the extent of change in left ventricular ejection fraction from rest to maximal exercise – to assessment of the functional severity of ischemia in a given individual (Borer et al. 1977, 1978, 1979, 1980; Kent et al. 1978). It seems intuitively reasonable that prognosis of the individual patient should depend directly on the functional severity of ischemia from which he or she suffers. Parenthetically, it is increasingly clear that coronary arteriography, as it is currently performed and analyzed, provides only a general guide to the severity of ischemia (Borer et al. 1979).

At a time when multiple constitutional, pharmacologic, and surgical approaches are available for the mangement of the patient with ischemic heart disease, selection and timing of therapy pose problems of ever-increasing sophistication. Since the solution of such problems involves determination of risk/benefit ratios for individual patients, it seems clear that fairly precise estimation of prognosis is required. In view of the limitations of coronary arteriography in the assessment of ischemia, the impracticality of performing coronary arteriography in all patients with clinically apparent coronary disease, and the well-demonstrated inadequacy of symptomatic or other clinical evaluation in indicating the severity of coronary disease or prognosis (Kent et al. 1979), the potential value of noninvasive radionuclide cineangiography in prognostication is of particular interest. Therefore, during the past 3½ years, we have performed a series of studies in an effort to elucidate the prognostic implications of results of radionuclide cineangiography in patients with known or suspected coronary artery disease. Selected aspects of the preliminary results of these studies are presented below.

* This work was supported in part by a grant from the Isadore Rosenfeld Heart Foundation

** He is an Established Investigator of the American Heart Association, and was supported in this work by the American Heart Association and the New York Heart Association

*** He is a New York Heart Association Research Fellow

Validity of Quantitation of Ejection Fraction During Exercise by Radionuclide Cineangiography

In order to accept the implication of radionuclide cineangiographic results, it is important first to demonstrate the quantitative accuracy of the method in the determination of left ventricular performance. While early after the development of the method we demonstrated its quantitative accuracy in the determination of ejection fraction at rest (Green et al. 1978), at that time no methods were readily available to permit comparative testing during exercise. With the recent application of computer-based digital techniques for obtaining contrast angiograms after intravenous administration of contrast medium (Goldberg et al. 1982a), such a technique now is available. In a study thus far involving 14 patients with coronary artery and/or cardiomyopathic diseases, we have found an excellent correlation ($r=0.81$, $p<.01$) between exercise ejection fractions obtained by radionuclide-based and contrast-based techniques in the same patient (Goldberg et al. 1982b). Correlation of the change in ejection fraction from rest to exercise was equally good when results of the two techniques were compared: $r=0.84$, $p<.01$ (Goldberg et al. 1982b). Thus, our data indicate the accuracy of radionuclide cineangiography in the determination of exercise ejection fraction data.

Prediction of Patients with Known High-Risk Lesions

Since determination of prognostic accuracy requires several years of gathering follow-up data, our initial efforts were cross-sectional. Among 250 patients with angiographically demonstrable coronary artery disease, but with symptoms generally at most moderately severe (i.e., not necessitating surgical therapy for acceptable symptom relief), we assessed the accuracy of radionuclide cineangiography in detecting patients with severe left main coronary artery stenosis (i.e., $\geq 75\%$ reduction in luminal diameter) or with severe lesions in the proximal portions of all three major coronary arteries (Phillips et al. 1982a). These lesions are known to be associated with particularly high short-term mortality risk, which can be mitigated in part by coronary bypass grafting. Our population was characterized by the absence of large prior infarctions; patients were excluded if resting ejection fraction was $<30\%$, since such patients are known to be at particularly high risk for death, and exercise stress in such patients is known to cause little variation in ejection fraction, irrespective of underlying coronary lesions. Our preliminary findings indicated that, among our typical urban catheterization population approximately 10% had severe left main lesions and approximately 20% had severe proximal three-vessel stenosis (Phillips et al. 1982a). Functionally, the group could be divided roughly into three parts: Approximately one-third of patients manifested little or no change in ejection fraction with exercise (i. e., either an increase, or a fall of $<5\%$ – the error of the method); slightly more than one-third manifested marked diminution in ejection fraction during exercise (i. e., $\geq 10\%$, more than two standard deviations different from the first group); and approximately one-third manifested changes midway between those of the other groups (i.e., fall of 5%–9% from rest to exercise) (Phillips et al. 1982a). Superimposing the functional results upon the anatomic findings, it was apparent that radionuclide cineangiography provided a very potent means of selecting patients with and without high-risk lesions: of the third of patients with little or no ejection fraction alteration with exercise, none had severe left main disease and only 6% had proximal three-vessel stenosis (Phillips et al. 1982a). However, of the more than one-third of patients with functionally severe ischemia (≥10% fall with exercise), more than 50% had one of the two anatomic indications of poor prognosis (Phillips et al. 1982a). Moreover, those patients with functionally severe ischemia without left main or proximal three-vessel disease generally were those patients with single-, double-, or triple-vessel disease involving at least a severe (≥75%) proximal stenosis of the left anterior descending coronary artery, also known to be generally associated with relatively higher risk for death (Phillips et al. 1982b). Interestingly, a clear functional gradient was apparent between patients with ≥75% left main coronary artery stenosis and the prognostically less severe 50%–74% stenoses (Phillips et al. 1981). These data indicated to us that radionuclide cineangiography during exercise was effective in detecting patients with anatomic abnormalities known to be associated with a particularly high short-term mortality risk, and suggested that the method might prove of independent value in stratifying patients according to prognosis, irrespective of catheterization data.

Direct Assessment of Prognosis

We recently undertook to determine the mortality pattern among the approximately 1200 patients with known or suspected coronary artery disease who had undergone radionuclide cineangiography during exercise in our laboratory in 1979–1980. Among 600 patients initially canvassed we found that almost two-fifths of those with resting ejection fraction <30% had died during the 18- to 36-month period since testing (Wallis et al., to be published). Moreover, the mortality risk ratio for patients with resting ejection fraction <30% versus those with resting ejection fraction ≥30% was 15:1 during this period (Wallis et al., to be published). However, while ejection fraction response during exercise was of no help in further stratifying the high-risk, <30% resting ejection fraction group, within the far larger, relatively low-risk group with less prior myocardial damage cardiac mortality risk was proportional to the extent of diminution in ejection fraction from rest to exercise at the initial study, varying from approximately 7% among those with severe (≥10%) fall in ejection fraction with exercise, to 2% among those with functionally moderate ischemia, to a significantly lower zero cardiac mortality among patients with no fall in ejection fraction during exercise (Wallis et al., to be published).

Conclusions

Our data, while preliminary, support the contention that radionuclide cineangiography during exercise may be of particular prognostic value in patients with coronary artery disease. If further assessment of our study cohort supports our preliminary data, it would appear that functional assessment of ischemia severity might properly be considered a mandatory part of the evaluation of patients with known or suspected coronary artery disease, in order to permit optimal selection and timing of therapy.

References

Borer JS, Bacharach SL, Green MV, Kent KM, Epstein SE, Johnston GS (1977) Real-time radionuclide cineangiography in the noninvasive evaluation of global and regional left ventricular function at rest and during exercise in patients with coronary artery disease. N Engl J Med 296:839

Borer JS, Bacharach SL, Green MV, Kent KM, Johnston GS, Epstein SE (1978) Effect of nitroglycerin on exercise-induced abnormalities of left ventricular regional function and ejection fraction in coronary artery disease: Assessment by radionuclide cineangiography in symptomatic and asymptomatic patients. Circulation 57:314

Borer JS, Kent KM, Bacharach SL, Green MV, Rosing DR, Seides SF, Epstein SE, Johnston GS (1979) Sensitivity, specificity and predictive accuracy of radionuclide cineangiography during exercise in patients with coronary artery disease: comparison with exercise electrocardiography. Circulation 60:572

Borer JS, Bacharach SL, Green MV, Rosing DR, Kent KM, Epstein SE, Johnston GS (1980) Radionuclide cineangiography during exercise: sensitivity and specificity in diagnosis of coronary artery disease. Adv Clin Cardiol 1:171

Goldberg HL, Borer JS, Moses JW, Fisher J, Carter J, Cohen B, Skelly NT (1982a) Intravenous digital subtraction left ventricular angiography: comparison with standard left ventricular cineangiography. Circulation [Suppl II] 66:227

Goldberg HL, Moses JW, Borer JS, Fisher J, Skelly NT, Cohen B (1982b) Exercise ventriculography utilizing intravenous digital subtraction angiography. Circulation [Suppl II] 66:191

Green MV, Brody WR, Douglas MA, Borer JS, Ostrow HG, Line BR, Bacharach SL, Johnston GS (1978) Ejection fraction by count rate from gated images. J Nucl Med 19:880

Kent KM, Borer JS, Green MV, Bacharach SL, McIntosh CM, Conkle D, Epstein SE (1978) Effects of coronary artery bypass on global and regional left ventricular function during exercise. N Engl J Med 298:1434

Kent KM, Rosing DR, Borer JS, Seides SF, Epstein SE (1979) The natural history of asymptomatic or mildly symptomatic patients with coronary artery disease. Clin Res 27:179A

Phillips P, Borer JS, Jacobstein J, Moses J, Goldstein JE, Kligfield P, Collins MB, Plancher K (1981) Comparative sensitivity of exercise ECG and RNCA in detecting left main disease. Clin Res 29:685A

Phillips P, Borer JS, Jacobstein JG, Plancher K, Carter J, Moses JW, Goldstein JE, Collins MB, Fisher J (1982a) Prognostically critical coronary stenoses: identification by radionuclide cineangiography. Am J Cardiol 49:991

Phillips P, Borer JS, Goldstein JE, Jacobstein JG, Moses JW, Fisher J (1982a) Proximal left anterior descending coronary stenosis: the functional equivalent of triple vessel disease? Am J Cardiol 49:957

Wallis J, Borer JS, Moses JW, Goldberg H, Fisher J, Holmes J, Goldstein J, Rosenfeld I (to be published) Radionuclide cineangiography during exercise: prognostic importance in coronary artery disease. J Am Coll Cardiol

The Prognostic Significance of Ventricular Arrhythmias After Acute Myocardial Infarction: Is It Independent of Left Ventricular Function?

F. M. Weld, J. T. Bigger, jr., J. Coronilas, L. M. Rolnitzky, and W. E. DeTurk

Department of Medicine, Division of Cardiology, Columbia University, 630 West 168th Street, New York, NY 10032, USA

Introduction

Ventricular arrhythmias in the convalescent phase of acute myocardial infarction are associated with an increased risk for cardiac death after hospital discharge, but whether ventricular arrhythmias exert this increased mortality risk independent of left ventricular function is not known. In order to answer this question we performed 24-h ambulatory (Holter) ECG recordings in patients two weeks after acute myocardial infarction, and analyzed the outcome with regard to both Holter arrhythmias and measures of left ventricular function. We found that both ventricular arrhythmias and left ventricular function are important determinants of survival following acute myocardial infarction, and that each exerts an independent risk force in the year after hospital discharge.

Methods

The diagnosis of acute myocardial infarction was made in the Coronary Care Unit when at least two of the following criteria were present: (a) chest pain for at least one-half hour; (b) elevation of serum creatine kinase to twice normal with MB fraction positive; (c) electrocardiographic Q waves diagnostic of myocardial infarction. After enrollment, items from the medical history, physical examination, and laboratory data were collected on forms and logged into a computerized data bank.

24-Hour Electrocardiographic Recordings

The Holter recording was obtained using modified leads V1 and V5 with an Avionics two-channel recorder. Of 558 patient records, 550 were of diagnostic quality and these constitute the basis of this study. Each 24-h tape was analyzed by a digital computer program, Columbia IV, which has a sensitivity of 97% and a specificity of 99.9% for detecting ventricular premature depolarizations (VPD) (Birman et al. 1978). At the end of the analysis the record was edited by the operator to remove false-positive and false-negative VPD. A statistical summary and electrocardiographic strips were prepared for review by a cardiologist. Strips included the 20 shortest and the 20 longest R-R and R-V intervals and ten samples of each of the following: (a) each VPD shape; (b) paired VPD; (c) ventricular tachycardia; (d) ventricular bigeminy; (e) shortest R-V/QT; (f) shortest R-V/R-R; and (g) shortest R-V interval. If the cardiologist found errors in the analysis, the electrocardiographic and annotated QRS files were reloaded from digital magnetic tape and reedited; this was required in approximately 15% of cases. VPD pairs were defined as two consecutive VPD regardless of rate. Ventricular tachycardia (VT) was defined as three or more consecutive VPD regardless of rate. Repetitive VPD was defined by the presence of either VPD pairs or VT.

Radionuclide Ejection Fraction

For the MPIP and MILIS study patients detailed below, a radionuclide ejection fraction was obtained by one of two techniques: A multiframe gated (MUGA) picture of the left ventricular radioactivity, comparing radioactive counts during systole to diastole, summated over a 20-min period; or a "first pass" technique with the Baird-Atomic System 77, which rapidly quantifies left ventricular function by comparing the changes in radioactivity between systole and diastole during the first pass of radioactivity through the chambers of the heart. As these studies were multicenter in nature, the exact equipment varied from institution to institution, but quality control was exercised at each place.

Low Level Exercise Test

Just prior to hospital discharge, patients walked on a treadmill according to the exercise protocol shown in Table 1, which consists of a 9-min pre-exercise period, three 3-min stages of exercise with a maximum energy expenditure of approximately 4 METs, and a 9-min recovery period. We identified VPDs from a continuous ECG record on paper, and separated VPDs occurring during this exercise protocol into "rest" VPDs and "exercise" VPDs, as shown in Tables 2 and 3. We defined "rest" VPDs as those occurring during the 9-min pre-exercise period and final 3 min of recovery, which is a total of 12 min. We defined "exercise" VPDs as those occurring during the exercise period and the first 3 min of recovery, which is a maximum of 12 min. We excluded VPDs in the middle 3 min of recovery from analysis.

Table 1. Low-level exercise test protocol

Stage	Treadmill			
	Incline (%)	Speed (mph)	Duration (min)	METs
Supine	–	–	9	1.0
0	0	1.7	3	2.3
½	5	1.7	3	3.5
1	10	1.7	3	4.6
Recovery	–	–	9	–

Left Ventricular Failure

We defined clinical left ventricular failure in the CCU as the presence of rales over one-quarter or more of both lung fields, or the presence of a third heart sound gallop.

Statistical Methods

Associations between ventricular arrhythmias and other clinical variables or outcome were evaluated using the χ^2 test with Yates' continuity correction (Snedecor and Cochran 1967). A p value of 0.05 or less was considered statistically significant. The strength of association was estimated with the odds ratio (Fleiss 1973). To determine whether ventricular arrhythmias had a significant and independent association with 1-year mortality when other important risk variables were controlled, we used log-linear and multiple logistic regression models (Cox 1970; Bishop et al. 1977).

Results

Clinical Characteristics of the Study Group

The baseline characteristics of a population are important in determining both subsequent mortality and the functional subclasses of death (arrhythmic, ischemic, and ventricular failure) (Moss et al. 1979; Taylor et al. 1980; Kleiger et al. 1981; Schulze et al. 1975, 1977; Schultz et al. 1977; Bigger 1979). Baseline characteristics may differ due to enrollment criteria (such as age limits), definition of myocardial infarction, permitted time lapse since index myocardial infarction, population demographics, physician referral patterns, hospital admission policies, regional of institutional patterns of drug use and surgery, prevalence of left ventricular dysfunction, and exclusion criteria relating to intervention trials. The clinical characteristics of the 550 patients enrolled in the Columbia-Presbyterian Medical Center postinfarction natural history study are given in Table 2.

Prevalence of Ventricular Arrhythmias after Acute Myocardial Infarction

Table 3 shows the prevalence of VPD after discharge from the CCU. Fifteen percent of patients had no VPD on their 24-h ECG record. About half of the patients had more than one VPD per hour, and one-quarter had more than ten VPD per hour. Approximately one-third of the patients had repetitive VPD (two or more consecutive VPD). The relationship between VPD features and mortality in the year after hospital discharge is shown in Table 4. Repetitive VPD proved more strongly related to mortality than either frequency or other complex VPD features, in accordance with previous data (Ruberman et al. 1981). It is partly for this reason that many investigators have chosen repetitive VPD as the feature to compare with left ventricular dysfunction in terms of predicting outcome.

Table 2. Clinical characteristics of postinfarction patients at the Columbia-Presbyterian Medical Center ($n = 550$, mean age 58 ± 9)

Characteristic	Number	Percent
Demographic		
Age >60	275	50
Male	423	78
Medical history		
Myocardial infarction	132	24
Angina pectoris	226	41
Cigarette smoking	385	70
Hypertension	270	49
Diabetes mellitus	109	20
Severity of infarction		
Left ventricular failure	143	26
Atrial fibrillation	57	10
VT/VFIB in CCU	234	43
Anterior infarction	215	39
Creatine kinase >1000	100	18
Enlarged heart (X-ray)	231	42
Discharge medication		
Digitalis	235	43
Diuretic	148	26
Antiarrhythmic	75	14
Beta-blocker	77	14
Nitrate	187	34

Table 3. VPD frequency and 1-year mortality following myocardial infarction

VPD frequency (VPD/h)	Patients no. (%)	Mortality no. (%)
<0.1	138 (25)	8 (6)
0.1–0.9	136 (25)	8 (6)
1–9.9	133 (24)	23 (17)
10–99	110 (20)	28 (25)
≥100	33 (6)	8 (24)
Total	550 (100)	75 (14)

Table 4. Relationship of complex VPD features to 1-year cardiac death after myocardial infarction ($n = 550$)

Characteristic	Patients no. (%)	Mortality no. (%)
VPD ≥10/h	143 (26)	36 (25)
Multiform	296 (54)	49 (17)
R-on-T	150 (27)	35 (23)
Pairs	168 (31)	42 (27)
Ventricular tachycardia	67 (12)	24 (36)

Ventricular Arrhythmias and Left Ventricular Dysfunction

In the past, one of the greatest problems in defining the relationship between ventricular arrhythmias and left ventricular dysfunction has been our inability to define either parameter with accuracy or precision. The development of reliable long-term ambulatory ECG recording techniques, coupled with quantitative computer detection methods, has recently provided research-grade long-term arrhythmia detection. The development and refinement of radionuclide angiography has given us an easily obtainable, relatively noninvasive quantitative measure of left ventricular function. These methods have been applied to postinfarction patients during the past 4 years, and the results of these studies are now becoming available.

A preliminary report by the Multicenter Investigation of the Limitation of Infarct Size (MILIS) study group related radionuclide ejection fraction (EF), repetitive VPD and 1-year cardiac death in a group of 388 patients (Table 5) (Mukharji et al. 1982). The lowest mortality was for the group with EF greater than 40% and no repetitive VPD; 65% of patients were in this group and their 1-year mortality was 2%. Twelve percent of patients had EF less than 40% and repetitive VPD, and the mortality in this subgroup was 25%, representing one-half of all deaths. A strong association between repetitive VPD and mortality was found in both the low and high EF groups, indicating a lack of multiplicative interaction between these two important variables. Log-linear and logistic regression analyses confirm this analysis and interpretation.

The Multicenter Post Infarction Program (MPIP) collected almost identical data in 765 patients. During 1 year of follow-up 85 cardiac deaths occurred. Though the MPIP findings are similar to those of the MILIS (Table 6), the magnitude of the increase in risk attributable to repetitive VPD was less in the MPIP study. Both of these studies indicate that repetitive VPD are more likely to occur in patients with low EF, but when the data are adjusted for left ventricular EF there is still an association between repetitive VPD and death.

Table 5. Mortality 1 year after infarction as a function of LV ejection fraction and repetitive VPD (Mukharji et al. 1982)

Ejection fraction	Repetitive VPD	Status		Total	Mortality (%)	Odds ratio
		Dead	Alive			
>40%	No	3	196	199	2	
	Yes	4	51	55	7	4.9
≤40%	No	6	81	87	7	
	Yes	12	35	47	25	4.4
	Total	25	363	388	6	

Table 6. Cardiovascular mortality 1 year after infarction as a function of LV ejection fraction and repetitive VPD (MPIP study)

Ejection fraction	Repetitive VPD	Status		Total	Mortality (%)	Odds ratio
		Dead	Alive			
≥40%	No	9	382	391	2	
	Yes	8	111	119	7	3.1
<40%	No	18	138	156	12	
	Yes	18	81	99	18	1.7
	Total	53	712	765	7	

Low Level Exercise Test: Ventricular Arrhythmias and Cardiac Failure

We also performed a standardized 9-min low-level treadmill exercise test (maximum level: Bruce stage I) in 325 patients who where ambulatory at the time of hospital discharge. Two simple changes in enrollment criteria (the ability to walk at the time of discharge and age less than 70 years) resulted in a reduction in mortality from 13.6% in the myocardial infarction population at Columbia-Presbyterian Medical Center to 8.3% in this subgroup of patients. Mortality was significantly higher among patients with any exercise VPD (20/137, 15%) than among patients with no exercise VPD (7/188, 4%). Among exercise patients with left ventricular failure (third heart sound gallop and/or rales extending over at least one-quarter of the posterior lung fields in the CCU), mortality was still significantly higher for patients with exercise VPD (15/73, 21%) than for patients with no exercise VPD (2/71, 3%).

Discussion

It has long been apparent that post-infarction ventricular arrhythmias are related to left ventricular dysfunction. A major question has been whether or not ventricular arrhythmias contribute to post-hospital mortality risk, independent of left ventricular dysfunction (Schulze et al. 1975, 1977; Schultz et al. 1977; Bigger 1979; Ruberman et al. 1981). A provocative preliminary study by Schulze et al. (1977) of 81 patients 2 weeks after myocardial infarction showed that all eight sudden deaths during 2–16 months of follow-up occurred among the 26 patients with both an ejection fraction (gated blood-pool scan) less than 0.40 and complex ventricular arrhythmias (repetitive VPDs, multiform VPDs, and/or R-on-T VPDs). On the basis of this small study, no definitive statement could be made concerning the independent contribution of arrhythmias and low ejection fraction to mortality risk. In a much larger study, involving 1739 men who survived myocardial infarction, Ruberman et al. (1981) made 1-h ECG recordings and followed up patients for as long as 5½ years. Men demonstrating complex ventricular arrhythmias (repetitive VPDs, multiform VPDs, R-on-T VPDs and/or bigeminal VPDs) were at 2.4 times the risk of sudden death for men without complex ventricular arrhythmias, after control for the influence of other clinical variables (including clinical congestive heart failure) in a Cox multivariate regression model for survival.

The data reviewed and presented in this paper confirm an association between ventricular arrhythmias and left ventricular failure in patients in the convalescent phase of acute myocardial infarction. This is true for both repetitive VPDs recorded with 24-h ambulatory ECG techniques and for simple VPDs recorded during a low level exercise test performed prior to hospital discharge. The association holds true for a wide range of measures of left ventricular failure, including low ejection fraction, X-ray cardiomegaly, X-ray pulmonary vascular congestion, pulmonary rales, third heart sound gallop, and decreased exercise time.

A most important conclusion is that ventricular arrhythmias and left ventricular failure contribute independently to mortality risk in the year after acute myocardial infarction. This means that a rational approach to intervention in patients after acute myocardial infarction should include measures directed at both arrhythmias and left ventricular failure. The data available at present do not suggest that intervention directed at either abnormality alone is sufficient to encompass both risk categories.

References

Bigger JT Jr (1979) New directions and new uses for risk stratification in the post-hospital phase of acute myocardial infarction. Am J Med 67:1

Birman KP, Rolnitzky LM, Bigger JT Jr (1978) A shape-oriented system for automated Holter ECG analysis. In: Computers in cardiology. IEEE Computer Society, Long Beach, p 217

Bishop YMM, Fienberg SE, Holland PW (1977) Discrete multivariate analysis: theory and practice. MIT Press, Cambridge, p 357

Cox DR (1970) The analysis of binary data. Methusen, London, p 1

Fleiss JL (1973) Statistical methods for rates and proportions. Wiley, New York, pp 14, 43

Kleiger RE, Miller JP, Thanavaro S, Marin TF, Province MA, Oliver GC (1981) Relationship between clinical features of acute myocardial infarction and ventricular runs two weeks to one year following infarction. Circulation 63:64

Moss AJ, Davis HT, DeCamilla J, Bayer LW (1979) Ventricular ectopic beats and their relation to sudden and nonsudden cardiac death after myocardial infarction. Circulation 60:998

Mukharji J, Rude RE, Poole K, Croft C, Thomas LJ Jr, Strauss HW, Roberts R, Raabe DS Jr, Braunwald E, Willerson JT, cooperating investigators, Multicenter Investigation of the Limitation of Infarct Size (MILIS) (1982) Late sudden death following acute myocardial infarction: importance of combined presence of repetitive ventricular ectopy and left ventricular dysfunction. (abstract) Clin Res 30:208A

Ruberman W, Weinblatt E, Frank CW, Goldberg JD, Shapiro S (1981) Repeated 1-hour electrocardiographic monitoring of survivors of myocardial infarction at 6-month intervals: arrhythmia detection and relation to prognosis. Am J Cardiol 47:1197

Schultz RA, Humphries JO, Griffith LSC, Ducci H, Achuff S, Baird MG, Mellits ED, Pitt B (1977) Left ventricular and coronary angiographic anatomy. Relationship to ventricular irritability in the late hospital phase of acute myocardial infarction. Circulation 55:839

Schulze RA, Rouleau J, Rigo P, Bowers S, Strauss HW, Pitt B (1975) Ventricular arrhythmias in the late hospital phase of acute myocardial infarction: relation of left ventricular function detected by gated cardiac blood pool scanning. Circulation 52:1006

Schulze RA Jr, Strauss HW, Pitt B (1977) Sudden death in the year following myocardial infarction. Relation to ventricular premature contractions in the late hospital phase and left ventricular ejection fraction. J Med 62:192

Snedecor GW, Cochran WG (1967) Statistical methods, 6 edn. Iowa University Press, Ames, p 51

Taylor GJ, Humphries JO, Mellits ED, Pitt B, Schule RA, Griffith LSC, Achuff SC (1980) Predictors of clinical course, coronary anatomy and left ventricular function after recovery from acute myocardial infarction. Circulation 62:960

Significance of Late Ventricular Potentials for the Identification of Patients at Risk of Sudden Death or Ventricular Tachycardia After Acute Myocardial Infarction*

G. Breithardt, M. Borggrefe, and L. Seipel

Med. Einrichtungen der Universität Düsseldorf, Klinik und Poliklinik, Klinik B, Moorenstrasse 6, 4000 Düsseldorf 1, FRG

The occurrence of sustained ventricular tachycardia or of sudden cardiac death after myocardial infarction is of great clinical significance. The prognosis after acute myocardial infarction depends on the extent of myocardial damage, the persistence of myocardial ischemia, and the occurrence of malignant ventricular arrhythmias. Both the frequency and type of ventricular ectopic beats are of prognostic significance. The detection of repetitive forms has a high sensitivity for identification of patients at risk. However, the clinical value of these ventricular arrhythmias with regard to the indication for antiarrhythmic therapy is limited by the fact that repetitive ventricular beats also occur in a large proportion of patients who do not develop ventricular tachycardia or sudden cardiac death. Thus, a large number of false-positive results limits the clinical usefulness of spontaneous ventricular arrhythmias if it must be decided which patient to treat with antiarrhythmic drugs.

Therefore, new methods that allow a clear identification of patients at risk of sudden cardiac death or of sustained ventricular tachycardia would be of clinical value. For this purpose, the noninvasive recording of late, fragmented ventricular potentials has recently been introduced (Berbari et al. 1978; Fontaine et al. 1978; Uther et al. 1978; Breithardt et al. 1980, 1981a; Hombach et al. 1980; Simson et al. 1980; Rozanski et al. 1981; Simson 1981). These low-amplitude signals can only be recorded by means of sophisticated techniques. They probably originate in areas of regional slow conduction in the border zone of old myocardial infarction (Daniel et al. 1971; Simson et al. 1981a, 1981c; El-Sherif et al. 1977a, b, c; Klein et al. 1981; Spielman et al. 1981). The presence of late potentials is closely correlated to the propensity to ventricular tachycardia and to the results of programmed ventricular stimulation in patients without reviously documented ventricular tachycardia (Breithardt et al. 1980, 1981a, 1981b, 1982; Simson 1981; Simson et al. 1980, 1981b; Hombach et al. 1980; Rozanski et al. 1981).

In previous studies these signals have been analyzed retrospectively. Whether they possess any prognostic significance for the identification of patients at risk of ventricular tachycardia, or even sudden death, after acute myocardial infarction was not clear. This was the purpose of the present prospective pilot study of 160 patients after recent acute myocardial infarction. Preliminary results have already been reported (Breithardt et al. 1981c).

* This study was supported by a grant from the Johann A. Wülfing Foundation and the *Sonderforschungsbereich 30 (Kardiologie)* of the *Deutsche Forschungsgemeinschaft*

Patients and Methods

The study population consisted of 160 patients. As sudden death after acute myocardial infarction is more frequent among younger patients, the upper age limit for entry into the study was 70 years. The patients were studied prospectively between 7 and 109 days (median 25.5 days) after onset of acute myocardial infarction. Patients were recruited from five hospitals and one rehabilitation center. Only patients who exhibited two of the following three abnormalities were included in the study: (a) prolonged chest pain typical of myocardial ischemia; (b) electrocardiographic changes including the development of new abnormal Q waves; and (c) an elevation of total creatine kinase to twice the normal level with a rise in the MB fraction. On the basis of the findings in the 12-lead ECG, the patients were classified as having either anterior wall (including anterior-lateral) or inferior wall (including inferior-lateral and true posterior) myocardial infarction. Those patients on whom no consensus on the site of myocardial infarction was obtained using this simple classification were categorized as a third group.

Noninvasive high-gain recording of the terminal portion of the QRS complex and of the onset of the ST segment was performed on all patients, using the previously described averaging technique (Breithardt et al. 1981a).

For 135 patients, long-term tape recordings of the ECG were available. With 34 patients 24-h Holter monitoring, using portable recorders (Medilog, Oxford), was done. Recordings were quantitatively evaluated on a special-purpose computer system (Pathfinder, Reynolds Medical Electronics, England). With another 101 patients, 10- to 20-h Holter ECGs were recorded using the Siemens Meditape system, which, however, only allows visual evaluation of arrhythmias on the oscilloscopic screen.

In order not to influence the management of the patients by the results of averaging, these were not communicated to the referring physicians. The point of the study was to correlate the outcome of the patients to the presence or absence of late potentials on precordial recordings. After discharge from the hospital, the patients were followed up by contact with the home physicians and with the patients themselves, either by telephone or by questionnaire. If necessary, further information was obtained from the hospital which a patient may have entered during follow-up, or from the relatives in case of death at home. By careful evaluation of all data, a decision was made - independent of the results of averaging - on whether death was sudden, had a noncardiac cause, or was due to reinfarction or heart failure. Sudden death was defined as death within minutes of the patient being in his or her usual state of health, and in the absence of any symptoms or signs that suggested the possibility of a new episode of acute myocardial infarction. Patients who were operated upon were withdrawn from the study at the time of cardiac surgery and regarded as alive.

Results

Mean age of the 160 patients studied was 56 ± 8.3 years (range 38–70 years); 124 patients were male. Sixty-seven patients (41.9%) had anterior wall infarction and 88 patients (55%) had inferior wall infarction, whereas in five patients the site of infarction was "undefined." Maximal LDH during the acute stage of myocardial infarction was 669±374.2 units/liter (mean±SD). In patients with anterior wall infarction it was 729±457.6 units/liter, and in those with inferior wall infarction, 631±305.1 units/liter.

Late potentials were recorded in 81 patients (50.6%). The distribution of late potentials with regard to the site of myocardial infarction and their length is shown in Table 1; mean duration of late potentials was 27±16.5 ms. An example is shown in Fig. 1.

Table 1. Incidence of late potentials and distribution according to site of myocardial infarction

	Duration				
	0	<20 ms	20–29 ms	30–39 ms	≥40 ms
Anterior wall infarction (%)	65.7	16.4	7.4	4.5	6.0
Inferior wall infarction (%)	37.5	23.9	11.3	12.5	14.8
Mean maximal LDH (units/liter)	615	622	675	752	835

In the 135 patients in whom Holter monitoring for 10–24 h was performed there was no significant correlation between the number of ventricular ectopic beats and the presence or duration of late potentials. If only those 34 patients with 24-h Holter monitoring and quantitative evaluation were considered, there was a tendency to more frequent ventricular ectopic beats in those with late potentials of 20 ms or more duration.

Follow-Up

Sufficient information on the course of the patients after discharge from the hospital was obtained for all 160 patients. The follow-up period was 7.5±3.2 months (mean±SD; maximum 15.8 months). In 136 patients (85%) the course after discharge was uneventful. Sudden cardiac death occurred in seven patients (4.4%) after 3.7±3.4 months (range 0.7–8.3 months). Sustained ventricular tachycardia was documented in four cases (requiring resuscitation in three) 2.9±1.3 months after myocardial infarction. The remaining types of events are listed in Table 2.

The incidence of sudden death or ventricular tachycardia was significantly greater in patients with late potentials of ≥20 ms duration, compared with patients without late potentials or with late potentials of <20 ms duration (Fig. 2).

Among the 23 patients with anterior wall infarction and documented late potentials, the incidence of sudden death ($n=2$) and ventricular tachycardia ($n=3$) together was 21.7% whereas it was significantly less among the 55 pa-

Table 2. Appearance of events during follow-up

	No. of patients	Months
Total follow-up	160	7.5 ± 3.2
Bypass surgery	8	7.7 ± 5.2
Sudden death	7	3.7 ± 3.4
Ventricular tachycardia	4	2.9 ± 1.3
Nonsudden cardiac death	4	3.2 ± 3.0
Noncardiac death	1	1.8
Uneventful	136	8.0 ± 2.7

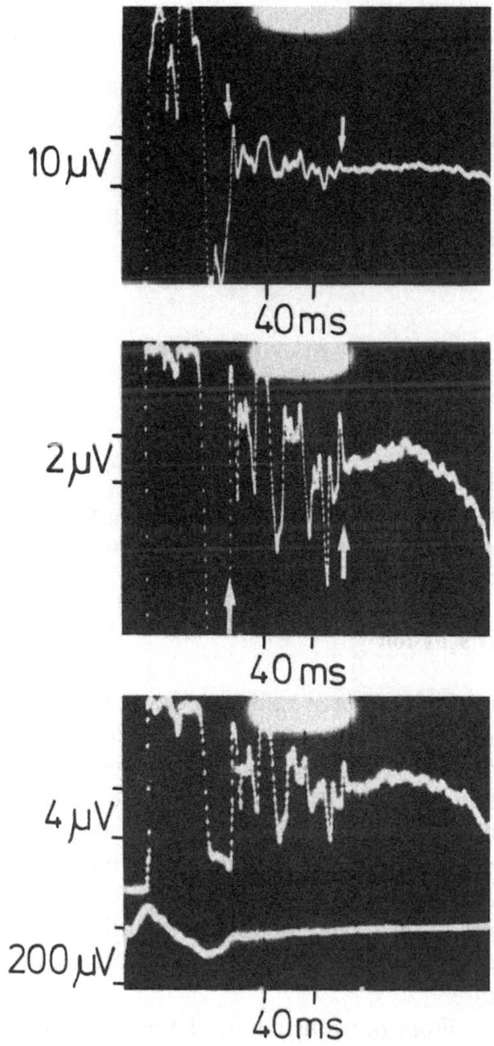

Fig. 1. A typical example of a long late potential in a patient with left ventricular anterior wall aneurysm

tients with inferior wall infarction, two with sudden death and one with ventricular tachycardia ($p<0.05$)

The management of the patients did not have a biasing influence on the results. Patients with and those without late potentials received antiarrhythmic drugs (16% vs. 16.5%), beta blockers (24.6% vs. 35%), sulfinpyrazone (18.5% vs. 13.9%), and oral anticoagulants (30.9% vs. 34.4%) with identical frequencies. Coronary angiography was performed in 25.9% of patients with and in 25% without late potentials; 45.7% of patients with and 53.2% of those without late potentials were referred to a cardiac rehabilitation center after the acute phase of myocardial infarction.

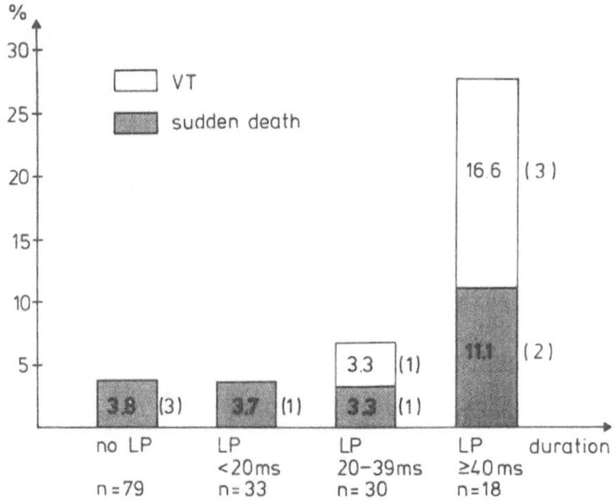

Fig. 2. Incidence of *sudden death* or ventricular tachycardia (*VT*) with regard to the absence or presence of late potentials (*LP*) and their duration

Discussion

In this prospective pilot study we were able to show that the recording of late ventricular potentials from the body surface using high-gain amplification, band-pass filtering, and noise reduction by averaging (Berbari et al. 1978; Fontaine et al. 1978; Uther et al. 1978; Breithardt et al. 1980, 1981a; Hombach et al. 1980; Simson 1981; Simson et al. 1980; Rozanski et al. 1981) is able to predict subsequent occurrence of symptomatic sustained ventricular tachycardia or sudden death after discharge from the hospital. Thus, averaging might be a promising technique for the identification of patients at risk of sudden cardiac death. Comparable prospective data have not yet been reported in the literature.

From previous studies (Breithardt et al. 1981a, b) it was apparent that the great majority of patients with late potentials had had a previous myocardial infarction. However, as these studies were mainly conducted retrospectively in selected patients with ventricular tachycardia after myocardial infarction, the prognostic significance of late potentials after myocardial infarction was obscure. Therefore, the present prospective pilot study was undertaken to determine: (a) the incidence of late potentials after myocardial infarction, and (b) the prognosis of patients after myocardial infarction with respect to the presence or absence of late potentials.

The results show that late potentials are a frequent finding after recent myocardial infarction. Half of the patients exhibited late potentials of varying duration at the end of or after the QRS complex, which suggests that in these cases there are areas of diseased tissue which lead to slow and fragmented regional activation. Furthermore, this study is the first to show that averaging might be able to predict the subsequent occurrence of sustained ventricular tachycardia in patients after recent myocardial infarction. All four patients who developed sustained ventricular tachycardia, three of whom had to be resuscitated, exhibited late potentials. In contrast, no patient without late potentials had an episode of documented symptomatic ventricular tachycardia. None of the patients who died suddenly or had ventricular tachycardia showed conduction abnormalities in their discharge ECGs. Thus, it seems justified to assume that the mode of sudden death in these patients was ventricular fibrillation. Whether the occurrence of sudden death in those patients with late potentials was related to primary reentrant arrhythmias remains unsettled. Sudden death in those without late potentials might be due to a new ischemic event leading to ventricular fibrillation. Though this hypothesis seems attractive, there is presently no way to determine the mechanism of the final arrhythmias leading to death in the individual case.

The incidence of late potentials was much greater in patients with inferior wall infarction (62.5%) than in patients with anterior wall infarction (34.3%). The reason for this difference cannot be given on the basis of this study. One possible explanation might be different activation times of various left ventricular sites. Since the inferoposterobasal areas of the left ventricle are activated late, a late potential from this site will clearly extend beyond the QRS. However, an electrogram of broad duration - perhaps even longer than from the inferior wall, which is associated with anterior infarction and begins early in the QRS - may not extend a great deal beyond the QRS because most of it is hidden within the QRS complex. This explanation is, in fact, probable according to data presented by Simson et al. (1981a). Another interesting finding which might be of practical importance was that the incidence of sudden death or sustained symptomatic ventricular tachycardia was much greater in those patients with late potentials and anterior wall infarction than in those with inferior wall infarction. Thus, averaging might have a greater predictive value in patients with anterior wall infarction.

Patients who have survived an episode of acute myocardial infarction are at high risk of subsequent sudden cardiac death after hospital discharge. Identification of these patients is still one of the major problems of clinical cardiology (Lown 1979). There seems to be sufficient evidence that most episodes of sudden cardiac death are due to ventricular fibrillation (Iseri et al. 1978). Multivariate statistical techniques have provided evidence that frequent, and above all complex, ventricular arrhythmias detected by long-term ECG recording

(Kotler et al. 1973; Moss 1980; Moss et al. 1977, 1979; Geltman et al. 1979; Ruberman et al. 1980; Califf et al. 1981) independently contribute to prognosis and are thus considered precursors of sudden death. However, some doubt has recently been cast on the usefulness of the long-term ECG for the identification of individual patients at risk of sudden death (Cats et al. 1979). Furthermore, the usefulness of spontaneous ventricular arrhythmias may be limited by their great spontaneous variability (Morganroth et al. 1978; Winkle 1978; Michelson and Morganroth 1980). In addition, long-term recording of the ECG during 24 h, though noninvasive, is time consuming with regard to both recording and evaluation, even if semiautomatic or automatic arrhythmia detection devices are used. In contrast, recording of late potentials would not have the disadvantage of spontaneous variability, as late potentials seem to be stable for many months (unpublished results). Unfortunately, in the present pilot study the results of Holter monitoring are too limited to allow any final conclusion with regard to the relationship between late potentials and spontaneous ventricular arrhythmias.

It is therefore impossible to state whether noninvasive recording of late potentials from the body surface can contribute, independent of spontaneous ventricular arrhythmias, to the identification of those patients at risk for sudden death or ventricular tachycardia. A larger prospective multicenter study is needed, using the averaging technique and 24-h ambulatory monitoring, in order to establish with more certainty the predictive value of late ventricular potentials after recent acute myocardial infarction. Furthermore, methods shoulds be devised to automatically determine the onset and end of a given late potential to avoid possible bias in assessment. This has recently been accomplished in our laboratory using a soft-ware program (Karbenn et al., to be published).

Summary

The prognostic significance of late ventricular potentials recorded from the body surface using high-gain amplification and signal averaging was assessed prospectively in 160 patients (mean age 56 ± 8.3 years) after recent acute myocardial infarction (median day of study 25.5).

Late potentials were recorded in 81 of the patients (50.6%); a duration of less than 20 ms was observed in 33 (20.6%), whereas late potentials of 20 ms duration or more were present in 48 (30%). Mean duration of late potentials was 27 ± 16.5 ms. There was no significant correlation to the frequency and type of spontaneous ventricular arrhythmias during 10- to 24-h Holter monitoring.

The follow-up period was 7.5 ± 3.2 months (mean $\pm$ SD; maximum, 15.8 months). In 136 patients (85%) the course after discharge was uneventful. Sudden cardiac death occurred in seven patients (4.4%) after 3.7 ± 3.4 months (range 0.7 to 8.3 months). Sustained ventricular tachycardia was documented in four cases, 2.9 ± 1.3 months after myocardial infarction, all patients having late potentials. The incidence of sudden death or ventricular tachycardia was significantly greater in patients with late potentials of ≥ 20 ms duration, compared with patients without late potentials or with late potentials of < 20 ms duration. Ventricular tachycardia or sudden death occurred in 21.7% of patients with late potentials and anterior wall infarction, compared with 5,4% in patients with late potentials and inferior wall infarction ($p < 0.05$).

This prospective multicenter pilot study therefore suggests that averaging might be a promising noninvasive technique for the identification of patients prone to ventricular tachycardia, or possibly even sudden death, after recent acute myocardial infarction.

Acknowledgements. We gratefully acknowledge the collaboration of the following hospitals: *Medizinische Klinik A* of the University of Düsseldorf (Prof. Dr. W. Schneider and co-workers); *Medizinische Kliniken C, D* and *E* (Prof. Dr. H. L. Krüskemper, Prof. Dr. C. Strohmeyer, Prof. Dr. H. Zimmermann and co-workers); Internal Department of the *Augusta-Krankenhaus,* Düsseldorf-Rath (Dr. M. Schwick and Dr. K. Knauer); Cardiological Department of the Marien Hospital, Wesel (PD Dr. K. Haerten, Dr. Schepers); Internal Department of the *St. Vinzenz Krankenhaus,* Essen-Stoppenberg (Dr. Y. Toker); Cardiological Department, *Rhein-Ruhr-Klinik,* Essen-Kettwig (Dr. L. L. Benesch, Dr. E. Hahnel).

References

Berbari EJ, Scherlag BJ, Hope RR, Lazzara R (1978) Recording from the body surface of arrhythmogenic ventricular activity during the ST segment. Am J Cardiol 41:697

Breithardt G, Becker R, Seipel L (1980) Non-invasive recording of late ventricular activation in man. Circulation [Suppl III] 62:320

Breithardt G, Becker R, Seipel L, Abendroth R-R, Ostermeyer J (1981a) Non-invasive detection of late potentials in man – a new marker for ventricular tachycardia. Eur Heart J 2:1

Breithardt G, Seipel L, Schwarzmaier J, Karbenn U (1981b) Clinical significance of ventricular late potentials. In: Hombach V, Hilger HH (eds) Signal averaging technique in clinical cardiology. Schattauer Stuttgart, pp 219–232

Breithardt G, Schwarzmaier J, Abendroth R-R, Borggrefe M, Seipel L (1981c) Prospective study on the incidence of late potentials in postmyocardial infarction patients. Circulation [Suppl IV] 64:328

Breithardt G, Borggrefe M, Karbenn U, Abendroth R-R, Yeh HL, Seipel L (1982) Prevalence of late potentials in patients with and without ventricular tachycardia – correlation to angiographic findings. Am J Cardiol 49:1932

Califf RM, Wagner GS, Rosati RA (1981) Prognostic value of ventricular arrhythmias (abstract). Am J Cardiol 47:397

Cats VM, Lie KI, van Capelle FJL, Durrer D (1979) Limitations of 24-hour ambulatory electrocardiographic recording in predicting coronary events after acute myocardial infarction. Am J Cardiol 44:1257

Daniel T, Boineau J, Sabiston D (1971) Comparison of human ventricular activation with canine model in chronic myocardial infarction. Circulation 44:74

El-Sherif N, Scherlag BJ, Lazzara R, Hope RR (1977a) Reentrant ventricular arrhythmias in the late myocardial infarction period. I. Conduction characteristics in the infarction zone. Circulation 55:686

El-Sherif N, Scherlag BJ, Lazzara R, Hope RR (1977b) Reentrant ventricular arrhythmias in the late myocardial infarction period. II. Patterns of initiation and termination of reentry. Circulation 55:702

El-Sherif N, Lazzara R, Hope RR, Scherlag BJ (1977c) Reentrant arrhythmias in the late myocardial infarction period. III. Manifest and concealed extra-systolic grouping. Circulation 56:225

Fontaine G, Frank R, Gallais Hamonno F, Allali I, Phan-Thuc H, Grosgogeat Y (1978) Electrocardiographie des potentiels tardifs du syndrome de post-excitation. Arch Mal Coeur 71:854
Geltman EM, Ehsani AA, Campbell MK, Schechtman K, Roberts R, Sobel BE (1979) The influence of location and extent of myocardial infarction on long-term ventricular dysrhythmia and mortality. Circulation 60:805
Hombach V, Höpp H-W, Braun V, Behrenbeck DW, Tauchert M, Hilger HH (1980) Die Bedeutung von Nachpotentialen innerhalb des ST-Segmentes im Oberflächen-EKG bei Patienten mit koronarer Herzkrankheit. Dtsch Med Wochenschr 105:1457
Iseri L, Humphrey SB, Siner EJ (1978) Prehospital brady-asystolic cardiac arrest. Ann Intern Med 88:741
Karbenn U, Breithardt G, Borggrefe M, Simson MB (to be published) Automatic identification of late potentials
Klein H, Werner P, Frank G, Bethge KP, Lichtlen PR (1981) Value of left ventricular endocardial catheter mapping in patients with ventricular arrhythmias. Eur Heart J [Suppl A] 2:42
Kotler MN, Tabatznik B, Mower MM, Tominaga S (1973) Prognostic significance of ventricular ectopic beats with respect to sudden death in the late postinfarction period. Circulation 47:959
Lown B (1979) Sudden cardiac death: the major challenge confronting contemporary cardiology. Am J Cardiol 43:313
Michelson EL, Morganroth J (1980) Spontaneous variability of complex ventricular arrhythmias detected by long-term electrocardiographic recording. Circulation 61:690
Morganroth J, Michelson EL, Horowitz LN, Josephson ME, Pearlman AS, Dunkman WB (1978) Limitations of routine long-term ambulatory electrocardiographic monitoring to assess ventricular ectopic frequency. Circulation 58:408
Moss AJ (1980) Clinical significance of ventricular arrhythmias in patients with and without coronary artery disease. Prog Cardiovasc Dis 23:33
Moss AJ, DeCamilla JJ, Davis HP, Bayer L (1977) Clinical significance of ventricular ectopic beats in the early posthospital phase of myocardial infarction. Am J Cardiol 39:635
Moss AJ, Davis HT, DeCamilla J, Bayer LW (1979) Ventricular ectopic beats and their relation to sudden and nonsudden cardiac death after myocardial infarction. Circulation 60:998
Rozanski JJ, Mortara D, Myerburg RJ, Castellanos A (1981) Body surface detection of delayed depolarizations in patients with recurrent ventricular tachycardia and left ventricular aneurysm. Circulation 63:1172
Ruberman W, Weinblatt E, Goldberg JD, Frank CW, Shapiro S, Chaudhary BS (1980) Ventricular premature complexes in prognosis of angina. Circulation 61:1172
Simson MB (1981) Use of signals in the terminal QRS complex to identify patients with ventricular tachycardia after myocardial infarction. Circulation 64:235
Simson M, Horowitz L, Josephson M, Moore EN, Kastor J (1980) A marker for ventricular tachycardia after myocardial infarction. Circulation [Suppl III] 62:262
Simson MB, Euler DE, Michelson EL, Falcone R, Spear JF, Moore N (1981a) Confirmation of a new technique for detecting slow ventricular activation on the body surface (abstract). Am J Cardiol 47:488
Simson M, Spielman S, Horowitz L, Josephson M, Harken A, Kastor J (1981b) Slow ventricular activation detected on the body surface in patients with ventricular tachycardia after myocardial infarction (abstract). Am J Cardiol 47:498
Simson MB, Euler D, Michelson EL, Falcone RA, Spear JF, Moore EN (1981c) Detection of delayed ventricular activation on the body surface in dogs. Am J Physiol 241 (363–369)
Spielman SR, Untereker WJ, Horowitz LN, Greenspan AM, Simson MB, Kastor JA, Josephson ME (1981) Fragmented electrical activity – relationship to ventricular tachycardia. Am J Cardiol 47:448
Uther JB, Dennett CJ, Tan A (1978) The detection of delayed activation signals of low amplitude in the vectorcardiogram of patients with recurrent ventricular tachycardia by signal averaging. In: Sandoe E, Julian DG, Bell JW (eds) Management of ventricular tachycardia – role of mexiletine. Excerpta Medica, Amsterdam, pp 80–82
Winkle RA (1978) Antiarrhythmic drug effect mimicked by spontaneous variability of ventricular ectopy. Circulation 57:1116

Prognosis in Patients with Mild Coronary Atherosclerosis

W. C. Sheldon, W. L. Proudfit, A. V. G. Bruschke, and J. S. Lim
The Cleveland Clinic Foundation, 9500 Euclid Avenue, Cleveland, OH 44106, USA

The introduction of coronary arteriography a quarter of a century ago permitted the recognition of coronary atherosclerosis and estimation of its prognosis based upon the presence and extent of atherosclerotic involvement, as well as on the degree of left ventricular dysfunction. After 25 years, however, there is a relative paucity of data regarding the prognosis of patients with less than severe coronary artery disease. This article is an attempt to summarize the pertinent literature describing the prognosis of patients with arteriographic evidence of mild to moderate involvement. The data are largely for patients studied by coronary arteriography in the 1960s. Less than severe coronary atherosclerosis, or mild to moderate disease, is defined as the presence of angiograph ic evidence of coronary artery narrowing not exceeding 50% of lumen caliber. Prognostic end points considered include mortality, myocardial infarction, and angiographic progression of disease.

Although not all reports distinguish between patients with normal coronary arteriograms and those with mild to moderate disease, there is a predominance of normals. Eight series from the literature describe patients with normal coronary arteriograms (Bemiller et al. 1973; Bruschke et al. 1973; Friesinger et al. 1970; Humphries et al. 1974; Kemp et al. 1973; Lim et al. 1974; Ljungberg et al. 1979; Proudfit et al. 1981; Storstein et al. 1981), five distinguish patients with mild-to-moderate abnormalities (Bruschke et al. 1973; Friesinger et al. 1970; Humphries et al. 1974; Lim et al. 1974; Ljungberg et al. 1979; Proudfit et al. 1981), and two (Mock et al. 1982; Oberman et al. 1972) describe patients with less than severe coronary atherosclerosis (less than 50%) without distinguishing those with normal coronary arteriograms (Table 1). In the Bruschke series from the Cleveland Clinic (Bruschke et al. 1973) there is some overlap of patients who are also included in other Cleveland Clinic series (Lim et al. 1974; Proudfit et al. 1981) which focused on younger patients. Among series of patients unselected by age or sex, the average age with normal coronary ateriograms ranged from 40 to 48 years, and the proportion of males ranged from 50% to 69%. The average duration of follow-up ranged from 21.7 months to more than 12 years. In the one series of specified patients unselected by age or sex with abnormal arteriograms, but less than severe disease, the mean age was 51 years, and 67% were men (Ljungberg et al. 1979). The duration of follow-up ranges from 5 to 12 years.

Table 1. Series of patients with normal to moderately abnormal coronary arteriograms

Series (References)		Combined				Normals				Abnormals[a]			
		$n=$	m̄ age (yrs)	Sex	Follow-up	$n=$	m̄ age (yrs)	Sex	Follow-up	$n=$	m̄ age (yrs)	Sex	Follow-up
Lim (1)	1961–66	261	<40	M	>5 yrs	231	<40	M	>5 yrs	30	<40	M	>5 yrs
Bruschke (2)	1964–65	500	45 M, 48 F	61% M	>5 yrs	342	NS	NS	>5 yrs	158	NS	NS	>5 yrs
Proudfit (3)	1961–68	761	<50	F	>10 yrs	644	<50	F	>10 yrs	117	<50	F	>10 yrs
Humphries (4, 5)	1960–67	121	41	62% M	5–12 yrs	102	NS	NS	5–12 yrs	19	NS	NS	5–12 yrs
Ljungberg (6)	1961–66	213	–	–	7–12 yrs	128	40	69% M	7–12 yrs	85	51	67% M	7–12 yrs
Kemp (7)	1964–70	–	–	–	–	200	47	50% M	3 yrs	–	–	–	–
Storstein (8)	1972–76	–	–	–	–	112	48	NS	2–7 yrs	–	–	–	–
Bemiller (9)	NS	–	–	–	–	37	43	57% M	1–7 yrs	–	–	–	–
Oberman (10)	1965–70	98	43	62% M	22 mos	–	–	–	–	–	–	–	–
CASS (11)	1975–79	5084	53	75% M	2–5 yrs	–	–	–	–	–	–	–	–

[a] Criterion of significance 50% diameter reduction (70% in CASS series)
NS, not stated; *M*, male; *F*, female

1 Lim et al. (1974)
2 Bruschke et al. (1973)
3 Proudfit et al. (1981)
4 Humphries et al. (1974)
5 Friesinger et al. (1970)
6 Ljungberg et al. (1979)
7 Kemp et al. (1973)
8 Storstein et al. (1981)
9 Bemiller et al. (1973)
10 Oberman et al. (1972)
11 Mock et al. (1982)

Table 2. Mortality in patients with normal to moderately abnormal coronary arteriograms[a]

Series (References)[b]	Normal n=	Normal Deaths	Normal Survival[c]	Abnormal n=	Abnormal Deaths	Abnormal Survival[c]		Combined n=	Combined Deaths	Combined Survival
Lim (1)								231	2 Cardiac 2 Noncardiac	98.4% (5-yr)
Bruschke (2)	342	0 Coronary 3 Sudden	99.4% Cardiac	158	3 Coronary	98% Cardiac 96.8% Cardiac	<30% lesion 30%–50% lesion	500	15 Noncardiac	–
Proudfit (3)	644	0 Coronary 7 Cardiac, other	100% Coronary 98.1% Gross	117	5 Coronary 3 Cardiac, other	97.6% Coronary 96.8% Coronary	<30% lesion 30%–50% lesion	761	25 Noncardiac	–
Humphries (4, 5)	102	0 Coronary 5 Noncoronary	100% Coronary 96% Gross	19	0 Coronary	100% Coronary				
Ljungberg (6)	128	0 Coronary 15 Cardiac, other 10 Noncardiac	87% (7-yr)	85	2 Coronary 8 Cardiac, other 5 Noncardiac	87% (7-yr)				
Kemp (7)	200	2 Noncoronary 2 Unknown	97%							
Storstein (8)	112	NS	95%							
Bemiller (9)	37	0 Coronary 1 Sudden	97% (4-yr)							
Oberman (10)								98	0 Coronary 1 Cardiac, other 2 Noncardiac	97% (2-yr)
CASS (11)								5084		97% (4-yr)

[a] See Table 1
[c] Five year gross survival except as noted

Survival

An attempt was made to classify the mode of death among those patients with less than severe coronary artery disease who died during the period of follow-up (Table 2). Several series included patients with congenital, valve, or myocardial disease, resulting in a rather variable incidence of cardiac mortality. While few series distinguished between coronary deaths and those due to other causes, there appears to be a slightly higher incidence of cardiac deaths generally, and coronary disease specifically among patients with mild to moderately abnormal arteriograms. Among seven series, in which 1565 patients with normal coronary arteriograms were distinguished, no deaths occurred that could be clearly ascribed by clinical or postmortem data to coronary atherosclerosis. Three sudden deaths occurred among patients with normal coronary arteriograms in Bruschke's series: two of these patients had conduction abnormalities, and one died possibly of a drug overdose. Among 379 patients with mild-to-moderate coronary atherosclerosis, 15 deaths were ascribed to coronary artery disease.

In three series in which mortality could not be related to patients with normal arteriograms or to those with mild-to-moderate coronary atherosclerosis (Lim et al. 1974; Mock et al. 1982; Oberman et al. 1972), coronary deaths did not occur in one, and were either not reported or not stated in the other two. Several cardiac deaths were attributed to noncoronary disease and a number of noncardiac deaths occured.

The 5-year *cardiac* survival was 98% in the Bruschke series with minimal (less than 30%) coronary atherosclerosis, and 94.7% with moderate (30%–50%) coronary artery involvement.

Myocardial Infarction

The history of myocardial infarction during the period of follow-up was addressed in several-series of patients with normal coronary arteriograms (see Table 3), and in three series distinguishing mild-to-moderate atherosclerosis (Bruschke et al. 1973; Lim et al. 1974; Proudfit et al. 1981). Although there may be come overlap between the Lim series and the Bruschke series, it appears that subsequent myocardial infarction is rare in patients with normal coronary arteriograms, having been reported in only 12 of 1566 patients followed up for 5–10 years, compared with 15 of 305 patients with mild-to-moderate disease, a sixfold increase in incidence.

Progression of Disease

Only three series examined progression of disease as documented by follow-up arteriography (see Table 4). Indication for restudy were usually new symptoms or ECG changes, resulting in a bias favoring the identification of progression, particularly in categories of patients with less than severe disease. This bias

Table 3. Myocardial infarction in patients with normal to moderately abnormal coronary arteriograms

Series (References)	Normal			Abnormal [a]		
	$n=$	No. with infarction	Interval	$n=$	No. with infarction	Interval
Lim (1)	231	3	25–48 mos.	30	2	78–83 mos.
Bruschke (2)	342	4	22–70 mos.	158	8	17–87 mos.
Proudfit (3)	644	0	–	117	5	9–119 mos.
Humphries (4, 5)	102	5	NS	–	–	–
Kemp (6)	200	0	–	–	–	–
Bemiller (7)	37	0	–	–	–	–

[a] Lesions <50%

1 Lim et al. (1974)
2 Bruschke et al. (1973)
3 Proudfit et al. (1981)
4 Humphries et al. (1974)
5 Friesinger et al. (1970)
6 Kemp et al. (1973)
7 Bemiller et al. (1973)

may have been offset by excluding patients whose deaths were possibly due to progression of disease, a complication perhaps more likely to have occurred among patients with more severe disease. Nevertheless, progression of disease was observed in only two of 13 patients who were restudied and had had normal angiograms initially, compared with 15 of 21 patients with mild-to-moderate disease at baseline, a fivefold increase in incidence. In another study of progression of coronary atherosclerosis, Kramer et al. (1983) observed an incidence of nonocclusive progression of disease of only 4.1% in patients with normal angiograms at baseline, compared with 21.3% among patients with mild-to-moderate (less than 50%) disease initially (Table 5). New occlusions occurred in only 1.2% of normals, compared with 7.3% of patients with mild-to-moderate abnormalities.

Table 4. Progression of disease in patients with normal to moderately abnormal coronary arteriograms

Series (References)	Normal			Abnormal [a]		
	No. restudied	No. with progression	Interval (months)	No. restudied	No. with progression	Interval (months)
Bruschke (1)	6	2	25–58	14	8	14–88
Proudfit (2)	–	–	–	7	7	40–123
Bemiller (3)	7	0	–	–	–	–

[a] Lesions <50%

1 Bruschke et al. (1973)
2 Proudfit et al. (1981)
3 Bemiller et al. (1973)

Table 5. Progression of diasease according to severity of disease at initial study (Kramer et al. 1983)

Initial severity (%)	No. of patients	Progression to > 100% *n*	(%)	Progression to occlusion *n*	(%)
0	2341	96	4.1	28	1.2
1-30	143	31	21.6	8	5.6
31-50	158	33	20.9	14	8.9
51-99	257	7	2.5	65	25.3

In summary, deaths from coronary artery disease are rare in patients with normal coronary arteriogram. The incidence of noncoronary cardiac deaths relates primarily to factors determining the indications for angiography (e.g., suspicion of congenital, valvular, or idiopathic heart disease, ventricular arrhythmias). The incidence of cardiac mortality ranges from 1% in 10 years among patients with normal coronary arteriograms, to 2% among patients with mildly abnormal coronary arteriograms (less than 30%), and 5% among patients with moderate (30%-50%) angiographic abnormalities at baseline. Subsequent myocardial infarction occurs six times more frequently among patients with mildly to moderately abnormal arteriograms, compared with normals at baseline during a follow-up period of 5-10 years. The appearance of significant coronary atherosclerosis is unusual in patients with normal baseline studies; occlusive or nonocclusive progression of disease occurs approximately five times more frequently in patients with mild-to-moderate baseline abnormalities than among normals.

A normal coronary arteriogram implies, but does not necessarily assure, the absence of atherosclerotic involvement. A normal coronary arteriogram is associated with a prognosis that is even more favorable than that for an unselected population of similar age and sex (Bruschke et al. 1973), and an arteriogram demonstrating mild to moderate disease not only identifies its presence, but a prognosis which is intermediate - better than that associated with severe disease, but less favorable than one based on a normal arteriogram.

References

Bemiller CR, Pepine CJ, Rogers AK (1973) Long-term observations in patients which angina and normal coronary arteriograms. Circulation 47:36-43

Bruschke AVG, Proudfit WL, Sones FM Jr (1973) Clinical course of patients with normal and slightly or moderately abnormal coronary arteriograms. Circulation 47:936-945

Friesinger GC, Page EE, Rose RS (1970) Prognostic significance of coronary arteriography. Trans Assoc Am Phys 83:78-92

Humphries JO, Kuller L, Ross RS, Friesinger GC, Page EE (1974) Natural history of ischemic heart disease in relation to arteriographic findings. Circulation 49:489-497

Kemp HG, Vokonas PS, Cohn PF, Gorlin R (1973) The anginal syndrome associated with normal coronary arteriograms. Am J Med 54:735-742

Kramer JR, Kitazume H, Proudfit WL, Mastuda Y, Goormastic M, Williams GW, Sones FM Jr (1983) Segmental analysis of the rate of progression in patients with progressive coronary atherosclerosis. Am Heart J 106:600

Lim JS, Proudfit WL, Sones FM Jr (1974) Selective coronary arteriography in young men. Circulation 49:1122–1126
Ljungberg S, Forsberg SA, Paulin S, Werko L (1979) Coronary arteriography in 486 patients – Arteriographic pathology and prognosis. Acta Med Scand 206:145–151
Mock MM, Ringqvist I, Fisher LD et al. (1982) Survival of medically treated patients in the coronary artery surgery study (CASS) registry. Circulation 66:562–568
Oberman A, Jones WB, Riley CP, Reeves TJ, Sheffield LT, Turner ME (1972) Natural history of coronary artery disease. Bull NY Acad Med 48:1109–1125
Proudfit WL, Welch CC, Siqueira C, Morcerf FP, Sheldon WC (1981) Prognosis of 1000 young women studied by coronary angiography. Circulation 64:1185–1190
Storstein O, Enge I, Erikssen J, Thaulow E (1981) Natural history of coronary artery disease studied by coronary arteriography. Acta Med Scand 210:53–58

Prognosis of Patients with Normal Coronary Arteries at Middle Age

G. G. Gensini

St. Joseph's Hospital Health Center, Msgr. Toomey Cardiovascular, Laboratory and Research Department, 301 Prospect Avenue, Syracuse, NY 13203, USA

The value of coronary arteriography in separating the real from the imaginary patient with coronary artery disease was promptly established soon after coronary arteriography became widely accepted. It led to the possibility of "curing" with a mere diagnostic test at least one-fifth of all patients suspected of having coronary artery disease, while it offered the appropriately aggressive treatment to those most likely to benefit from it. However, the opportunity of stratifying patients according to the severity of their prognosis did not materialize as easily.

How reliable is coronary arteriography in identifying normal coronary arteries? How does one define mild coronary disease, or, for that matter, moderate, severe, or life-threatening coronary artery disease? Once we had freed ourselves from the burden of utilizing pain as an important factor in the assessment of severity, and once we had agreed to consider the degree of coronary luminal narrowing and the quality of left ventricular dysfunction in the assessment of prognosis, how were we to proceed?

The current method of grading coronary disease as single-, double-, and triple-vessel involvement was suggested as the simplest solution to a very complex problem. It was immediately successful, to the surprise of those who had suggested it. This simplistic approach became the key in practically every study of coronary artery disease, yet today everyone agrees to the need for a better way of achieving a more meaningful patient stratification.

For instance, in a recent editorial, Selzer (1982) criticized the current classification of coronary artery disease severity, which is utilized in all randomized trials on the surgical versus medical therapy of coronary artery disease. He pointed out that this classification of single-, double-, and triple-vessel disease allows the inclusion in each subgroup of a mixture of patients with both favorable and unfavorable prognoses and provides, at best, only marginal discrimination between medically and surgically treated patients. In my book entitled "Coronary arteriography" (Gensini 1975) and subsequently in a chapter on coronary arteriography in Braunwald's textbook "Heart disease" (Gensini 1980) I identified these shortcomings. I described a system which takes into consideration the geometrically increasing severity of lesions, the cumulative effect of multiple obstructions, the significance of their locations, the modifying influence of the collaterals, the size and quality of the distal vessels, and the importance of the status of myocardial function. The basis of this system is the hypothesis that the severity of ischemic heart disease must be regarded as the consequence of the functional significance of the vascular narrowing and the extent of the area perfused by the involved vessel or vessels; however, the presence of an effective collateral circulation may modify the functional significance of a severe obstruction or occlusion. The severity of the lesion, identified as 0% (or normal), 25%, 50%, 75%, 90%, 99%, or 100% occluded, is given a geometrically larger number, i.e., 0, 1, 2, 4, 8, 16, or 32, expressing the geometrically increasing reduction of coronary blood flow (Fig. 1). This value is then multiplied by a factor expressing the size of the dependent territory perfused by that artery (Fig. 2). After the separate scores for each segment of the arteries have been calculated they are added together to produce severity scores for each artery, which are then for the entire coronary system. The severity score may vary from 0, i.e., normality, to over 20 for the most severe and diffuse type of coronary artery disease.

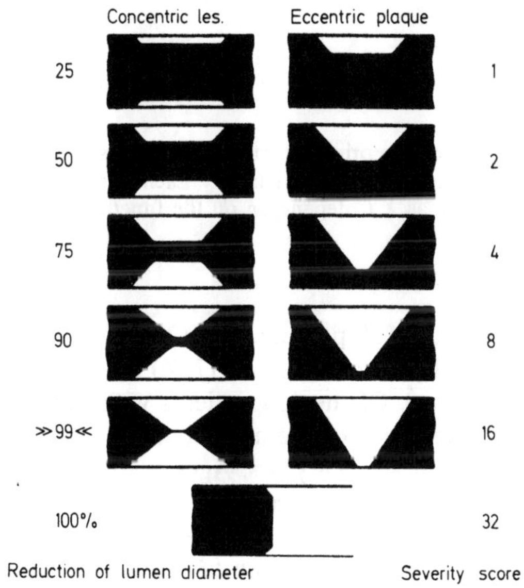

Fig. 1. The roentgenographic appearance of *concentric lesions* and *eccentric plaques* resulting in (*left*) degrees of obstruction, or complete occlusion (*100%*). Also (*right*) the relative severity of these lesions, using a score of geometric increments, progressing according to the increased reduction of lumen diameter

This method of stratifying patients with normal or diseased arteries was applied to 2000 patients studied between 1964 and 1974. All patients received a questionnaire concerning their health and functional capacity. In case of a patient's death, his or her family was requested to indicate date, place, and cause of death, if known. Of these patients, 1737 either replied or were later reached by telephone; 263 were lost to follow-up. We concentrated on the first group of 830 patients who had been follwoed up for 6–13 years and were found to have either normal or diseased coronary arteries, without any other complicating features.

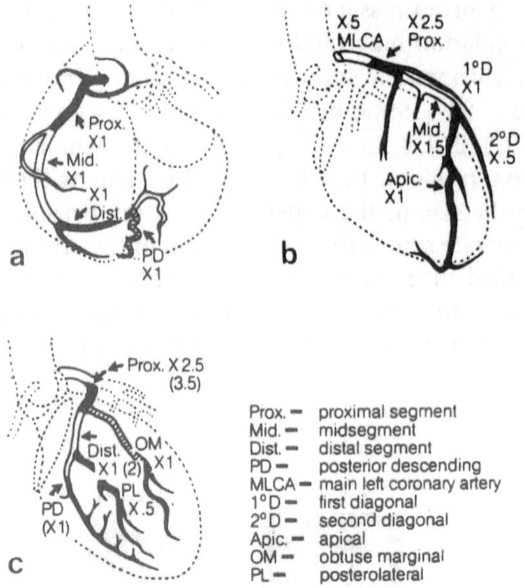

Fig. 2a–c. The principal vascular segments of **a** the right coronary artery, **b** the left anterior descending, and **c** the circumflex. Each segment identification is followed by a multiplying factor, such as *X 1*, depending on the functional significance of the area supplied by the segment

Of the 830 patients, 189 (23%) had GACS = 0 and were classified as "normal." The remaining 641 (77%) had coronary artery disease (CAD), based on GACS > 0. Of the 189 patients with normal coronary arteries, 51% were men. The mean age of the normal group was 46.5, the median 47, and the standard deviation was 9.4 years. Ages in this group ranged from 26 to 72 years.

Of the 641 patients who had evidence of CAD based on GACS > 0, there were 84%. The mean age of the group with CAD was 52.1, the standard deviation 8.3, and the median 53 years. Ages ranged from 25 to 85 years.

Substantial efforts were made to follow the survival times of all patients, and survival information was available on 750. The remaining 80 patients (9.6%) were lost to follow-up. Survival time was defined as the length of time between coronary angiography and death.

The first step in the statistical analysis was to investigate whether or not there were any prognostic factors for survival, i.e., variables that appeared to be good predictors. The Cox proportional hazards model was used to relate covariates to survival time. This procedure may be viewed as similar to multiple regression analysis.

Survival curves were obtained via the Kaplan-Meier technique for the SDTML classification scheme, including those patients with less involvement than any of the others as a group denoted "little," and including the "normals" (GACS = 0).

These curves confirm the results of the statistical analysis in indicating the lack of usefulness of the standard classification scheme in predicting survival.

The "little" group is hardly distinguishable from the "normals" over 60 months. The "single" group separates nicely from the other groups of diseased patients as early as 10 months. However, the triple and main left groups have interwined survival curves over 50 months, after which those of the double and triple groups are interwined. The crossing and interwining of curves is indicative of nonproportional hazards.

The statistical evidence, both visual and from formal hypothesis tests, indicates that the standard SDTML classification scheme is not useful in predicting survival, but that the GACS and age are very relevant for the entire group of patients.

Our investigation revealed that no cardiac deaths occurred among the 189 patients with normal coronary arteries during a period of follow-up that ranged initially from 6 to 13 years and now extends, for some patients, to nearly 20 years. Six deaths were found, three as the result of malignancies and three because of traffic accidents. Twenty patients were reexamined because of persistent chest pain, and only one patient with normal coronary arteries did develop classical CAD after 7 years of observation.

Thus, our conclusion that the finding of normal coronary arteries and normal left ventricular function in a middle age patient is an excellent predictor for survival seems to be firmly proven by the weight of statistical evidence and of long-term follow-up.

On the other hand, we were profoundly troubled by a group of patients with normal coronary arteries, abnormal ECG, and left ventricular motion abnormalities, such as regional akinesis or dyskinesis, clearly indicative of past myocardial infarctions.

Recently, during the application of our protocol for thrombolitic treatment of the evolving myocardial infarction, we encountered a most interesting case that appears to resolve the dilemma of myocardial infarction in patients with no apparent obstruction or occlusion of coronary artery disease. A 44-year-old white man with a history of classical diaphragmatic myocardial infarction suffered 2 years before was admitted to our emergency room with a history of crushing chest pain, nausea, and diaphoresis of 90 min duration. An ECG on admission demonstrated a wide current of injury over the lateral leads. The opacification of the right coronary artery made 120 min after the onset of pain demonstrated – to our surprise – a perfectly patent dominant vessel. The opacification of the LAD showed a patent LAD and an occluded Rcx.

Within 20 min of streptokinase infusion the Cx began to clear. A huge, sausage-like thrombus was seen outlined and the artery became essentially free of obstruction within 60 min from the beginning of the infusion.

A left ventriculogram performed at the end of the procedure demonstrated that the area of akinesis was mainly localized to the diaphragmatic segment, the site of the old infarction. This case appears to indicate that in predisposed individuals an occluding thrombus may suddenly appear in a slightly irregular – occasionally ectatic – coronary artery. The thrombus may disappear spontaneously but late, leaving behind an area of necrosis, or at a much earlier time because of thrombolytic treatment, thereby leaving intact or minimally injured myocardium.

The case just described probably represents the exception to the rule – namely that if you have reached middle age and have normal coronary arteries, have frequent checkups to uncover malignancy and drive carefully!

References

Gensini GG (1975) Coronary arteriography. Futura, Mount Kisco

Gensini GG (1980) Coronary arteriography. In: Braunwald E (ed) Heart disease. A textbook of cardiovascular medicine, vol 2. Saunders, Philadelphia, p 363

Selzer A (1982) On the limitation of therapeutic intervention trials in ischemic heart disease: A clinician's viewpoint. Am J Cardiol 49:252

Follow-Up of Patients with Left Ventricular Aneurysm and Nonsurgical Therapy

J. Jehle, M. Heerdt, P. Spiller, A. Krian, and F. Loogen

Med. Einrichtungen der Universität Düsseldorf, Klinik und Poliklinik, Klinik B, Moorenstrasse 5, 4000 Düsseldorf, FRG

The indication for surgical or medical treatment of patients with postinfarction aneurysm of the left ventricle is not clearly defined, except in patients with congestive heart failure or life-threatening arrhythmias (Blümchen et al. 1978; Faxon et al. 1982; Otterstad et al. 1981; Schulte et al. 1979). Figure 1 shows that the mortality of patients medically treated does not differ significantly from that of patients surgically treated over a 5-year observation period, when patients with life threatening arrhythmias are excluded.

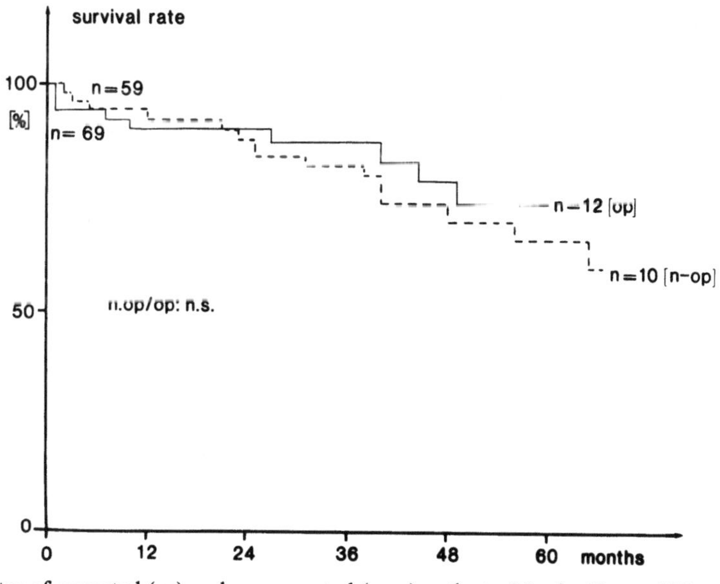

Fig. 1. Survival rates of operated (*op*) and nonoperated (*n-op*) patients. No significant difference over a 5-year observation period

The aim of this study was to identify a group of patients with aneurysm of the left ventricle by using clinical, angiographic, and hemodynamic paramters. We tried to determine whether the prognosis was better with surgical or with medical treatment.

The results of a total of 128 patients were retrospectively analyzed. The patients were assigned to two groups: 69 had been treated surgically (op group)

and 59 had been treated medically (n-op group). There was no signficant difference in mean age (op group: 49 years, ranging from 22 to 69; n-op group: 47 years, ranging from 29 to 67) or in mean observation time (op group: 35 months, ranging from 0 to 91; n-op group: 40 months, ranging from 2 to 108). The decision to operate was based on clinical and hemodynamic findings.

The data for surviving and deceased patients reveal no differences concerning the clinical symptoms of angina and/or dyspnea between the two groups. The mean values for the surviving and deceased patients of the two groups are shown in Fig. 2. Only patients who died because of myocardial failure were considered. The end-diastolic pressure (PLVED) was significantly higher only in the deceased patients who had been treated medically. No difference was found in the op group. The chamber volumes were higher in the deceased patients of both groups. Ejection fraction decreased significantly only in the medically treated patients who died. The size of the aneurysm, estimated angiographically (c_A/c_{ED}), did not differ significantly. The findings show that the function of the contracting part of the ventricle was better in the surviving patients. This is true for the circumferential fiber-shortening velocity of a basal diameter but only in the medically treated group.

	OP			N-OP		
	surv. n=67	death n=5	p<	surv. n=43	death n=14	p<
PLVED [mmHg]	20,0± 8,4	20,6± 8,0	n.s.	14,6± 7,1	22,3± 12,2	0,01
EDVI [ml/m2]	140 ± 44	200 ± 50	0,005	141 ± 41	175 ± 60	0,025
ESVI [ml/m2]	92± 39	135± 46	0,025	91± 38	131 ± 62	0,005
EF [%]	36± 9	34± 12	n.s.	37± 13	29± 14	0,05
V_{CFb} [s-1]	0,80± 0,40	0,81± 0,32	n.s.	1,00± 0,39	0,72± 0,30	0,02
C_A/C_{ED} [%]	38± 10	42± 13	n.s.	36± 9	40± 12	n.s.
Exercise [Watt]	—	—	—	89± 30	59± 40	0,02
$\overline{P}_{PA}$ (30-60Watt) [mmHg]	—	—	—	34± 11,2	46± 9,9	0,05

Fig. 2. Table of hemodynamic parameters of surviving and deceased patients of the operated (*op*) and nonoperated (*n-op*) patients. In the n-op group there was significantly better left ventricular function at rest (*PLVED, EF,* V_{CFb}) and during exercise ($\overline{P}_{PA}$, exercise capacity) of the surviving patients. Chamber volumes (*EDVI, ESVI*) were increased in the patients of both groups who subsequently died

Exercise tests using flotating catheters and measurements of pulmonary pressure were performed only with the medically treated patients. At an exercise level of 30-60 watt, achieved by all patients, those who subsequently died had a significantly higher increase in mean pulmonary pressure than did those who survived. In addition, the average exercise capacity of patients who died was even lower.

As no judgement of prognosis is possible for the individual patient because of the great scatter of all these parameters, we divided the nonoperated patients into two subgroups. The group with an indication for surgery (kons-op) had clinical and hemodynamic findings identical to those of the operated group, and consisted of 28 patients. The group without indication for surgery (kons) had less angina and dyspnea, higher exercise capacity, and less impairment of left ventricular function than was found in the op group, and consisted of 31 patients.

Figure 3 shows that there was no difference in angina pectoris between patients of the op group and patients of the kons-op group who refused surgery. Patients of the kons group show less distinct angina than do those of the other two groups. Similar results were found concerning dyspnea.

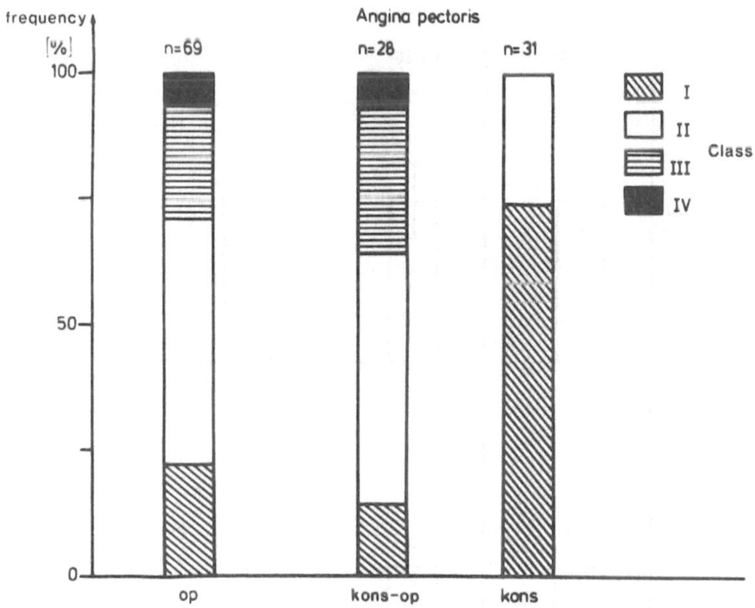

Fig. 3. Frequency of angina pectoris (classification according to NYHA) in the operated (*op*) and medically treated patients, either with indication (*kons-op*) or without indication (*kons*) for surgery. The symptoms were less distinct in the kons group than in the op and kons-op groups; there was no significant difference between these two groups

Figure 4 shows the intraventricular pressures in the three groups. No difference was found in average systolic peak pressure. End-diastolic pressure was almost identical in the op and kons-op groups, whereas in the kons group average end-diastolic pressure was significantly lower. In all groups, however, an increase in end-diastolic pressure was seen.

There was no significant difference in end-diastolic volume among the three groups (Fig. 5). Ejection fraction and the function of the contraction part of the ventricle were better in the kons group than in the other two groups, but this difference was not statistically significant (Fig. 5). The size of the aneurysm was not significantly different in all three groups.

Figure 6 shows the results of exercise tests in some of the patients who were examined by this method. The average exercise capacity did not differ significantly between the op group and the kons-op group, but was higher in the kons group. The mean pulmonary artery pressure at this maximal exercise level was smaller in the kons group in spite of the higher work load. No difference at lower work load was found between the op group and the kons-op group.

Thus, there was a group of patients treated medically with clinical and hemodynamic results almost identical to those of the operated patients (Faxon et al. 1982; Jehle et al. 1981). Figure 7 shows the prognosis of these patients in comparison with that of the operated patients and of patients with less impairment of ventricular function. In a 4-year observation period there was a significantly higher survival rate for the operated patients than for the patients of the

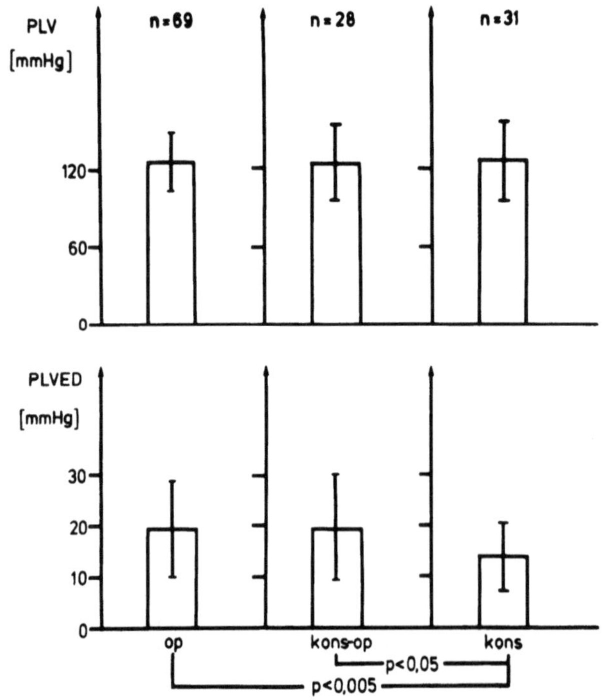

Fig. 4. Peak systolic (*PLV*) and end-diastolic (*PLVED*) pressure in the operated (*op*) and medically treated patients, either with indication (*kons-op*) or without indication (*kons*) for surgery. There was no significant difference in PLV among the three groups. PLVED was decreased in the kons group, but there was no difference between the op group and the kons-op group on the average

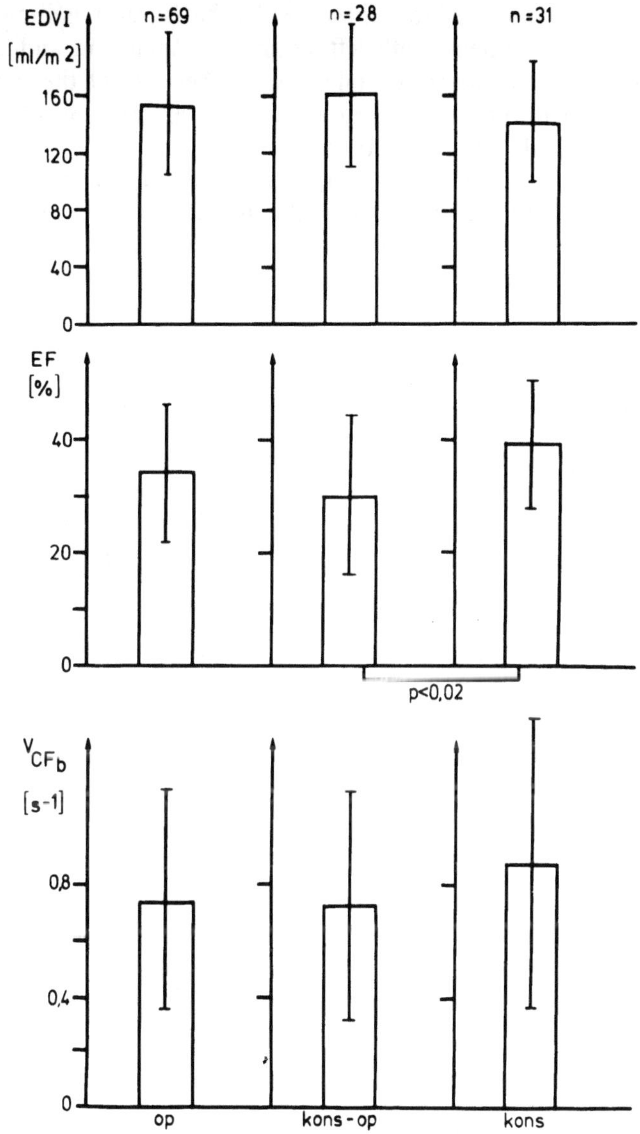

Fig. 5. End-diastolic volume (*EDVI*), ejection fraction (*EF*), and circumferential fiber-shortening velocity (V_{CFb}) of a basal diameter in the operated (*op*) and medically treated patients, either with indication (*kons-op*) or without indication (*kons*) for surgery. There were no significant differences in parameter averages between groups

kons-op group. No significant difference was found between the op group and the kons group. All deceased patients were included in this analyis except those who died of extracardial causes. This means that patients with so-called sudden death are also included, such death probably being caused by arrhtyhmias. In the op group four patients died perioperatively due to myocardial failure. In the kons-op group 50% of patients died during observation. In the kons group, however, only two patients died - suddenly, as far as we know.

We conclude from these results that surgery is indicated in a certain subgroup of patients with left ventricular aneurysm and certain clinical, angiographic, and hemodynamic findings because of the improved prognosis. Patients with life-threatening arrhythmias are not considered (Faxon et al. 1982; Jehle et al. 1981; Schulte et al. 1979).

We conclude that surgery – that is, aneurysmectomy with or without revascularization – is indicated in the individual patient with severe symptoms, because of the improvement after operation (Jehle et al. 1981; Otterstadt et al. 1981), or with increased end-diastolic pressure (more than 20 mmHg), in-

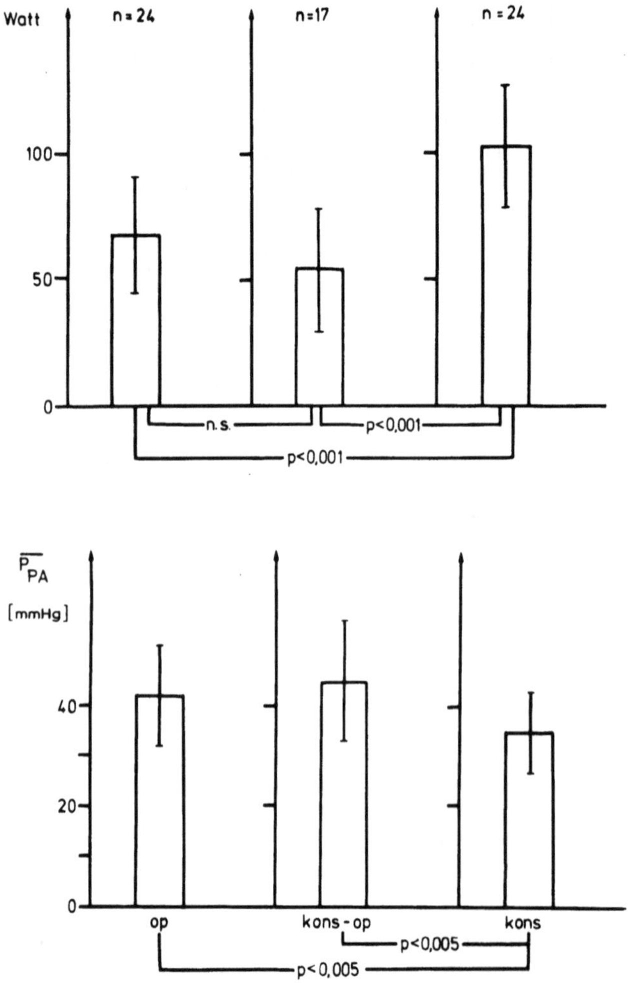

Fig. 6. Exercise capacity (*watt*) and mean pulmonary artery pressure ($\overline{P_{PA}}$) in the operated (*op*) and medically treated patients, either with indication (*kons-op*) or without indication (*kons*) for surgery. There was a significantly higher exercise capacity in the kons group, but a smaller increase in $\overline{P_{PA}}$ during this exercise level. There was no significant difference in either parameter between the op group and the kons-op group

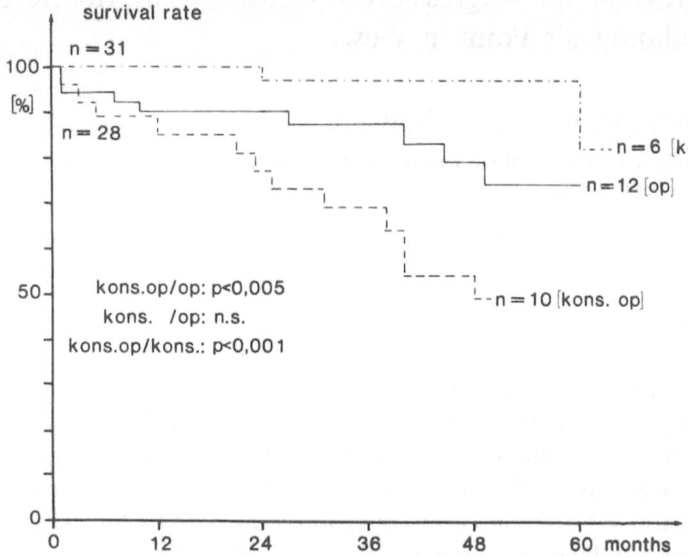

Fig. 7. Survival rates of the operated (*op*) and medically treated patients, either with indication (*kons-op*) or without indication (*kons*) for surgery. The rate was significantly lower for the kons-op group than for the other two other during a 4-year observation period. No significant difference between the op group and the kons group was observed

creased end-diastolic volume (more than 200 ml/m^2), decreased ejection fraction (less than 30%), decreased circumferential fiber-shortening velocity of a basal diameter as a parameter of the function of the residual contracting ventricle (less than 0.7 s^{-1}), and increased mean pulmonary artery pressure during exercise (more than 40 mmHg at 30–60 watt), because of the bad prognosis of these patients without operation, and in some cases because of the improved ventricular function and exercise tolerance that can be expected with it (Jehle et al. 1981).

References

Blümchen G, Heid HP, Scharf-Bornhofen E, Reidemeister JCh (1978) Langzeitbeobachtungen bei 27 Patienten mit nichtoperierten linksventrikulären Aneurysmen. Z Kardiol 67:736

Faxon DP, Ryan TJ, Davis KB, McCabe CH, Myers W, Lesperance J, Shaw R, Tong TGL (1982) Prognostic significance of angiographically documented left ventricular aneurysm from the coronary artery surgery study (CASS). Am J Cardiol 50:157

Jehle J, Heerdt M, Spiller P, Loogen F, Krian A, Schulte H-D (1981) Klinische und hämodynamische Befunde bei linksventrikulärem Aneurysma vor und nach chirurgischer Therapie. Z Kardiol 70:870

Otterstad JE, Christensen O, Levorstad K, Nitter-Hauge S (1981) Long-term results after left ventricular aneurysmectomy. Br Heart J 45:427

Schulte H-D, Bircks W, Ostermeyer J, Seipel L (1979) Surgery for life-threatening ventricular tachyarrhythmias associated with ventricular aneurysm. J Thorac Cardiovasc Surg 27:124

Progression and Regression of Coronary Arteriosclerosis – A Pathologist's Point in View

M. Stolte, D. Wittek, and B. Braun
Städtische Krankenanstalten, Pathologisches Institut, Kulmbacher Strasse 23, 8580 Bayreuth, FRG

Introduction

From animal experiments it is known that lipid accumulations in the intima can regress completely; also that mural thrombi and endothelial damage can be dissolved or diminished through organization and retraction (Table 1). The main mechanisms of progression and regression in the clinically relevant morphological substrate of coronary heart disease can be logically derived on the basis of histological examinations. While edema, necrosis, plaque, hemorrhage and mural thrombi make the stenosis worse, opposing morphological processess can lead to partial regression. (Woolf 1982, Stolte 1981).

Table 1. Mechanisms of progression and regression of coronary arteriosclerosis

Progression		Regression
Lipid accumulation	→	Back-diffusion Resorption
Mural thrombus	→	Lysis Organization Retraction
Atheroma:		
Edema	→	Resorption
Hemorrhage Necrosis Mural thrombus	→	Organization Retraction

The most dramatic and most important progression is occluding thrombosis. But why do many coronary stenoses remain static for many years, and why, in other cases, do thrombotic occlusions occur?

Material and Methods

We have studied the possible mechanisms of progression of coronary arteriosclerosis in three groups:

In a postmortem study we analyzed the causes of progression in 23 coronary stenoses bridged by means of a venous bypass graft (Braun 1980). In a second study we subjected 168 successfully bypassed coronary stenoses to pre- and postoperative angiographic assessment (Braun 1980). In a third postmortem angiographic and histological study of 60 coronary thromboses we tried to determine the mechanisms of thrombogenesis (Wittek 1983).

Results and Discussion

Model of Coronary Stenosis Bridged by Means of an ACB

Classical pathology teaches that thrombogenesis involves a hemodynamic factor, a blood factor, and a wall factor. In the model of a coronary stenosis successfully bridged by means of an aortocoronary bypass (ACB) the hemodynamic factor is present; nevertheless, clinical statistics show that, angiographically, 50% of these stenoses remain patent (Stürzenhofecker et al. 1978, Schmuziger et al. 1979).

We subjected 23 stenoses bridged by means of an ACB, to angiographic, macroscopic, and histological examinations in an attempt to discover causes for occlusion. Only six of the 23 cases revealed progression. The morphometric analysis of the degree of the bridged stenosis showed that progression is more common as the degree of the stenosis increases (Table 2).

Table 2. Progression of coronary arteriosclerosis in stenoses, successfully bridged by means of an ACB, as related to the degree of the stenosis

Stenosis (%)	Progression ($n = 23$)	
	No	Yes
<70	8	–
70–90	8	4
>90	1	2

Table 3. Relationship between the form and the histological quality of 23 coronary stenoses bridged by means of an ACB

Stenosis	Histologically quality	
	Sclerosis	Atheroma
Excentric	5	11
Concentric	6	1

The form of the stenosis is also of importance; progression occurs in eccentric, but not in concentric, stenoses. Of the 23 stenoses, there were 16 eccentric and seven concentric; only six of the eccentric showed progression and none of the concentric did.

The form provided indirect information as well, about the possible histological quality of the coronary stenosis: at the back of the eccentric stenosis there is usually an atheroma, in the case of concentric stenoses, in contrast, mainly rigid sclerosis (Table 3). Indeed, the breakdown of the cases by histological quality shows that scleroses and atheromas with a predominantly sclerotic component rarely develop a thrombosis, while most cases of thrombosis occur in atheromas (Table 4). The fact that not all atheromas become thrombotic is due to the varying thickness of the plaque cap: with increasing thickness of this plaque cap occlusion becomes rarerer (Table 5).

Table 4. Relationship between the histological quality of coronary stenoses bridged by an ACB and the frequency of progression

Histological quality	Progression ($n=23$) No	Yes
Sclerosis	7	1
Sclerosed atheroma	4	1
Atheroma	6	4

Table 5. Relationship between the thickness of the plaque cap of an atheroma and the occurrence of a progression of arteriosclerosis in coronary stenoses bridged by an ACB

Thickness of plaque cap (mm)	Progression No	Yes
<0.1	–	2
>0.1	10	3
Sclerosis	6	1

The observation that even in atheromas with a broad plaque cap, partial atheroma necroses accompanied by hemorrhage can also be found led to the following hypothesis for the morphogenesis of such thromboses. Not only stasis and rupture of the plaque cap due to an increased transmural pressure can cause a thrombosis to develop; a reduced perfusion and a diminished supply of blood to the vessel wall can lead to partial necrosis with edema, hemorrhage, and rupture of the plaque cap (see Fig. 1).

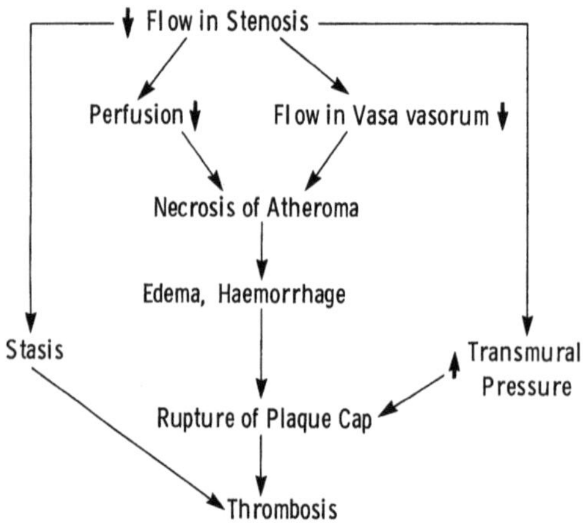

Fig. 1. Hypothesis for the morphogenesis of a thrombosis in a coronary stenosis, bridged by means of an ACB

Pre- and Postoperative Angiographic Assessment

In order to see whether these results translated to the clinical situation, we subjected 168 bypassed coronary stenoses to pre- and postoperative angiographic assessment and found that 45.2% of them revealed a progressive course. The length of the stenosis had little influence on progression; 52.9% of the short ones did not show progression, 47.1% did; 42.2% of the long stenoses did not, 57.8% did.

As the degree of stenosis increases, the rate of progression also increases. The finding in the group with <70% cannot be taken into account (see Table 6), as this group comprised only ten cases.

Table 6. Relationship between the degree of stenosis and the progression of arteriosclerosis in 168 bypassed coronary stenoses

Stenosis (%)	Progression (%)	
	No	Yes
<70	30.0	70.0
70–90	55.5	44.5
>90	33.3	66.7

As in the postmortem cases, it was again seen that progression can be expected, in particular with eccentric stenoses where 80.4% progressed; 63.4% of concentric stenosis did not progress.

Analysis of Coronary Thromboses

Can these results be reproduced in thrombotic stenoses that have not been bridged by means of an ACB? Or, is – as in the case of ACB – a thrombosis merely a result of a collateral flow, and thus merely a secondary phenomenon?

In an attempt to find an answer to this question, we made a postmortem study of 60 coronary thromboses (serial sections and morphometry). The initial results showed that the hypothesis of the significance of collateral flow in the development of coronary thrombosis was not correct, for, in the case of fresh thrombotic occlusions, the collateral flow is usually not increased.

The morphometric analysis showed that the degree of the stenosis in which a thrombosis developed was usually more than 70%, although even noncritical stenoses can develop thrombotic occlusions (Table 7).

Table 7. Relationship between the degree of coronary stenosis and the development of a thrombotic occlusion

Stenosis (%)	Thrombosis (%)
<70	17,1
>70	82,9

Table 8. Frequency of the different forms of coronary stenosis in thrombotic occlusions

Form of stenosis	Thrombosis	
Eccentric	32.6%	89.1%
Mainly eccentric	56.5%	
Concentric	10.9%	

It was again found that the form of the stenosis is an important prognostic parameter: 89.1% of the stenoses in which a thrombosis developed were eccentric, or predominantly eccentric (see Table 8).

The analysis of the histology of the underlying coronary atherosclerosis showed that the decisive parameter of progression is the histological quality of the stenosis, since an atheroma presented in almost 94% of cases.

The consequence of these findings in the following hypothesis of the causes of progression and regression in clinically relevant coronary atherosclerosis (Fig. 2): As a result of an increase in pressure, either from the inside or the outside - here we might consider a spasm, for parts of the media are still intact - the plaque of an atheroma can rupture. Then develops either a mural thrombosis or an occluding thrombosis, which may be permeated by parts of the ateromatous pool. But even in cases with a rupture of the plaque cap and mural or even occluding thrombosis, a sometimes astonishing angiographic regression may be possible in particular through the embolization of the atheromatous pool or the thrombosis.

Figure 3 shows a stenosis of the left main stem in a patient who died due to an extensive anterior and lateral wall infarction. Histologically the stenosis

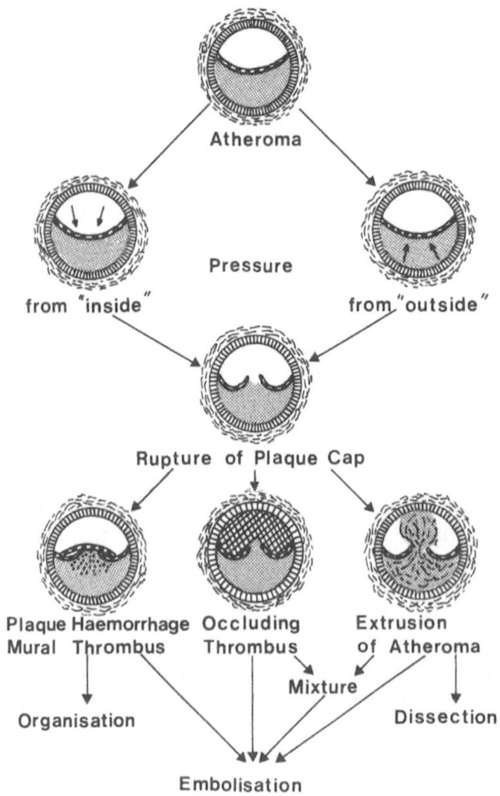

Fig. 2. Hypothesis of the main mechanisms of progression of clinically relevant coronary atherosclerosis

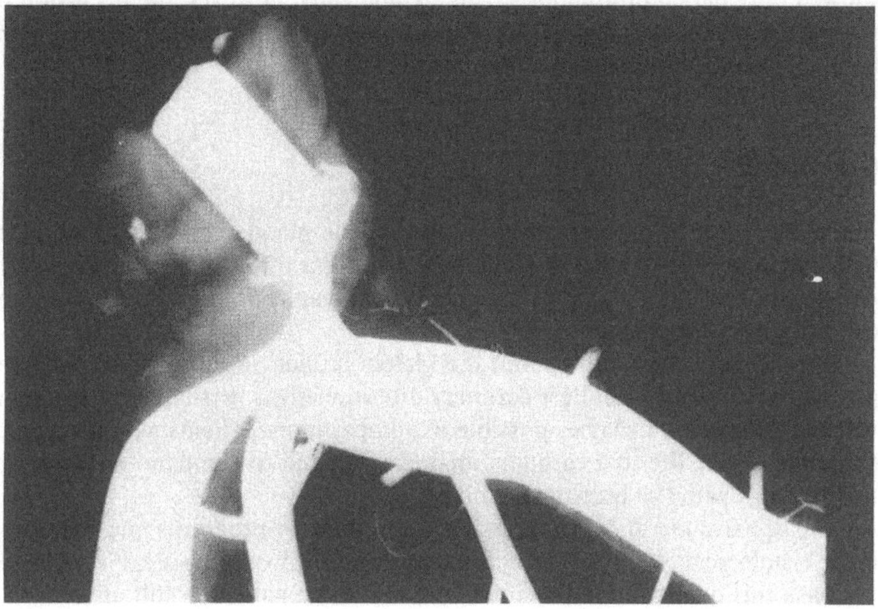

Fig. 3. Postmortem angiography of the left coronary artery with a stenosis of the left main stem

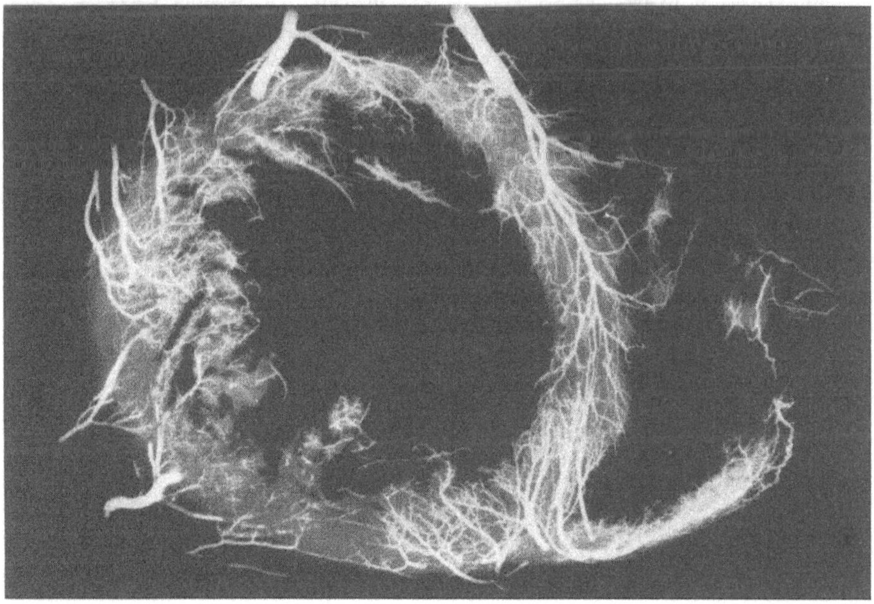

Fig. 4. Postmortem angiography of a slice of the heart with occlusion of some peripheral branches of the coronary ateries; same case as in Fig. 3

showed only parietal thrombosis. Angiographically, however, the occlusion of several peripheral branches of coronary arteries proved to contain thromboembolic or embolic atheromatous material (Fig. 4).

Conclusions

The main factor in progression is rupture of the plaque cap of an atheroma, with extrusion of the atheromatous pool and/or a thrombosis. But even here embolization of the "pool," or thrombolysis, organization, and recanalization can bring about regression.

We still know very little about the factors influencing progression and regression of clinically manifest coronary arteriosclerosis. Perhaps this situation will change when it becomes possible to autopsy more patients who have been subjected during life to a coronary angiography, and to compare the postmortem findings with the intravitam finding.

The decisive factor for progression - and thus for prognosis and therapy - is the histological quality of the coronary stenosis. It would be ideal if we could establish this quality by indirect methods while the patient is still alive.

References

Braun B (1980) Ursachen der Progression der Koronararteriensklerose in der durch einem aorto-koronaren Bypass überbrückten Stenose. Inaugural-Dissertation, Erlangen

Schmuziger M, Roskamm H, Stürzenhofecker P, Hahn CH, Stolte M (1979) Is revascularisation limited to good quality and high caliber vessels? In: Roskamm H, Schmuziger M (eds) Coronary heart surgery. A rehabilitation measure. Springer, Berlin Heidelberg New York

Stolte M (1981) Anatomie und Pathologie der Koronararterien, Konsequenzen für Klinik und Praxis. Perimed, Erlangen

Stürzenhofecker P, Schmuziger M, Rentrop P, Roskamm H, Stolte M, Pietsch K (1978) Faktoren, die die Verschlußhäufigkeit eines aortokoronaren Bypass bestimmen. Verh Dtsch Ges Kreislaufforsch 44:214

Wittek D (1983) Koronarthrombose: angiographische, histologische und morphometrische Untersuchungen. Inaugural-Dissertation, Erlangen

Woolf N (1982) Pathology of atherosclerosis. Butterworth, London

Progression of Coronary Atherosclerosis in Nonoperated Patients: Relation to Risk Factors

J. R. Kramer, H. Kitazume, W. L. Proudfit, Y. Matsuda, G. W. Williams, and F. M. Sones, jr.

The Cleveland Clinic Foundation, Department of Cardiology, 9500 Euclid Avenue, Cleveland, OH 44106, USA

Important determinants of progression have recently been described by Bruschke and colleagues (1981). Careful analysis of sequential coronary cineangiograms obtained in 256 nonoperated patients with significant coronary atherosclerosis showed time to be the most important determinant of progression. In addition, the initial severity of disease could be correlated to progression, whereas risk factors at first study could not. If progressive coronary atherosclerosis occurs in relation to time and initial severity of disease independently of risk factors, "secondary prevention" by risk-factor modification may not be possible. We studied 302 patients to determine the relation of progression to risk factors.

Methods

Methods of patient selection, technique of film review, definitions, and a discussion of the biases involved in studying progression have been reported previously (Kramer et al. 1981, 1983). A data base of 385 patients with two cardiac catheterizations is presented. After exclusions, 302 patients were studied by comparing 26 arterial segments at first and second study.

Results

The 277 men and 25 women, aged 29 to 68 years, with 50% or more narrowing of the lumen in at least one coronary artery at first study were restudied at least 2 months later (mean interval = 36.8 months). Of these, 20 patients (7%) were restudied electively, 136 (45%) because of persistent angina pectoris, and 146 (48%) because of an intervening clinical event.

At second study, 136 men (49%) and 12 women (48%) met preestablished angiographic criteria for progression. Progressive changes were found in one vessel in 102 patients (69%), in two vessels in 40 patients (27%), and in three vessels in six patients (4%). Time was a major determinant of progression: nonprogression patients had a mean interval between studies of 29.3 ± 22.3 months, whereas in progression patients the mean interval was 44.2 ± 31.5 months ($p < 0.001$). When the interval between studies was less than 2 years, 42 of 113 patients (37%) exhibited progression, but when the interval exceeded 5 years, progression was noted in 46 of 60 patients (77%, $p < 0.0005$).

Left ventriculography showed evidence of new segmental impairment at second study in 105 patients: 78 patients (74%) met criteria for progression ($p < 0.0001$). Analysis of risk factors at first study was not helpful in predicting who would have new segmental impairment at second study. In patients with progression and an interval of less than 2 years between studies there was a mean drop in systolic blood pressure of 9 mm Hg at second study. Twelve of the 42 patients (35%) in this group had electrocardiographic evidence of an interval myocardial infarction.

Risk factors obtained at the time of first study, including family history, weight, smoking habits, diabetes, blood pressure, and cholesterol and triglyceride levels, were evaluated and could not be related to progression. For example, cholesterol and triglyceride levels at first study are shown in relation to the number of patients with progression at second study (Tables 1 and 2). No significant correlation is evident. Analysis of the same risk factors at second study (improved, worsened, or unchanged) showed no relation to progression. As an example, cholesterol levels at first and second study were compared and related to the number of patients with progression at second study (Table 3). Again, no significant correlation could be made.

Table 1. Relation of cholesterol at first study to progression

Cholesterol levels (mg/dl)	Nonprogression (no. of patients)	Progression (no. of patients)	Total
<100			
101–150	2	2	4
151–200	28	15	43
201–250	64	68	132
≤250	94 (53%)	85 (47%)	179 (59%)
>250	43 (50%)	53 (50%)	106 (35%)
251–299	36	32	68
300–349	10	15	25
350–399	4	6	10
>399	3	0	3
Unknown	7 (41%)	10 (59%)	17 (6%)

Table 2. Relation of triglycerides at first study to progression

Initial study (mg/dl)	Nonprogression (no. of patients)	Progression (no. of patients)	Total
<50			
51–100	9	16	25
101–135	15	14	29
≤135	24 (44%)	30 (56%)	54 (18%)
>135	91 (55%)	75 (45%)	166 (55%)
136–200	47	37	84
>200	44	38	82
Unknown	39	43	82 (27%)

Table 3. Relation of cholesterol at first and second studies to progression

Cholesterol ≤250 mg/dl first study	Cholesterol ≤250 mg/dl second study	Cholesterol status at second study	Nonprogression (no. of patients)	Progression (no. of patients)	Total
Yes	Yes	Unchanged: normal	61 (53%)	54 (47%)	115 (38%)
No	No	Unchanged: abnormal	23 (45%)	28 (55%)	51 (17%)
No	Yes	"Better"	29 (58%)	21 (42%)	50 (17%)
Yes	No	"Worse"	24 (57%)	18 (43%)	42 (14%)
Unknown	Unknown	-	17 (39%)	27 (61%)	44 (14%)

All risk factors at first and second study were known in 124 patients. Multiple logistic regressions were performed in this group using age, sex, interval between studies, risk factors at first study, and risk factors at second study. Only the interval between studies was significantly related to progression ($p = 0.0002$).

Discussion

Time is a strong determinant of progression. In comparison, risk factors at first and second study - whether unchanged, improved, or worsened - do not appear to influence progression. If this is the case, therapeutic interventions to control risk factors in the patient who already has disease may not be effective in preventing progressive coronary atherosclerosis. However, there continue to be strong indications for controlling some risk factors for reasons other than prevention of coronary atherosclerosis. For example, the treated hypertensive patient is less likely to suffer stroke, and the smoker who stops is less likely to develop carcinoma of the lung. In contrast, recommendations for dietary intervention to control lipids in the patient with mild to moderate elevation of serum cholesterol may have to be reexamined (Food and Nutrition Board 1980). In addition, the search for important unknown risk factors should continue.

Acknowledgements. We appreciate the editorial suggestions of Ms. Shannon J. Henry and thank Mrs. Jo Rolph for preparation of the manuscript.

References

Bruschke AVG, Wijer TS, Kolsters W, Landmann J (1981) The anatomical evolution of coronary artery disease demonstrated by coronary arteriography in 256 nonoperated patients. Circulation 63:527–536

Food and Nutrition Board (1980) Toward healthful diets. Harper AE, Chairman. National Academy of Sciences, Washington DC

Kramer JR, Matsuda Y, Mulligan JC, Aronow M, Proudfit WL (1981) Progression of coronary atherosclerosis. Circulation 63:519–526

Kramer JR, Kitazume H, Proudfit WL, Matsuda Y, Williams GW, Sones FM (1983) Progression and regression of coronary atherosclerosis: relation to risk factors. Am Heart J 105:134–144

Progression of Coronary Arteriosclerosis in Nonoperated Patients

P. Stürzenhofecker, K. Peters, E. Steinmann, P. Betz, and H. Roskamm
Rehabilitationszentrum für Herz- und Kreislaufkranke, Südring 15, 7812 Bad Krozingen, FRG

Introduction

Coronary arteriosclerosis is a progressive disease. Degree and speed of progression in man can only be assessed by repeated angiography. There are only a few systematic studies with repeated angiography performed independent of the development of symtoms and signs in the patients (Palac et al. 1981; Rafflenbeul et al. 1979; Stürzenhofecker et al. 1981). Most studies were done on operated patients and on nonoperated patients with clinical deterioration (Bemis et al. 1973; Ben-Zwi et al. 1974; Bruschke et al. 1981; Gensini and Kelly 1972; Gensini et al. 1974; Kramer et al. 1981; Marchandise et al. 1978; Moccetti et al. 1976; Nash et al. 1974, 1977). Our study also belongs to the latter category.

The data on coronary heart disease patients who had undergone recatheterization because of symptomatic deterioration were studied to answer the following questions:

1. What is the incidence, localization, and extent of progression of arteriosclerosis?
2. Is progression of arteriosclerosis predictable from the coronary morphology shown by the first coronary angiogram?
3. Can progression of arteriosclerosis be predicted from clinical data and exercise parameters, including hemodynamics?

Patients and Methods

Between 1973 and 1982, 219 patients (aged 28–63, mean age 49 years) had undergone reangiography because of progression of symptoms. Complete clinical and angiographic data on these patients were available at the time of both the first and the second angiographies. The time interval between the first and second angiography ranged from 3 months to 9 years, the mean interval being 2.8 years. After the second angiography 115 patients underwent surgery.

In a retrospective study the 219 angiograms were reviewed by three experienced angiographers. Measurements of the luminal diameter (20 coronary artery segments) were performed in at least two projections. Degree of stenosis was defined by the most severe reduction of the lumen diameter in any given projection.

Progression was assumed if there was a difference of at least two grades, according to the AHA classification of stenoses (AHA Committee Report 1975), or if a subtotal occlusion had developed into a total occlusion. Clinical and exercise variables and angiographic data were computerized and statistically analyzed.

Results

Progressive changes of coronary morphology were seen in 130 patients (59.3%) at the time of the second angiography.

At the time of the first angiography, distribution of coronary disease was equal in the progressive and in the nonprogressive group as analyzed by a coronary score (Fig. 1). Progression in one vessel occurred in 70 patients, in two vessels in 38, and in three vessels in 22.

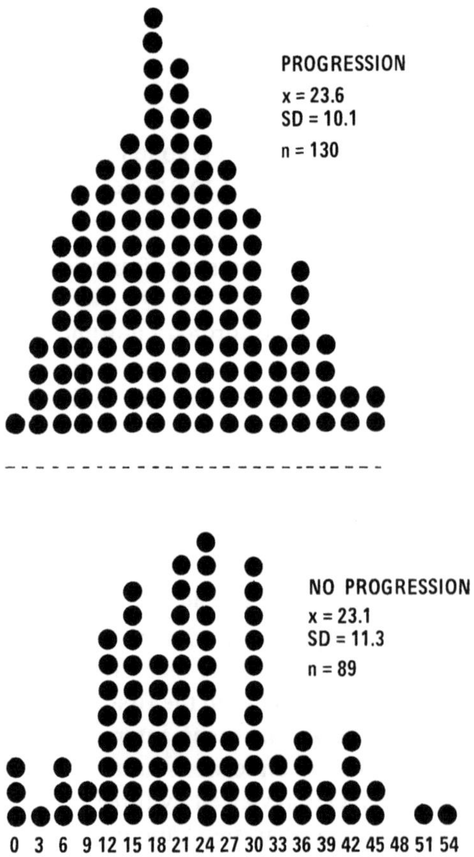

Fig. 1. Individual values of a coronary score (Kaltenbach 1975) derived from the first angiogram in 130 patients with progression and in 89 patients without progression. There is no significant difference between the two groups

Progressive changes were equally distributed among the main coronary artery branches, the proximal segment of the right coronary artery showing a slightly higher frequency of progression.

Progression was rather rare in the left main coronary artery (Fig. 2). Of 4380 coronary artery segments in 219 patients, 282 (6.4%) showed progression in the second angiogram. Of 3384 segments not originally stenosed 144 (4.3%) segments showed progression, and of 996 originally stenosed segments 138 (14%) showed progression, 81% were unchanged, and 5% showed regression (Fig. 3).

Of a total of 282 segments that showed progression in the second angiogram, 144 had been judged as not stenosed according to the first angiogram, and 30 of these 144 even showed progression to total occlusion. The remaining 60 total occlusions occurred in originally stenosed segments (Fig. 4).

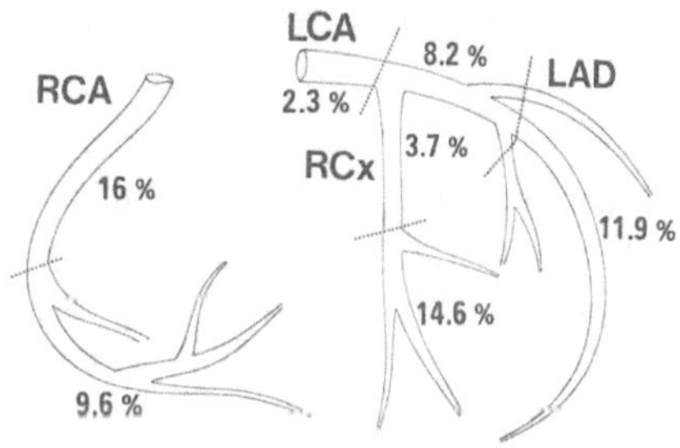

Fig. 2. Incidence of progression in various segments of the coronary arteries

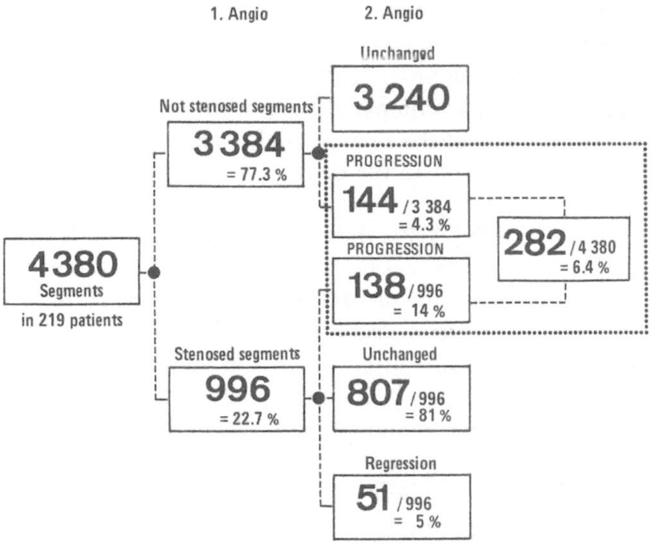

Fig. 3. Incidence of progression in segments not originally stenosed, and of progression and regression in originally stenosed segments of the coronary arteries. In the second angiogram stenoses distal of the occlusion could not be evaluated; they were assumed to be unchanged

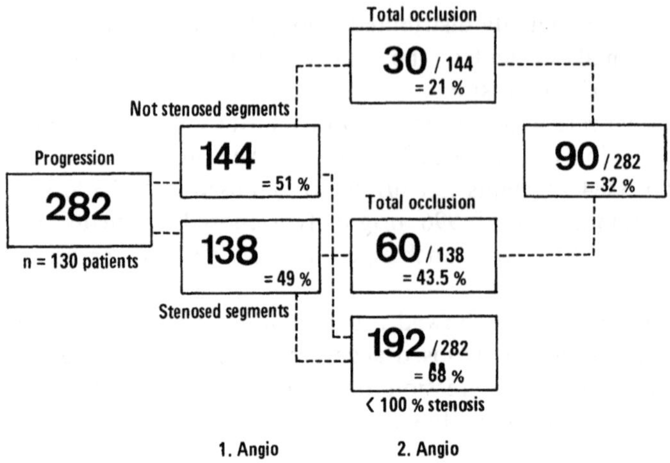

Fig. 4. Status of 282 coronary artery segments in 130 patients which were stenosed or even totally occluded in the second angiogram

The 30 total occlusions that occurred in previously nonstenotic segments were an unexpected and surprising result; Fig. 5 shows an example. The total number of progressions in 282 segments of 130 patients is shown in Fig. 6. Again it can be seen that new occlusions can occur in originally normal or minimally stenosed vessels and from different grades of stenoses seen in the first angiogram. There were many progressions from a low degree to a high degree of stenosis. In 71 of the 130 patients, segmental progression resulted in the involvement of additional vessels. There were six progressions to one-vessel disease, 27 progressions to two-vessel disease, and 38 progressions to three-vessel disease.

Concentric stenoses were relatively rare and showed little tendency to progression (11%) as compared with diffuse and eccentric stenoses (20%) (Fig. 7).

At the time of the second angiography, the maximal exercise tolerance was significantly lower in the progression group; other statistically significant differences between the two groups were found for maximal pulmonary capillary wedge pressure (PCP_{max}) and maximal cardiac index (see Table 1). Only in the progression group was there a significant increase in maximal PCP, and a significant decrease in cardiac index at maximal exercise.

Using a logistic regression model (Cox 1970), the univariate analysis showed significant differences in the alteration from the first to the second study (delta = Δ) for Δ maximal cardiac index, Δ maximal PCP, Δ time and Δ maximal exercise tolerance (Table 2). In the multivariate stepwise analysis with the logistic regression model only the following variables were independent: Δ maximal cardiac index, Δ maximal PCP, and Δ time (Table 2).

Using these parameters in the model, 85% of progression patients and 65% of nonprogression patients could be predicted correctly, yielding a totally correct prediction of 75%.

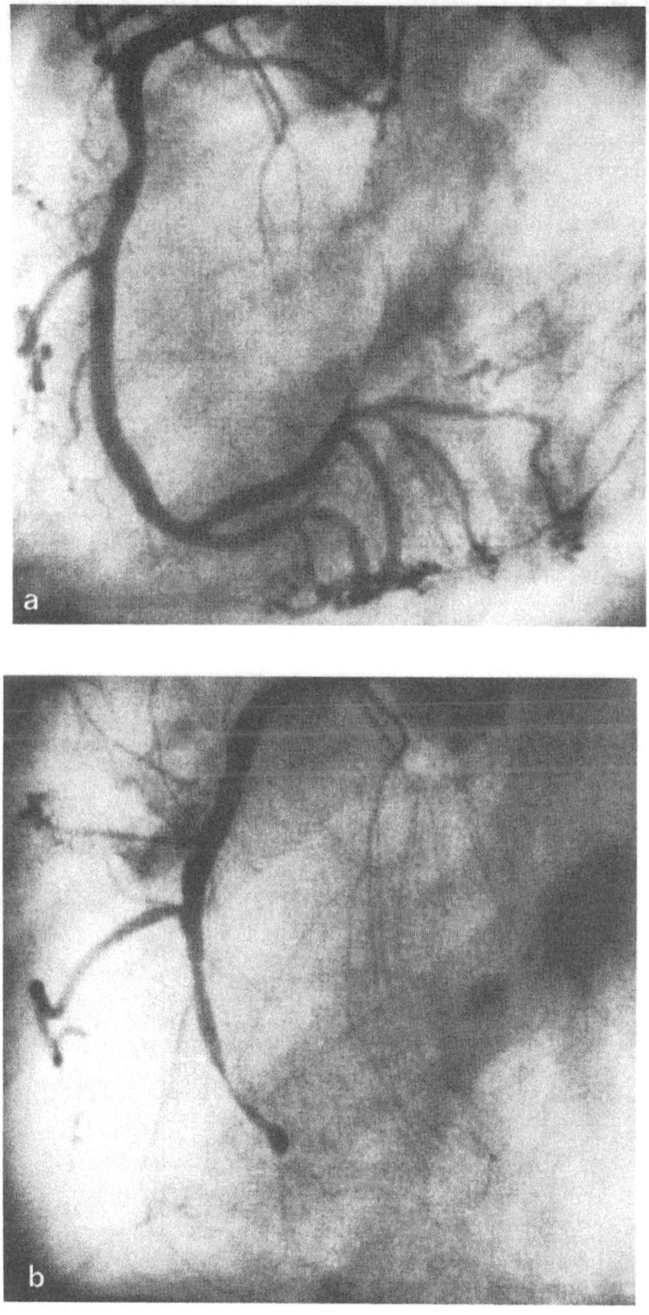

Fig. 5a, b. Right coronary artery in left anterior oblique projection in **a** the first angiography and **b** the second. The second angiogram was performed 75 months after the first. A total occlusion developed from a nonstenosed vessel with minimal wall irregularities

Table 1. Exercise parameters at the time of the first and second angiography in patients without and with progression of coronary arteriosclerosis

		No change $n=97$		Progression $n=93$
Maximal exercise tolerance (watts)	*1.*	*85.0*[b]	*ns*	*89.5*[b]
	2.	73.9	$p<0.05$	63.2
AP-free exercise tolerance (watts)	*1.*	*59.2*[b]	*ns*	*62.1*[b]
	2.	45.8	ns	37.1
ST-segment depression (mV)	*1.*	*0.13*	*ns*	*0.16*
	2.	0.17	ns	0.20
PCP_{max} (Torr)	*1.*	*24.3*	*ns*	*22.2*[b]
	2.	23.4	$p<0.02$	27.4
Maximal cardiac index (liters/min/m^2)	*1.*	*7.2*	$p<0.1$	*7.7*[b]
	2.	7.0	$p<0.001$	5.8
Maximal heart rate (beats/min)	*1.*	*119.0*[a]	*ns*	*121.7*[b]
	2.	111	ns	108
Maximal blood pressure (Torr)	*1.*	*180*	*ns*	*180*[a]
	2.	180	$p<0.03$	170

Data in italics refer to first study, those in roman type to second.
[a] $p<0.01$
[b] $p<0.001$

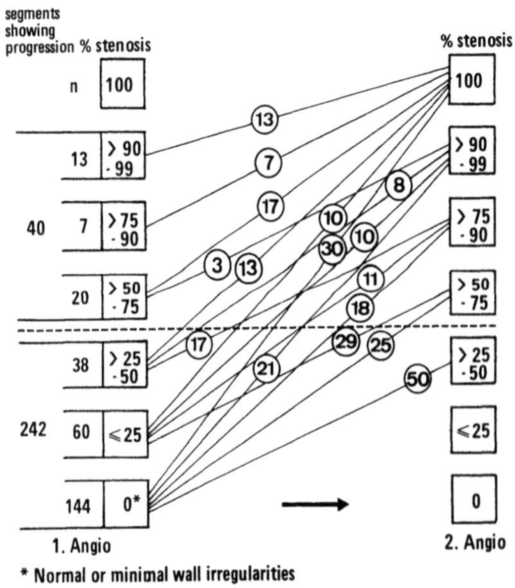

Fig. 6. Degree of stenosis at the time of the first and second coronary angiography in 130 patients who showed progression of at least two grades according to the AHA classification, or total occlusion, in 282 segments

Table 2. Predictors of progression in a univariate and multivariate analysis during stepwise logistic regression

Variables	Univariate	Multivariate
Δ Cardiac index	$p<0.0000$	$p<0.0001$
Δ PCP_{max}	$p<0.0007$	$p<0.02$
Δ Time	$p<0.0025$	$p<0.01$
Δ Maximal exercise tolerance	$p<0.005$	ns

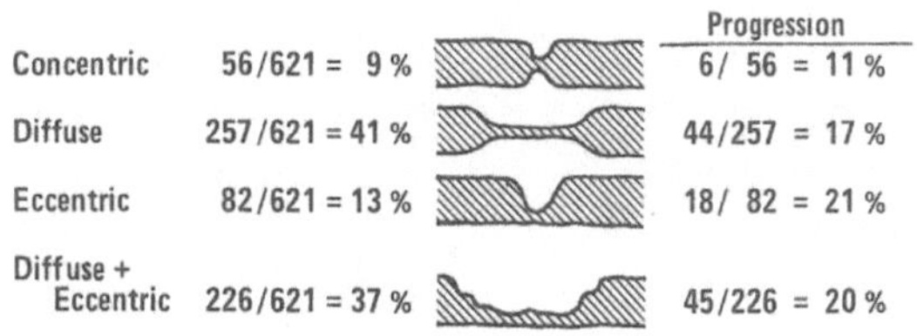

Fig. 7. Incidence of progression in relation to morphology of stenosis at the time of the first angiogram

Figure 8 shows the maximal exercise tolerance and cardiac index during maximal exercise for those patients who showed progression to anatomically defined indications for surgery, such as new three-vessel disease, new two-vessel disease with new high-degree proximal LAD stenosis, and new left main coronary artery disease. In most of these patients there was a decrease in maximal exercise tolerance, and in nearly all patients a decrease in maximal cardiac index. In the individual patient, however, progression cannot be excluded if functional variables do not change.

Conclusions

Of course, one must be well aware of the limitations of a retrospective study in a selected group of patients. Nevertheless, the above data may allow the following conclusions.

There were 130 patients (59%) who showed progressive changes in a total of 282 segments, which were equally distributed in the main coronary artery branches.

Progression occurred from all degrees of stenoses in the first angiogram; even total occlusions derived from segments that were not stenosed according to the first angiogram.

Concentric stenoses showed a lower frequency of progression than did eccentric and diffuse stenoses.

Deterioration of function (decrease in maximal exercise tolerance, increase in pulmonary wedge pressure, and decrease of cardiac index during maximal

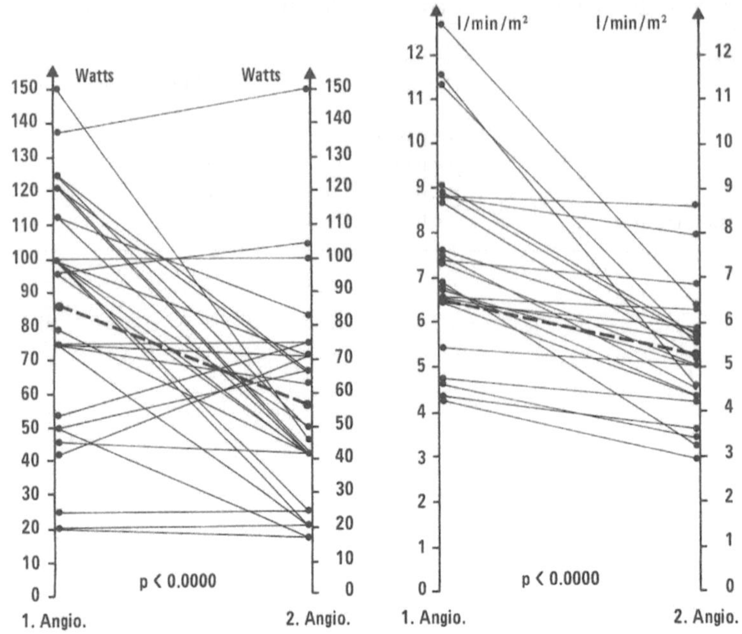

Fig. 8. Maximal exercise tolerance (*left*) and maximal cardiac index (*right*) in patients with progression of coronary artery disease to anatomically defined new indications for bypass surgery

exercise) is more pronounced in the progression group. But even a progression to anatomically defined new indications for bypass surgery is possible without changes in exercise parameters.

References

AHA Committee Report (1975) A reporting system on patients evaluated for coronary artery disease. Circulation 51:7-402

Bemis CE, Gorlin R, Kemp HG, Herman MV (1973) Progression of coronary artery disease. A clinical arteriographic study. Circulation 47:455-464

Ben-Zvi J, Hildner FJ, Javier RR, Fester A, Samet D (1974) Progression of coronary artery disease. Cinearteriographic and clinical observations in medically and surgically treated patients. Am J Cardiol 34:295-301

Bruschke AVG, Wijers TS, Kolsters W, Landmann J (1981) The anatomic evolution of coronary artery disease demonstrated by coronary arteriography in 256 nonoperated patients. Circulation 63:527-536

Cox DR (1970) The analysis of binary data. Methuen, London

Gensini GG, Kelly AE (1972) Incidence and progression of coronary artery disease. An angiographic correlation in 1263 patients. Arch Intern Med 129:814-827

Gensini GG, Esente P, Kelly A (1974) Natural history of coronary disease in patients with and without coronary bypass graft surgery. Circulation [Suppl II] 49/50:98-101

Kaltenbach M (1975) Quantitative Bewertung koronarangiographischer Befunde mit Hilfe eines Punktesystems (score). Z Kardiol 64:597-606

Kramer JR, Matsuda Y, Mulligan JC, Aronow M, Proudfit WL (1981) Progression of coronary atherosclerosis. Circulation 63:519–526
Marchandise B, Bourassa MG, Chaitman BR, Lesperance J (1978) Angiographic evaluation of the natural history of normal coronary arteries and mild coronary atherosclerosis. Am J Cardiol 41:216–220
Moccetti T, Lichtlen P, Schönbeck M, Steinbrunn W (1976) Progression of coronary artery disease based on cineangiographic data. In: Lichtlen PR (ed) Coronary angiography and angina pectoris, Thieme, Stuttgart, p 88
Nash DT, Caldwell N, Ancona D (1974) Accelerated coronary artery disease arteriographically proved. Analysis of risk factors. NY State J Med 74:947–950
Nash DT, Gensini GG, Simon H, Arno T, Nash SD (1977) The erysichthon syndrome. Progression of coronary atherosclerosis and dietary hyperlipidemia. Circulation 56:363–365
Palac RT, Hwang MH, Meadows WR, Croke RP, Pifarre R, Loeb HS, Gunnar RM (1981) Progression of coronary artery disease in medically treated patients 5 years after randomization. Circulation [Suppl II] 64:17–21
Rafflenbeul W, Smith LR, Mantle JA, Rackley CE, Russel RO Jr (1979) Quantitative coronary arteriography. Coronary anatomy of patients with unstable angina pectoris reexamined 1 year after optimal medical therapy. Am J Cardiol 43:699–707
Stürzenhofecker P, Samek L, Droste C, Gohlke H, Petersen J, Roskamm H (1981) Prognosis of coronary heart disease and progression of coronary arteriosclerosis in postinfarction patients under the age of 40. In: Roskamm H (ed) Myocardial infarction at young age. Springer, Berlin Heidelberg New York, p 82

Progression of Coronary Artery Disease Between 10 and 12 Years After Coronary Artery Bypass Graft Surgery*

M. G. Bourassa, M. Enjalbert, L. Campeau, and J. Lespérance

Institut de Cardiologie de Montréal, 5000 est, rue Bélanger, Montréal, Québec, H1T 1C8, Canada

Repeat coronary arteriography was performed approximately 1, 6, and 11 years after coronary artery bypass graft surgery at our institution in a group of unselected patients. The long-term attrition rate of saphenous vein bypass grafts and the influence of graft and native coronary artery changes on the late clinical course of these patients have been previously reported (Campeau et al. 1978, 1979, 1982; Enjalbert et al. 1982), or will be the subject of further analysis. The purpose of this report is to study the rate and extent of angiographic progression of coronary disease in the grafted and ungrafted arteries of these patients and to correlate progression of coronary disease with age, sex, risk factors, severity of preexisting disease, and left ventricular function.

Material and Methods

Patient Population

Angiographic studies were performed within 1 month after surgery in 400 of the 500 patients who underwent coronary artery bypass graft surgery at our institution before 1973 (Table 1).

Table 1. Angiographic studies after saphenous vein aortocoronary bypass surgery (Montreal Heart Institute)

Time after surgery	No. of patients studied (from first 500)	No. of grafts studied
Within 1 month (10–21 days)	400	721
At approximately 1 year (6–18 months)	200	352
At approximately 6 years (54–88 months)	108	202
At approximately 11 years (114–153 months)	82	143

* Work supported in part by the J. L. Lévesque Foundation and the Montreal Heart Institute Research Fund

Among these 400 cases, 200 patients underwent repeat angiography approximately 1 year after surgery. They were recruited from two near-consecutive series: a first series of 104 of our first 138 patients, and a second series of 96 patients, selected from patients 379–480, studied following modifications in surgical techniques.

We then studied 108 patients - recruited from both prospective series - angiographically, approximately 6 years after surgery, and 82 of these patients recently underwent repeat angiography approximately 11 years after surgery.

Coronary Arteriography

Coronary arteriography was performed by a percutaneous transfemoral approach using preformed polyethylene catheters (Bourassa et al. 1969); craniocaudal and caudocranial sagittally angulated views of the left coronary artery were routinely filmed (Lespérance et al. 1974). The same technique and the same projections were used for the baseline and follow-up angiograms.

The films were of good quality and the repeat studies were always compared with the baseline coronary arteriogram. The films were read on two side-by-side projectors, by two angiographers working to reach a consensus.

The coronary arteries were divided into 16 major segments; each major artery had five segments and the left main coronary artery had one segment (Principal Investigators of CASS and their Associates 1981).

Obstructions of the coronary arteries were defined as the linear percentage of narrowing of the diameter of the vessel compared with the diameter of the nearest normal segment. The estimated percentage of obstruction was derived from the angiographic view showing the greatest reduction in diameter for the vessel in question. A confidence code was recorded for each lesion and segments with a low confidence level, usually those distal to new or old occlusions, were excluded. When multiple lesions were present on the same segment of the artery, only the most severe lesion was considered.

Significant progression of obstructive disease was defined as: (a) any progression to total occlusion; (b) a change of at least 20% in lesions greater than 50%; (c) a change of at least 30% in lesions greater than 20% but less than 50%; (d) a change of at least 50% for normal segments (Bourassa et al. 1981).

Left Ventriculography

Left ventricular wall motion was evaluated from the 30° right anterior oblique ventriculogram. The cardiac silhouette was divided in the usual manner into five segments and each segment was scored by a point system (Principal Investigators of CASS and their Associates 1981). Normal left ventricular contraction was coded 1, moderate hypokinesis 2, severe hypokinesis 3, akinesis 4, and dyskinesis 5. The left ventricular contraction score was the sum of the total number of points. Thus, normal left ventricular contraction had a score of 5 and abnormal contraction a score of 6 or more.

Results

Rate and Extent of Progression of Disease in Grafted and Ungrafted Coronary Arteries

Among ungrafted coronary arteries with preexisting stenoses greater than 20% before bypass surgery, 9% showed significant progression of disease at 1 year, 33% at 6 years and 47% at 11 years (Table 2).

Table 2. Progression of disease in the native coronary arteries

	No. of preoperative occlusions	Progression of preexisting stenosis Time after surgery		
		Between 6 and 18 months	Between 5 and 7 years	Between 10 and 12 years
Ungrafted arteries	18	5/53–9%	14/43–33%	25/53–47%
Grafted arteries				
With patent grafts	44	37/84–44% $p<.001$	35/58–60% $p<.05$	28/46–61% NS
With closed grafts	8	4/7–57% $p<.001$	9/14–64% $p<.05$	42/45–94% $p<.05$

In contrast, the rate of disease progression in grafted coronary arteries was markedly accelerated during the first year after bypass surgery; 44% of preexisting stenoses in arterial segments proximal to patent grafts and 57% in segments proximal to occluded grafts showed progression of disease, as compared with 9% in ungrafted coronary arteries. Most of these proximal stenoses, however, progressed to total occlusion and there was little additional progression at 6 years after surgery.

At 11 years there was no significant difference in the rate of progression of disease between arteries with patent grafts and ungrafted arteries. On the other hand, coronary arteries with occluded grafts showed a very significant increase in the rate of progression of disease proximal to the graft between 6 and 11 years after bypass surgery. This coincided with a marked increase in graft occlusion, from 14 to 45 occluded grafts, during this period and these results may indicate that there was a more rapid progression of arteriosclerosis in these patients.

Relation of Progression to Severity of Preexisting Coronary Arteriosclerosis

Progression of disease in the native coronary arteries 11 years after bypass surgery was not different when single or multivessel disease was present at baseline coronary arteriography. This was true for both grafted and ungrafted coronary arteries. When the various coronary artery segments were considered, the difference in the rate of progression was again not statistically significant (Table 3).

Table 3. Progression related to severity of disease on the baseline coronary arteriogram

Baseline arteriogram	Arterial segments with progression			
	Ungrafted arteries	Difference	Grafted arteries	Difference
Single-vessel disease	11/32–34%		12/16–75%	
Multivessel disease	35/71–49%	n.s.	93/127–73%	n.s.
Normal segments	27/382–7%	$p<.05$	62/452–14%	$p<.05$
Stenosis <90%	33/94–35%	$p<.05$	101/172–59%	n.s.
Stenosis ≥90%	10/15–67%		15/24–63%	

Significant progression of coronary disease 11 years after bypass surgery was much less frequent in normal segments on the baseline coronary arteriogram than in segments with a preexisting stenosis: 7% versus 40% ($p<.05$) for ungrafted arteries and 14% versus 60% ($p<.05$). for grafted.

In grafted arteries all preexisting stenoses progressed at approximately the same rate. In nongrafted arteries, stenoses with ≥90% reduction in lumen diameter progressed more rapidly than stenoses <90%: 67% versus 35% ($p<.05$)

Relation of Progression to Alterations in Left Ventricular Function

Left ventricular function was evaluated by measurements of left ventricular end diastolic pressure and by visual inspection of left ventricular wall motion from the 30° right anterior oblique ventriculogram in this study (Table 4). The sum and severity of regional wall motion abnormalities were used to compute a left ventricular contraction score, as previously described.

Table 4. Progression related to alterations in left ventricular function in nongrafted arteries

	Left ventricular end diastolic pressure (mmHg)		Difference	Left ventricular score ≥6		Difference
	Pre-operative	At 11 years		Pre-operative	At 11 years	
No progression	13±5	14±6	n.s.	10 (33%)	13 (41%)	n.s.
Progression	15±6	19±10	$p<.05$	16 (40%)	24 (60%)	$p<.05$

Preoperative left ventricular end diastolic pressure and contraction score were not related to progression of coronary disease. However, 11 years after surgery, progression of disease was associated with a rise in left ventricular end diastolic pressure and a higher incidence of left ventricular wall motion abnormalities. These changes were probably more a consequence than a determinant of disease progression.

Relation of Progression to Age, Sex, and Coronary Risk Factors

Age, sex, a family history of premature (before age 55) coronary artery disease, and prior myocardial infarction at the time of baseline angiography were not predictive of disease progression in grafted and ungrafted coronary arteries (Table 5).

Table 5. Progression related to clinical characteristics of 71 patients at baseline in nongrafted arteries

	Progression	No progression	Difference
Age (years)	48±7	51±9	n.s.
Sex (men/women)	33/7	28/3	n.s.
Family history	24 (60%)	16 (52%)	n.s.
Prior myocardial infarction	14 (35%)	10 (32%)	n.s.

Coronary risk factors such as cigarette smoking, systemic hypertension, and diabetes at the time of baseline angiography and at 11 years, and the degree of improvement or deterioration of these factors with time did not influence progression of disease in grafted and ungrafted coronary arteries (Table 6).

Table 6. Progression related to risk factors in nongrafted arteries

		Progression	No progression	Difference
Cigarette smoking	- Preoperative	30 (75%)	22 (71%)	n.s.
	At 11 years	16 (40%)	12 (39%)	n.s.
Hypertension	- Preoperative	5 (12%)	3 (10%)	n.s.
	At 11 years	3 (8%)	2 (6%)	n.s.
Diabetes	- Preoperative	2 (5%)	1 (3%)	n.s.
	At 11 years	2 (5%)	1 (3%)	n.s.
Serum cholesterol	- Preoperative	270±64	258±47	n.s.
(mg/dl)	At 11 years	262±58	247±52	n.s.
Serum triglycerides	- Preoperative	172±85	158±62	n.s.
(mg/dl)	At 11 years	156±47	142±48	n.s.

Finally, total serum cholesterol and triglycerides before surgery, at 11 years, and changes in serum cholesterol and triglyceride levels with time were not related to progression or absence of progression of coronary disease in grafted and ungrafted coronary arteries (Table 6).

Conclusions

From these repeat angiographic studies we can draw the following conclusions.

Approximately 11 years after bypass surgery, progression of coronary disease is as frequent in nongrafted arteries as in grafted arteries with patent grafts. However, progression of disease is much more frequent in grafted arteries with occluded grafts, and most such arteries become occluded during this time interval.

As emphasized in previous reports (Aldridge and Trimble 1971; Gensini et al. 1974; Frick et al. 1975; Bourassa et al. 1978), the rate of progression of coronary disease is different in grafted and ungrafted arteries. In ungrafted arteries, progression appears to be more gradual and can be estimated at approximately 5% per year. In grafted arteries, progression is accelerated during the first year after surgery and decreases thereafter. However, in arteries with occluded grafts, there is a renewed outbreak between 5 and 10 years following surgery, which coincides with a high incidence of graft occlusion, suggesting that arteriosclerosis progresses more rapidly in these patients.

The rate of progression of coronary disease is not different in patients with single or multiple vessel disease on the baseline coronary angiogram. However, progression of preexisting stenoses on the baseline angiogram is much more frequent than the appearance of new stenoses. Progression of obstructive disease is related to the severity of the preexisting stenosis only in ungrafted arteries and only in segments with a preexisting stenosis equal to or greater than 90% in luminal diameter.

Progression of coronary disease is related to alterations in left ventricular function between the baseline study and the repeat angiogram at 11 years. However, this deterioration of left ventricular function appears to be much more a consequence than a determinant of progression of coronary disease.

Finally, progression of coronary disease between the baseline and follow-up angiogram at 11 years does not appear to be influenced by age, sex, or coronary risk factors, nor by improvement or deterioration of risk factors during this time period.

References

Aldridge HE, Trimble AS (1971) Progression of proximal coronary artery lesions to total occlusion after aorto-coronary saphenous vein bypass grafts. J Thorac Cardiovasc Surg 62:7–11

Bourassa MG, Lespérance J, Campeau L (1969) Selective coronary arteriography by the percutaneous femoral artery approach. Am J Roentgenol 107:377–383

Bourassa MG, Lespérance J, Corbara F, Saltiel J, Campeau L (1978) Progression of obstructive coronary artery disease 5 to 7 years after aortocoronary bypass surgery. Circulation 58 [Suppl I]: 100–106

Bourassa MG, Ryan TJ, Goulet C, Abramowitz BA, Lespérance J, Faxon DP, Enjalbert M, McCabe CH (1981) Early progression of coronary disease in patients assigned to medical therapy (abstract). Circulation 64 [Suppl IV]: 83

Campeau L, Lespérance J, Corbara F, Hermann J, Grondin CM, Bourassa MG (1978) Aortocoronary saphenous vein bypass graft changes 5 to 7 years after surgery. Circulation 58 [Suppl I]: 170–175

Campeau L, Lespérance J, Hermann J, Corbara F, Grondin CM, Bourassa MG (1979) Loss of the improvement of angina between 1 and 7 years after aortocoronary bypass surgery. Correlations with changes in vein grafts and in coronary arteries. Circulation 60 [Suppl I]: 1–5

Campeau L, Enjalbert M, Lespérance J, Bourassa MG (1982) Arteriosclerosis and late closure of aortocoronary saphenous vein grafts: sequential angiographic studies at 1 year, 5-7 years and 10-12 years after surgery (abstract). Circulation 66 [Suppl II]: 94

Enjalbert M, Campeau L, Lespérance J, Bourassa MG (1982) Clinical course 6 to 12 years after aortocoronary bypass surgery in patients having atherosclerotic saphenous vein grafts at routine 5-7 year postoperative angiography (abstract). Circulation 66 [Suppl II]: 222

Frick MV, Valle M, Harjola PT, Korhola O (1975) Changes in native coronary arteries after coronary bypass surgery. Am J Cardiol 36: 744-750

Gensini GG, Esente P, Kelly A (1974) Natural history of coronary disease in patients with and without coronary bypass surgery. Circulation 49 [Suppl II]: 98-102

Lespérance J, Saltiel J, Petitclerc R, Bourassa MG (1974) Angulated views in the sagittal plane for improved accuracy of cinecoronary angiography. Am J Roentgenol 121: 565-574

Principal Investigators of CASS and their Associates (1981) Killip T, Fisher LD, Mock MB (eds) National heart, lung, and blood institute coronary artery surgery study. Circulation 63 [Suppl I]: 1-81

Progression and Regression of Disease in the Native Coronary Circulation and Bypass Graft Surgery

R. W. Brower, P. W. Serruys, and P. G. Hugenholtz

Department of Cardiology, Thoraxcenter, P.O. Box 1738, 3000 DR Rotterdam, The Netherlands

Introduction

There is relatively little information on the progression and regression of disease in bypass grafts over a long period after coronary artery bypass graft surgery. This study was undertaken to document angiographically demonstrable changes in bypass status, the relation to the disease in the native coronary arteries, and the clinical factors possibly affecting this process.

This study was made possible by the existence of a large data bank designed for the 3-year follow-up of patients after bypass grafting (Brower et al. 1980). The pertinent aspects of this data bank are that it specifies recatheterization at 1 and 3 years after bypass surgery with complete scoring of the coronary angiogram and bypass status. A complete physical examination and history are also obtained at these points. The development in this laboratory of a coronary scoring system to quantify the extent of coronary artery disease and its changes over the follow-up period has been previously reported (Leaman et al. 1981). This method has also been applied here to address the aims of this study.

Methods

The selection criterion for this study was the availability in Rotterdam of selective graft and coronary angiograms at 1 and 3 years after coronary artery bypass graft surgery (CABG). All patients were also evaluated before surgery. A total of 221 patients met this criterion. All were adults, mean age 52 years; 96% were men. On the basis of clinically available information on medical therapy and functional class, these patients did not differ from those refusing recatheterization but seen in the outpatient clinic as part of the routine follow-up after CABG.

The purpose of the coronary score developed by Leaman et al. (1981) was to quantitate the severity of underlying coronary artery disease (CAD) before surgery and the effectively untreated disease remaining after CABG. The different coronary vessels carry different volumes of blood to the left ventricle, and the coronary score was derived to take this into account.

The left coronary artery carries approximately 5 times the amount of flow to the left ventricle, compared with the right coronary artery (Kalbefleisch and Hort 1977; Dwer et al. 1973; Ross et al. 1964). It has also been shown that in the usual right-dominant coronary system, the flow in the left coronary artery is 66% into the left anterior descending, and 33% into the circumflex coronary artery (Kalbefleisch and Hort 1977). Thus, the left anterior descending carries approximately 3.5 times and the circumflex 1.5 times as much blood as does the right coronary artery. This, then, was the basis for assigning different weighting values to the various coronary arteries. The coronary arteries were subdivided into segments according to the scheme devised by the American Heart Association (Report of the Ad Hoc Committee for Grading of Coronary Artery Disease). The right coronary artery does not supply blood to the left ventricle until it reaches the posterior descending branch, so only the segment with the most severe disease was analyzed. However, the left anterior descending and circumflex coronary arteries were further subdivided and weighting factors were assigned to each segment. As shown in Fig. 1, different weighting factors were assigned in the event of left dominanee.

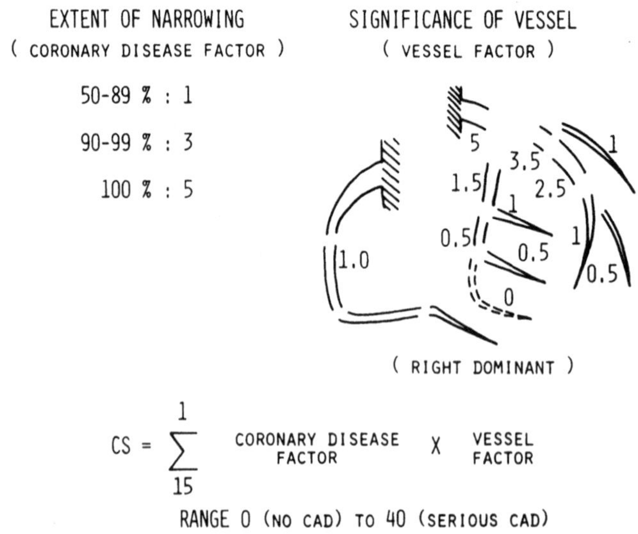

Fig. 1. Coronary score (*CS*) formulated to give a single number representing the severity of coronary artery disease (*CAD*) as it affects perfusion to the left ventricle, as described by Leaman et al. (1981). A value of zero represents no coronary artery disease, while 40 represents very serious three-vessel disease

The degree of stenosis was also considered in deriving the coronary score. If the vessel was totally occluded, the coronary artery segment value was multiplied by 5.0. If there was a 90%–99% occlusion (luminal diameter narrowing), it was multiplied by 3.0; for a 50%–90% obstruction, it was multiplied by 1.0. The segmental scores were then added to derive the total coronary score. A score of zero would indicate no obstructive coronary artery disease, and the higher the score, the greater the obstruction. The role of coronary collaterals has been previously studied and they were found not to effect the outcome of surgery (Brower et al. 1982).

In deriving the postoperative coronary score, a vessel segment was considered normal if it was supplied by a patent aortocoronary bypass graft that was free of occlusive disease. If the aortocoronary bypass graft was occluded, the score was derived from the degree of disease in the native coronary system; that is, the score was derived as if no graft had been placed.

Statistical analysis included the Student's paired *t*-test, χ^2 test, or analysis of variance (ANOVA) where appropriate. The lower limit for significance was taken as $p = 0.05$, two-sided distribution.

Results

There were 221 patients who met the inclusion criteria of angiography at 1 and 3 years. The coronary score (native and corrected for grafting) is summarized in Table 1. For the sake of clarity these data are also shown in Fig. 2.

Table 1. Coronary score before surgery and 1 and 3 years after surgery in 221 patients

	Mean 95% confidence	p[a]
Preop, native coronary arteries	14.2±1.02	–
1 year postop, native coronary arteries	18.1±1.12	.00001
1 year postop, corrected for grafting	5.3±0.76	.00001
3 years postop, native coronary arteries	20.7±1.29	.00001
3 years postop, corrected for grafting	7.2±1.06	.00001

[a] Student's *t*-test with respect to preoperative coronary score

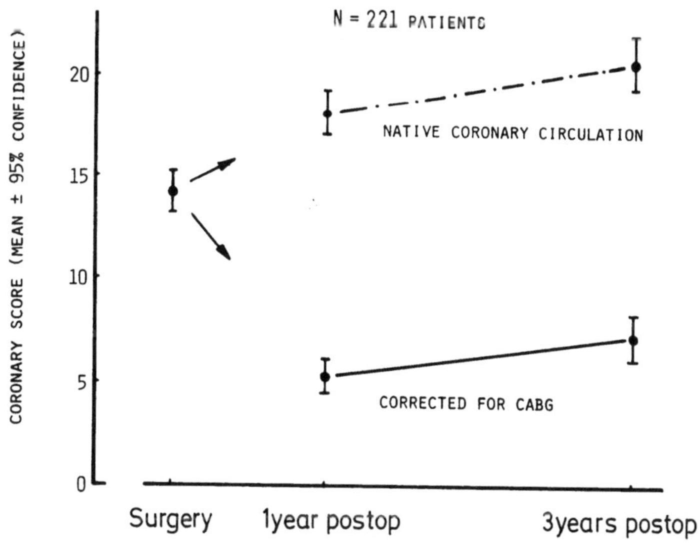

Fig. 2. Coronary score in the native circulation and corrected for bypass grafting before surgery, and 1 and 3 years after. *Vertical bars* represent the mean±95% confidence limits for the mean in 221 patients

At surgery the mean coronary score (CS) was 14.2±1.02 (mean±95% confidence interval for the mean = $1.96 \times SD/N^{1/2}$). One year after surgery the corrected coronary score falls to 5.3±0.76. This is not zero because some grafts had already occluded (patency rate at one year is 79.6%), and not all disease could be effectively bypassed in any case. Nevertheless, this drop does represent an important change for the better in anatomic severity of disease.

From 1 to 3 years there is some progression on the average (1.9 = 7.1 − 5.3) in the CS. The patency rate at 3 years is 76.5%; i.e., 3.1% more grafts occluded during the 2-year interval between follow-ups, giving a graft loss rate of 1.6% of grafts per year. Were this rate to continue indefinitely, about half the grafts would be occluded 20 years after surgery. During this period the CS in the native circulation increased by 2.1, or 40%. It is thus clear that the increase in the corrected CS is due primarily to progression of disease in the native coronary circulation.

It is interesting to note that if the dashed line connecting the 1- and 3-year native CS (Fig. 2) is extrapolated to the time of surgery, it projects a CS 2.6 units above that measured at the time. This may be ascribed to damage inflicted on the coronary arteries as a result of the operaton itself, or indirectly by the establishment of new perfusion pathways.

Returning to the apparent progression of disease corrected for grafting, it is apparent that should the line be extended into the future it would eventually intersect the level of the CS prior to surgery. While little confidence can be attached to such a long-term extrapolation, this point can be calculated to be about 10 years after surgery. This is probably an overly pessimistic estimation of the event, as the majority of disease progression is known to occur early in follow-up.

The actual graft status 1 and 3 years after surgery for these patients is summarized in Fig. 3. There were 570 grafts scored, giving a revascularization rate of 2.6 grafts per patient. As stated above, patency rate at 1 year was 79.6%, and at 3 years 76.5%. Comparing the graft data at 3 years with that at 1 year, the majority of grafts (83.5%) show no change within the scoring limits adapted for

1 Year \ 3-Year follow-up	Normal	< 50%	50%–90%	91%–99%	100%
Normal	309	31	5	1	10
< 50%	15	34	6	1	4
51% $\frac{|}{n}$ 90%	3	8	18	1	2
91% $\frac{|}{n}$ 99%	0	1	1	1	4
100%	0	0	1	0	114

Fig. 3. Summary of status of 570 grafts at 1 and 3 years after surgery. Five classes of occlusion are shown: 100% occlusion, 91%–99% occlusion, 50%–90% occlusion, less that 50% obstruction, and normal graft. Entries on the *diagonal* represent stability in graft status (476, 83.5%) from 1 year to 3 years. Entries above the diagonal represent progression of disease (65, 11.4%), while entries below the diagonal represent regression (29, 5.1%)

this study. While 11.4% of grafts were coded as progressing in severity of occlusion by one or more classes, 5.1% were classed as regressing by one or more classes.

In view of the known observer variability in scoring angiograms (see Discussion) it can be debated how much of this 5.1% represents true regression as opposed to observer variability. Studies conducted in our laboratory suggest that an observer variability of 5% is optimistic, though not unreasonable. However, as these angiograms have all been reviewed at least twice, we feel that these results do reflect actual regression of disease.

Although regression of disease can occasionally be demonstrated in a minority of grafts, it is clear that the graft status in the vast majority is stable, while in 11% of the grafts there is progression.

While ancillary to the primary aim of this report, it is pertinent to ask whether the usually sited risk factors for coronary artery disease are associated with progression or regression of disease in the bypass graft. A summary of several conventional and nonconventional risk factors is given in Table 2; results for cholesterol, smoking, use of anticoagulants, presence of hypertension, and preoperative coronary score are shown. There were no significant correlations found for any of these risk factors. It is particularly interesting to note that the preoperative coronary score had no bearing on disease in the bypass graft. This most clearly indicates the decoupling of conventional risk factors in coronary artery disease from later development of disease in the graft.

On reflection, this approach to the problem is an oversimplification. These risk factors are equally present for all the patient's grafts, yet it is a common observation that only one graft will show progression of disease while the others are stable or regress. The data presented in Table 2, therefore, only confirm

Table 2. Risk factors as related to coronary artery disease, presented for grafts which show progression of disease, stability, and progression. Analysis of variance or χ^2 contingency table used for statistical analysis

	Number of grafts			*p*
	Progression	Stable	Regression	
Cholesterol (M ± SD) m*M*/liter	52 (7.88 ± 2.01)	353 (7.60 ± 2.03)	23 (8.42 ± 2.00)	n.s.
Smoking				
Yes	30	206	12	
No	35	270	17	n.s.
Use of anticoagulants				
Yes	29	197	17	
No	36	279	12	n.s.
Hypertension				
Yes	22	154	12	
No	43	322	17	n.s.
Pre-op Coronary score (M ± SD)	14.5 ± 8.0	16.1 ± 7.8	12.0 ± 7.7	n.s.

that the conventional wisdom about risk factors in coronary artery disease does not apply to the graft itself. Other factors not identified in this report play a more decisive role.

Discussion

It has been argued that progression/regression of disease is sufficiently gradual that only small changes are likely to be detected over a 1- to 3-year follow-up period. Therefore, some investigators have adopted a system of subjective scoring, using many more classes with the idea of increasing the resolution of the observation. There is a limit to which this can be done, however, which is related to the inter- and intraobserver variability. Work in this area has been done, and provides some guidelines (Sanmarco et al. 1978; Zir et al. 1976; Detre et al. 1975), but no report has taken the analysis to its logical conclusion and recommended an optimal scoring system commensurate with the "signal-to-noise ratio" of the diagnostic technique and experienced observer. The above-cited reports all employ a coronary map of about the same number of segments as we used, but most use only two or three classes of disease as opposed to our five. For example, Sanmarco reports a 95% consistency in an expert panel when scoring the presence or absence of a significant lesion (70% area stenosis = 50% diameter stenosis) (Sanmarco et al. 1978). Only two classes clearly provide too low a resolution for studies of disease progression, but they do have an excellent reproducibility. In the same study it was reported that the average standard deviation of the difference was 14%, which is somewhat better than that determined by Zir et al. (1976). Thus, if one allows ± one SD for each class of disease, three classes are indicated: 50%, 50%–75%, and 75%–100%. Since we used five classes to achieve a higher resolution at the low and high ends of the scale, it would appear that we were already at the limit of observer variability. A few more classes could conceivably have been added, especially in the 50%–90% range, but to triple (15 classes) or even double (ten classes) this number would be pointless.

Machine scoring may be a useful adjunct, but a thorough and independent analysis of this reproducibility and failure mode is unavailable. Nor have radiographic standards been established or consistently applied in the multitude of adjustments and parameters where variability also contributes to variability in the objective measurement.

Returning to the data reported here, a number of conclusions are apparent. The majority of bypass grafts which occlude do so in the first year after bypass grafting. Afterwards, there is a much slower graft-attrition rate, but one which – if continued at a steady rate – would result in half of all grafts occluded in 20 years. A far more significant factor appears to be the progression of disease in the native circulation, part of which is bypassed and part of which is not. Between 1 and 3 years after CABG we find that most grafts are stable, there is progression of disease in 11%, and regression in 5%. Regression of disease in the graft is infrequent, but can occasionally be demonstrated. Those factors known to be risk factors for coronary artery disease do not appear to have a bearing on progression or regression of disease in the graft.

Summary

Angiographically demonstrable changes in bypass status and their relation to the disease in the native coronary arteries were studied in 221 patients, 1 and 3 years after coronary artery bypass graft surgery. The extent of coronary artery disease was scored according to the recommendations of the American Heart Association, and quantified following the method of Leaman. Patency in 570 grafts at 1 year was 79.6%, and at 3 years 76.5%.

The majority of grafts (83.5%) show no change, 11.4% progress in disease by one or more classes, and 5.1% regress. The coronary score (CS) before surgery is 14.2 ± 1.92 (mean ± 95% confidence) and drops to 5.3 ± 0.76 at 1 year when corrected for patent bypass grafting. The CS remains greater than zero (no effective disease left unbypassed) because of early graft closure and the existence of untreated or untreatable lesions. By 3 years the CS increases to 7.2, owing primarily to progression of disease in the native coronary circulation.

The majority of bypass grafts which occlude do so in the first year after grafting. Afterwards there is a much slower graft-attrition rate, but one which if continued at a steady rate would result in half of all grafts occluded in 20 years. Between 1 and 3 years the majority of grafts are stable. Regression of disease in the graft is infrequent, but can occasionally be demonstrated. Those factors known to be risk factors for coronary artery disease do not appear to have a bearing on progression or regression of disease in the graft.

Acknowledgements. The authors gratefully acknowledge the assistance of H. J. ten Katen in preparing the drawings and performing the data bank searches for this study. The study was supported as project 4c by the Interuniversity Cardiology Institute.

References

Brower RW, ten Katen HJ, Meester GT (1980) Interim data processing in the Netherlands study on coronary artery bypass graft surgery. Comput Biomed Res 13:87–101

Brower RW, ten Katen HJ, van der Brand M (1982) Do coronary collaterals influence the outcome of bypass graft surgery? J Thorac Cardiovasc Surg 30:259–264

Detre KM, Wright E, Murphy ML, Takaro T (1975) Observer agreement in evaluating coronary angiograms: Circulation 52:979–986

Dwer EM, Dell RB, Cannon PJ (1973) Regional myocardial blood flow in patients with residual anterior and inferior transmural myocardial infarction. Circulation 48:924

Kalbefleisch H, Hort W (1977) Quantitative study on the size of coronary artery supplying areas postmortem. Am Heart J 94:183–188

Leaman DM, Brower RW, Meester GT, Serruys P, van der Brand M (1981) Coronary artery atherosclerosis: severity of the disease, severity of angina pectoris, and compromised left ventricular function. Circulation 63:285–292

Report of the Ad Hoc Committee for Grading of Coronary Artery Disease (1975) A reporting system on patients evaluated for coronary artery disease. Council on Cardiovascular Surgery. Circulation 51:7–402
Ross R, Ueda K, Lichtlen PR, Rees JR (1964) Measurement of myocardial blood flow in animals and man by selective injection of radioactive inert gas into the coronary arteries. Circ Res 15:28–41
Sanmarco ME, Brooks SH, Blankenhorn DH (1978) Reproducibility of a consensus panel in the interpretation of coronary angiograms. Am Heart J 96:430–437
Zir LM, Miller SW, Dinsmore RE, Gilbert JP, Harthorne JW (1976) Interobserver variability in coronary angiography. Circulation 53:627–632

The Influence of Medical and Surgical Therapy on Progression of Coronary Artery Disease - Insights From a Randomized Study

R. T. Palac, M. H. Hwang, W. R. Meadows, H. S. Loeb, C. Gohlke-Bärwolf, R. Pifarre, and R. M. Gunnar

Department of Medicine, Section of Cardiology, Loyola University Stritch School of Medicine, Maywood, IL, and the Veterans Administration Medical Center, Hines, IL, USA

Controversies of efficacy (McIntosh and Garcia 1978) arising since the introduction of myocardial revascularization using saphenous vein grafts by Favaloro (1968) in 1967 have, for the most part, been resolved (Frye and Frommer 1982). Most rational interpretations of longevity studies have indicated the efficacy of this surgery in prolongation of life (Gunnar et al. 1980). The question of the effect of bypass grafting on native coronary disease progression has not yet been definitively answered, however, in spite of the many studies reported to date (Aldridge and Trimble 1971; Bourassa et al. 1973, 1978; Malinow et al. 1973; Maurer et al. 1974; Frick et al. 1975; Itscoitz et al. 1975; Robert et al. 1978; Levine et al. 1975; Glassman et al. 1974; Griffith et al. 1973; Benchimol et al. 1974; Gensini et al. 1974), and the influence of risk factors on this progression needs further study. The major shortcomings of previous studies have been that they were not prospective and that they lacked appropriately matched medically treated patients as a control group.

In this paper we discuss insights gained with regard to coronary artery disease progression over 4–6 years in patients with chronic angina assigned randomly to medical or surgical treatment. We also report on the influence of risk factors on progression of atherosclerosis in these patients.

Patients and Methods

Between 1970 and 1974 at Hines Veterans Administration Hospital, 148 patients with chronic stable angina were assigned randomly to medical or surgical treatment groups after informed consent was obtained. All patients were catheterized at the hospital, had surgically bypassable disease, and were considered by consensus to be good candidates for surgical treatment.

As part of the study protocol patients were requested to undergo repeat coronary arteriography 5 years after randomization. Symptomatic status did not determine who was restudied.

Of 71 patients randomly chosen for surgery, 67 consented to undergo surgery. Nine died before being eligible for restudy, and 32 of the remaining 58 patients (55%) underwent follow-up angiography 66 ± 10 months after randomization.

Of 77 patients randomly chosen for medical treatment, 24 died and 16 crossed over to surgery before the follow-up study. Of the remaining 37 patients 26 (70.3%) were restudied 63 ± 9 months after randomization.

When the prerandomization characteristics of both groups of patients were compared there were no differences between surgically or medically treated patients (Table 1). Additionally, the symptomatic status, as reported in the New York Heart Association classification, was similar in patients who agreed to restudy, but not in those who refused restudy, in either group (Table 2).

Table 1. Prerandomization characteristics for medically treated ($n=26$) and surgically treated ($n=32$) patients in study groups

	No. medically treated (%)	No. surgically treated (%)
Age	52.7±12.8	50.0±11.1
NYHA II	8 (31)	14 (44)
III	16 (61)	17 (53)
IV	2 (08)	1 (03)
Hypertension Systolic >150 and/or diastolic ≥95	15 (58)	15 (47)
Cholesterol ≤250	14 (54)	17 (53)
>250	11 (42)	14 (44)
Diabetes	4 (15)	4 (13)
Family Hx CAD	15 (58)	22 (68)
Previous MI	14 (54)	16 (50)
Hx of smoking	17 (65)	21 (66)

NYHA, New York Heart Association classification; *CAD*, coronary artery disease; *MI*, myocardial infarction

Table 2. Changes in NYHA classification at 5 years; comparison of patients who refused recatheterization with those who consented to it

	Medically treated (%)			Surgically treated (%)		
	I	S	W	I	S	W
Catheterization[a]	19.3	61.5	11.5	43.8	37.5	15.6
Refused catheterization[a]	27.2	54.6	9.1	50.0	42.4	3.8

I, improved; *S*, stable; *W*, worse
[a] Not all patients available at 5 years

Coronary angiography was performed using either Sones' (Sones and Shirey 1962) or Judkins' (Judkins 1968) technique. The coronary arteries were selectively cannulated and angiography was routinely obtained in multiple views. Our cardiac catheterization laboratory was equipped with a standard Phillips cine X-ray machine which was not changed or modified during the study. Sublingual nitroglycerin was not routinely used unless the patient had an anginal attack during the procedure.

The arteriograms were reviewed independently by two observers, and stenoses were graded using a modification of a system used at the Montreal Heart

Institute. Obstructions were graded on a scale of 0–5, which 0 being no stenosis; grade 1, stenosis of ≤50%; grade 2, 51%–75%; grade 3, 76%–90%; grade 4, 91%–99%; and grade 5, total obstruction.

A complete analysis of the arteriogram was facilitated by dividing the coronary tree into 15 segments (Fig. 1). Each segment was analyzed and its stenoses were graded. Discrepancies in the grading of a stenosis were resolved during a joint review of the angiogram by both observers.

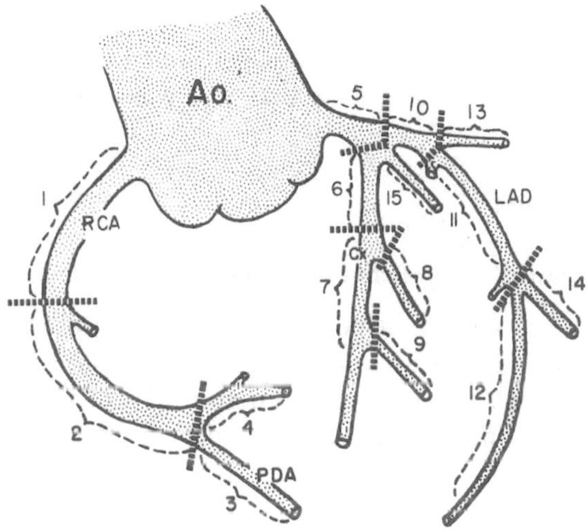

Fig. 1. Division of coronary tree into segments used for analysis of disease progression

A segment was considered grafted if it received a graft or was perfused by a graft. For example, if segment 1 had a critical stenosis (Fig. 1), and a graft was placed to segment 2, then segments 1, 2, 3, and 4 would be considered grafted. If the critical stenoses were in segment 2, then segments 2, 3, and 4 would be considered grafted.

Disease progression was also analyzed in each major trunk artery, i.e., the left anterior descending, the left circumflex, and the right coronary artery. For the purposes of this analysis, the left main coronary artery was considered part of the left anterior descending coronary artery. Thus, there were 78 arteries in our 26 medical patients and 96 arteries in our 32 surgical patients. Of the 96 arteries in the surgical group, 57 received bypass grafts.

Patients were followed-up clinically at 6-month intervals. Fasting serum triglycerides and cholesterol were drawn at least once a year from most of the patients in the study group. The average triglyceride and cholesterol level for each patient was determined. Triglycerides were analyzed using a fluorometric technique (Noble and Campbell 1970) until 1979, when an enzymatic method (Bucolo and David 1973) was introduced. Our laboratory did comparative studies on 230 samples and found excellent comparability with a correlation coefficient of 0.98. Cholesterol was analyzed using the cholesterol-oxidase enzymatic method. Both assays are performed according to procedures found in the Manual of Laboratory Operations, Lipid Research Clinic Program, DHEW Publication #(NIH) 75-628. Pure standards were used. Incidence of smoking and diabetes mellitus were determined at the 5-year clinic visit and used in our risk factor analysis. Diabetes was considered present if a patient had a fasting blood sugar ≥110 mg% or a 2-h postprandial blood sugar ≥140 mg%. Blood pressures were averaged on three consecutive clinic visits nearest to the fifth year anniversary of surgery, and hypertension was considered present if systolic blood pressure was ≥140 mmHg or diastolic blood pressure ≥95 mmHg.

Statistical analysis was performed using the χ^2 test with the Yates correction. A P value greater than 0.05 was considered not significant.

Results

Overall Progression in Coronary Segments and Arteries

There was no difference in incidence of progression between the surgical and medical patients when progression of disease in all coronary segments is considered. Progression occurred in 23% of the 396 segments in the surgical patients and 22% of the 312 segments in the medical patients (n.s.) (Fig. 2). When

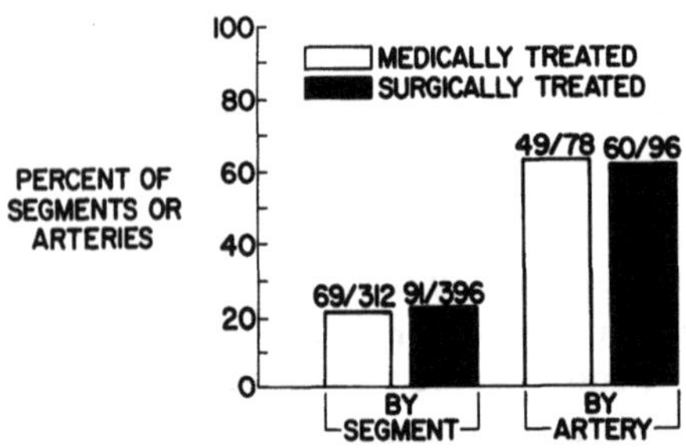

Fig. 2. Comparison of overall progression by segment and artery in surgically and medically treated patients

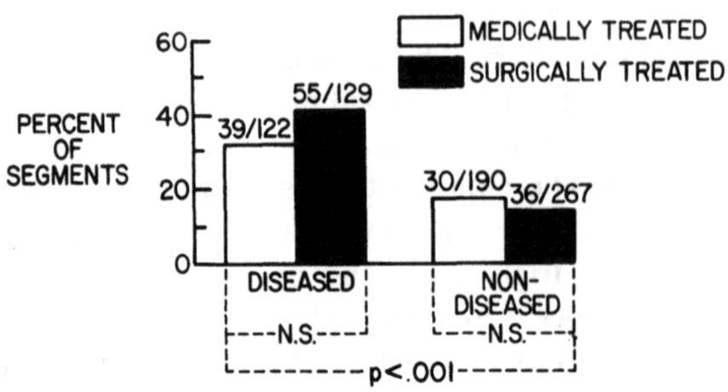

Fig. 3. Comparison of progression in diseased and nondiseased coronary segments

a similar comparison was made between major trunk arteries, progression was similar, 62% in the surgical patients and 63% in the medical patients (Fig. 2). Progression of disease in segments initially diseased was similar in both surgical and medical patients - 55 of 129 (41%) versus 39 of 122 (32%). Also, segments initially free of disease had a low incidence of progression in both the surgical and medical patients - 36 of 267 (13%) versus 30 of 190 (16%) (Fig. 3).

It is also apparent that when all patients are considered together progression of disease is significantly higher in segments initially diseased - 94 of 251 (37%) - than in segments initially free of disease - 66 of 457 (14%) - ($p < 0.001$).

The Influence of Saphenous Vein Grafting on Progression

The effect of aortocoronary grafting on progression of disease was evaluated in the surgical group (Fig. 4); 23% of the 177 grafted segments and 22% of the 217 nongrafted segments had progressed (n.s.). This compares favorably with the 22% incidence of progression in the medically treated patients (NS). When this same analysis was performed on major trunk arteries, the incidence of progression was 70% in grafted arteries versus 51% in nongrafted arteries (Fig. 4; n.s.).

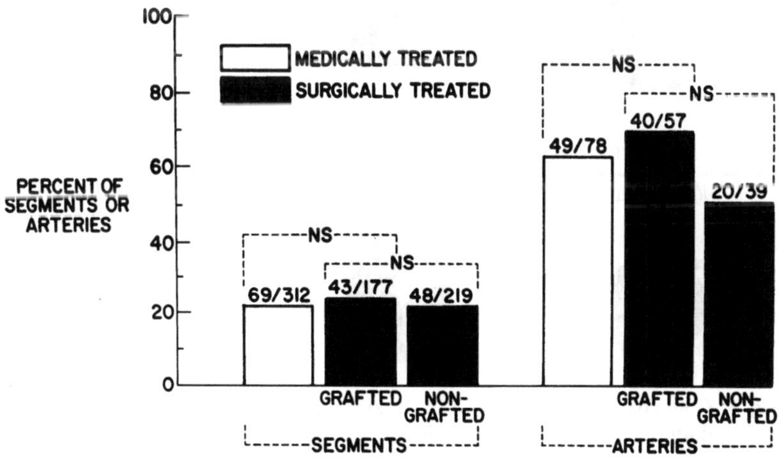

Fig. 4. The effects of grafting on coronary disease progression in segments and arteries

This was essentially the same as 63% incidence of progression in the medical group. The effect of graft status on the incidence of progression was evaluated; 21% of 29 segments supplied by an occluded graft had progressed, compared with 25% of 148 segments supplied by a patent graft (n.s.; Table 3). The incidence of progression of disease in segments proximal to graft anastomoses was 37%, compared with 13% in segments distal to the graft anastomoses ($p < .01$).

We felt that a logical analysis would be made if proximal segments of grafted arteries, usually significantly diseased, were compared with diseased segments in the medical patients, and if distal segments of grafted arteries, usually free of disease, were compared with nondiseased segments in the medical patients. As is seen in Fig. 5, 37% of 81 proximal segments in the surgical patients had progressed, compared with 32% of 122 diseased segments in the medical patients (NS). Similarly, 13% of 96 distal segments in the surgical patients showed progression, compared with 16% of 190 segments in the medical patients (NS).

Table 3. Progression of disease in occluded and patent grafted segments

	Total no. of segments	Progression	No progression
Occluded	29	6 (21%)	23 (79%)
Patent	148	37 (25%)	111 (75%)

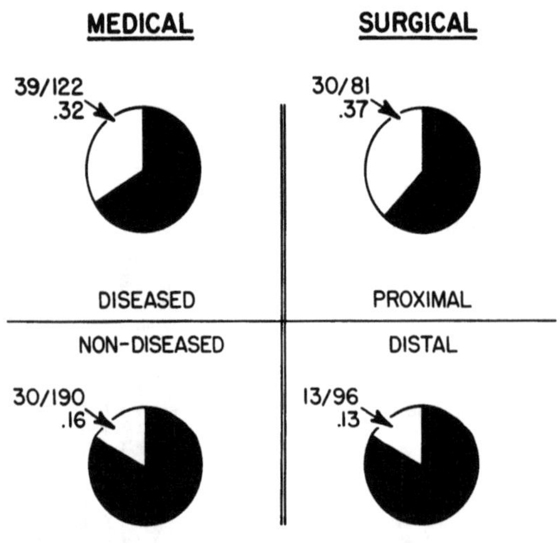

Fig. 5. Comparison of progression in proximal and distal protions of grafted arteries versus diseased and nondiseased segments in medical patients

Progression to New Total Occlusion

The incidence of new total occlusion was similar in both groups, occurring in 8% of 365 segments in the surgical patients and 6% of 287 segments in the medical patients. Progression to new total occlusion occurred predominantly in those segments already diseased, 22% of 98 segments and 15% of 97 segments in the surgical and medical patients respectively, compared with 3% of 267 and 1% of 190 nondiseased segments in the surgical and medical patients respectively ($p < .01$; Fig. 6).

The Effect of Risk Factors on Disease Progression

A univariate analysis of the effects of coronary disease risk factors on progression of disease was performed for all study patients. This was accomplished by comparing the number of segments that showed significant progression in patients with a certain risk factor with the number in patients without that particular risk factor. As shown in Fig. 7, there was no difference in incidence of progression in patients with hypertension, hypertriglyceridemia, smoking, or a family history of coronary disease, and in those without these risk factors. In patients with diabetes mellitus (fasting blood sugar ≥110 mg% or 2-h postprandial blood sugar ≥140 mg%), progression occurred in 29% of 161 segments, compared with 21% of 547 segments in patients without diabetes ($p < .01$). Likewise, in patients with elevated cholesterol levels (≥280 mg%) progression occurred in 30% of 159 segments, compared with 20% of 549 segments in patients with cholesterol levels <280 mg% ($p < .01$; Fig. 7).

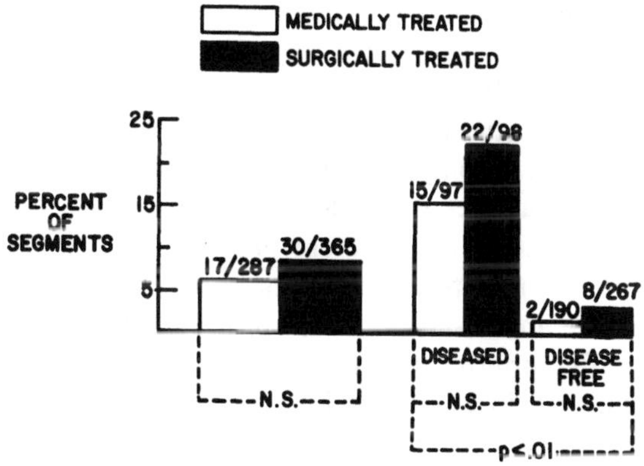

Fig. 6. Progression to new total occlusion in medical and surgical patients

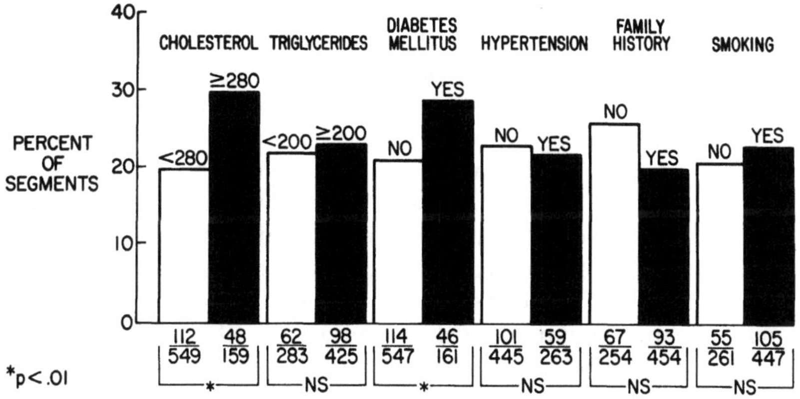

Fig. 7. Relationship of risk factors to percentage of segments which showed progression in all patients. *Diabetes mellitus,* fasting blood sugar ≥110 mg% or 2-h postprandial blood sugar ≥140 mg%; *hypertension,* systolic blood pressure >140 mmHg or diastolic blood pressure ≥95 mmHg; *family history,* of coronary disease; *smoking,* at 5-year followup

Discussion

When existing studies of native coronary disease progression in surgically treated patients are analyzed, it is important to realize that many biases can be introduced by the study design. Most studies of coronary disease progression are comprised of patients who underwent recatheterization for resurgence or worsening of anginal symptoms, which has a tendency to bias the results toward finding higher rates of progression (Aldridge and Trimble 1971; Malinow et al. 1973; Maurer et al. 1974; Frick et al. 1975; Itscoitz et al. 1975; Robert et al. 1978; Levine et al. 1975; Glassman et al. 1974; Griffith et al. 1973; Benchimol et al. 1974; Gensini et al. 1974; Ben-Zvi et al. 1974; Nitter-Hauge and Levorstad 1980). In this study, as previously reported (Palac et al. 1981), the patients were catheterized regardless of their symptomatic status, and progression rates should therefore reflect what could be expected in patients symptomatic with angina treated surgically, and in those treated medically, who survive for 5 years. It is important to note that a significantly higher number of our medical patients died (Loeb et al. 1979) prior to repeat cardiac catheterization, and it is logical to assume that this represented progression of disease. Hence, the progression rates reported for our medical survivors might be lower than those that actually occurred.

Most studies of progression of coronary disease in surgically treated patients have compared grafted and nongrafted vessels. As has been pointed out by Bourassa et al. (1978) and Itscoitz et al. (1975), although this comparison is simple, there are inherent problems with this type of analysis, resulting from the fact that proximal portions of grafted arteries have localized critical stenoses, and distal portions are usually free of disease. On the other hand, nongrafted arteries tend to be either diffusely diseased or normal. Any analysis of this sort does not take into account that lesions in different stages of development with possibly different rates of progression are being compared. This was pointed out by Bruschke et al. (1981), who found higher rates of progression in stenoses of greater diameter narrowing. Others (Rosch et al. 1976; Shub et al. 1981), however, have disagreed with this finding. An ideal study of the effects of bypass surgery on native coronary disease progression would have patients randomly assigned to medical and surgical treatment groups, each group having long-term follow-up studies with repeat coronary angiography at narrowly defined intervals. Progression of disease could then be compared for the two treatment groups. There have been a few attempts to do this retrospectively (Gensini et al. 1974; Ben-Zvi et al. 1974; Nitter-Hauge and Levorstad 1980); however, they suffer from a variety of other problems, such as differences in distribution of coronary risk factors, extent of coronary disease, and length of follow-up. We feel that our study does not suffer from many of the biases previously mentioned and that it should accurately reflect the incidence of native coronary disease progression after 5 years, in symptomatic patients with coronary disease treated surgically or medically.

There are major difficulties in comparing studies of coronary progression because different definitions for progression are used, and because some studies have analyzed progression in multiple coronary segments whereas others have used major coronary trunks. In this study we used both types of analysis and arrived at the same conclusions.

During the time of the study, 4–6 years, 95% of our patients had angiographic progression in at least one coronary segment. This is consistent with the work of Bruschke et al. (1981); they elegantly demonstrated that the single most important determinant of coronary disease progression is the lenght of follow-up, with greater than 90% of the patients who were followed up for longer than 5 years demonstrating progression.

Previous studies have shown a high incidence of progression of disease early after surgery, primarily in proximal portions of grafted vessels (Aldridge and Trimble 1971; Bourassa et al. 1973, 1978; Malinow et al. 1973; Maurer et al. 1974; Frick et al. 1975; Itscoitz et al. 1975; Robert et al. 1978; Levine et al. 1975; Glassman et al. 1974; Griffith et al. 1973; Benchimol et al. 1974). This progression usually involved new total occlusion at the site of a previous stenosis. This phenomenon of new occlusion has been attributed to stasis of blood with subsequent thrombosis, occurring because of loss of pressure gradient across a stenosis that has a graft implanted distal to it. However, these studies compared grafted and nongrafted arteries in a group of surgically treated patients. Gensini et al. (1974), who compared operated patients with a matched medical control group, concluded that progression in surgically treated patients represents the natural history of coronary disease rather than a consequence of bypass grafting. We feel that our study, because of its randomized design, helps to resolve this controversy.

In surgically or medically treated patients with stable angina after 5 years, the overall incidence of progression was similar whether we analyzed progression by segments or by major coronary arteries. Using the major-trunk-artery approach in our surgical patients we found a 70% incidence of progression in grafted arteries and a 51% incidence in nongrafted arteries, which is in general agreement with previous reports (Bourassa et al. 1978; Seides et al. 1978; Tyras et al. 1979) and does not differ significantly from the 63% incidence of progression in our medically treated patients. When we compared the incidence of progression in individual coronary segments, being careful to separate grafted segments from nongrafted, there was very little discrepancy in incidence of progression. We cannot comment on the high frequency of proximal progression seen early after bypass grafting, but caution must be taken in concluding that bypass grafting accelerates the rate of progression of proximal stenoses, because there is no matched medical control group. This is especially true in light of the recent report of rapidly progressive coronary disease in medically treated patients (Bourassa et al. 1981). Based on our study, we must conclude that at 5 years the incidence of progression in surgically treated patients varies little from the natural progression of coronary disease.

The question of the influence of coronary risk factors on the rate of coronary disease progression is very controversial. Some authors found no relationship between risk factors and progressive coronary narrowing (Shub et al. 1981; Kramer et al. 1981); others found a higher incidence of coronary disease progression in patients who were hyperlipidemic (Ben-Zvi et al. 1974; Bemis et al. 1973). Kuo et al. (1979) reported stabilization of coronary disease in patients with type-II hyperlipoproteinemia who were aggressively treated. Rosch et al. (1976) did not find any relationship between individual risk factors and rate of coronary disease progression; however, they did find that the presence of multiple risk factors was associated with a higher incidence of disease progression. In our study we found a higher incidence of progression in patients who had diabetes mellitus or an elevated cholesterol level, greater than 280 mg%. It is apparent that the results of these studies are conflicting; however, it seems justified to modify and treat risk factors aggressively in patients with coronary disease because there is enough evidence from the previously mentioned studies to imply that presence of multiple risk factors may influence the rate of coronary disease progression. Although one might conclude that this is not as important after aortocoronary grafts are placed, we have previously reported the association of hyperlipidemia and progressive graft atherosclerosis (Palac et al. 1982).

What other insights on the effects of aortocoronary bypass can be gained from this study? We found a significantly greater incidence of progression in segments with pre-existing disease (37%) than in nondiseased segments (14%; $p < .001$). Thus, the likelihood of new lesions forming within 5 years in a coronary segment angiographically free of disease is very low. However, this rate of progression - 14% - is substantially higher than progression rates reported from other studies of medically treated patients in whom all coronary arteries were normal at initial catheterization (Gensini et al. 1974; Marchandise et al. 1978).

Graft patency did not appear to affect the incidence of progression of disease as has been shown by some (Griffith et al. 1973). Among our surgical patients, progression of disease was greater in segments proximal to the graft anastomosis than in distal segments; this is consistent with previous reports (Aldridge and Trimble 1971; Bourassa et al. 1973, 1978; Glassman et al. 1974). However, when proximal segments in the surgical patients were compared with diseased segments in the medically treated patients there was no difference in the incidence of progression. Thus, it can be concluded that after 5 years segments proximal to grafts behave similarly to diseased segments in medically treated patients.

Finally, the number of new total occlusions in medically treated patients was similar to that in surgically treated patients. Although the clinical importance of new total occlusion is not discussed in this paper, in contradistinction to the surgical patient, in whom clinical consequences of native artery occlusion are related to graft status, an alternate direct route of blood supply around a new occlusion is not present in the medically treated patient. Thus, new occlusion may result in infarction and death, which is evidenced by the significantly higher mortality among our medical patients (Loeb et al. 1979).

References

Aldridge HE, Trimble AS (1971) Progression of proximal coronary lesions to total occlusion after aortocoronary saphenous vein bypass grafting. J Thorac Cardiovasc Surg 62:7
Bemis CE, Gorlin R, Kemp HG, Herman MV (1973) Progression of coronary artery disease. Circulation 47:455
Benchimol A, Harris CL, Fleming H, Desser KB (1974) Progression of obstructive coronary artery disease after implantation of aortocoronary saphenous vein bypass grafts. J Thorac Cardiovasc Surg 68:257
Ben-Zvi J, Hildner FJ, Javier RP, Fester A, Samet P (1974) Progression of coronary artery disease. Cine-arteriographic and clinical observations in medically and surgically treated patients. Am J Cardiol 34:295
Bourassa MG, Goulet C, Lespérance J (1973) Progression of coronary arterial disease after aortocoronary bypass grafts. Circulation 48 [Suppl III]:127
Bourassa MG, Lespérance J, Saltiel J, Corbara F, Campeau L (1978) Progression of obstructive coronary disease 5 to 7 years after aortocoronary bypass surgery. Circulation 58 [Suppl I]:100
Bourassa MG, Ryan TJ, Coulet C, Abramovitz BA, Lespérance J, Faxon DP, Enjalbert M, McCabe CH (1981) Early progression of coronary disease in patients assigned to medical therapy. Circulation 64 [Suppl IV]:83 (abstract)
Bruschke AVG, Wijers TS, Kolsters W, Landmann J (1981) The anatomic evolution of coronary artery disease demonstrated by coronary arteriography in 256 nonoperated patients. Circulation 63:527
Bucolo G, David H (1973) Quantitative determination of serum triglycerides by the use of enzymes. Clin Chem 19:476
Favaloro RG (1968) Saphenous vein autograft replacement of severe sequential coronary artery occlusion. Operative technique. Ann Thorac Surg 5:334
Frick MH, Valle M, Harjola PT, Korhola O (1975) Changes in native coronary arteries after coronary bypass surgery. Am J Cardiol 36:744
Frye RL, Frommer PL (1982) Consensus development conference on coronary artery bypass surgery: medical and scientific aspects. Circulation 65 [Suppl II]:1-129
Gensini GG, Esente P, Kelly A (1974) Natural history of coronary disease in patients with and without bypass surgery. Circulation 50 [Suppl II]:98
Glassman E, Spencer FC, Krauss KR, Weisinger B, Isom OW (1974) Changes in the underlying coronary circulation secondary to bypass grafting. Circulation 50:293
Griffith LSC, Achuff SC, Conti CR, Humphries JO, Brawley RK, Gott VL, Ross KS (1973) Changes in intrinsic coronary circulation and segmental ventricular motion after saphenous vein coronary bypass graft surgery. N Engl J Med 288:589
Gunnar RM, Loeb HS, Palac R, Pifarre R (1980) Improved survival in patients with chronic angina pectoris treated surgically: report of a randomized prospective study of aortocoronary bypass from Hines, Illinois. In: Hurst JW (ed) Update II - The heart. McGraw-Hill, New York, p 205
Itscoitz SB, Redwood DR, Stinson EB, Reis RL, Epstein SE (1975) Saphenous vein bypass grafts: long-term patency and effect on the native coronary circulation. Am J Cardiol 36:739
Judkins MP (1968) Percutaneous transfemoral selective coronary arteriography. Radiol Clin North Am 6:467
Kramer JR, Matsuda Y, Mulligan JG, Aronow M, Proudfit WL (1981) Progression of coronary atherosclerosis. Circulation 63:519
Kuo PT, Hayase K, Kostis JB, Moreyra AE (1979) Use of combined diet and colestipol in long-term (7-7½ years) treatment of patients with type II hyperlipoproteinemia. Circulation 59:199
Levine JA, Bechtel SJ, Gorlin R, Cohn PF, Herman MV, Cohn LH, Collins JJ Jr (1975) Coronary artery anatomy before and after direct revascularization surgery: clinical and cinearteriographic studies in 67 selected patients. Am Heart J 89:561

Loeb HS, Pifarre R, Sullivan H, Palac R, Croke RP, Gunnar RM (1979) Improved survival after surgical therapy for chronic angina pectoris. One hospital's experience in a randomized trial. Circulation 60 [Suppl I]: 22

Malinow MR, Kremkau EL, Kloster FE, Bonchek LI, Rosch J (1973) Occlusion of coronary arteries after vein bypass. Circulation 47: 1211

Marchandise B, Bourassa MG, Chaitman BR, Lespérance J (1978) Angiographic evaluation of the natural history of normal coronary arteries and mild coronary atherosclerosis. Am J Cardiol 41: 216

Maurer BJ, Oberman A, Holt JH, Kouchoukos NT, Jones WB, Russel RO Jr, Reeves JJ (1974) Changes in grafted and non-grafted coronary arteries following saphenous vein bypass grafting. Circulation 50: 293

McIntosh HS, Garcia JA (1978) The first decade of aortocoronary bypass grafting, 1967–1977. A review. Circulation 57: 405

Nitter-Hauge S, Levorstad K (1980) Does aortocoronary saphenous vein bypass surgery change the native coronary arteries? Acta Med Scand 207: 189

Noble RP, Campbell FM (1970) Improved accuracy in automated fluorometric determination of plasma triglycerides. Clin Chem 16: 166

Palac RT, Hwang, MH, Meadows WR, Croke RP, Pifarre R, Loeb HS, Gunnar RM (1981) Progression of coronary artery disease in medically and surgically treated patients 5 years after randomization. Circulation 64 [Suppl II]: 17

Palac RT, Meadows WR, Hwang MH, Loeb HS, Pifarre R, Gunnar RM (1982) Risk factors related to progressive narrowing in aortocoronary vein grafts studied 1 and 5 years after surgery. Circulation 66 [Suppl II]: 40

Robert EW, Guthaner DF, Wexler L, Alderman EL (1978) Six-year clinical and angiographic follow-up of patients with previously documented complete revascularization. Circulation 58 [Suppl I]: 194

Rosch J, Antonovic R, Trenouth RS, Rahimtoola SH, Sim DN, Dotter CT (1976) The natural history of coronary artery stenosis. Radiology 119: 513

Seides SF, Borer JB, Kent KM, Rosing DR, McIntosh CL, Epstein SE (1978) Long-term anatomic fate of coronary artery bypass grafts and functional status of patients five years after operation. N Engl J Med 298: 1213

Shub C, Vliestra RE, Smith HC, Fulton RE, Elveback LR (1981) The unpredictable progression of symptomatic coronary artery disease. Mayo Clin Proc 56: 155

Sones FM, Shirey EK (1962) Cine coronary arteriography. Mod Concepts Cardiovasc Dis 31: 735

Tyras DH, Ahmad N, Kaiser GC, Barner AB, Codd JE, Willman VL (1979) Ventricular function and the native coronary circulation five years after myocardial revascularization. Ann Thorac Surg 27: 547

Progression of Coronary Artery Disease: A Prospective Angiographic Study of Medical and Surgical Patients

M. H. Frick, M. Valle, and P.-T. Harjola
Helsinki University Central Hospital, Haarmaninkatu 4, 00290 Helsinki 29, Finnland

Introduction

Progression of coronary artery disease has been studied retrospectively in patients subjected to coronary bypass surgery (Alderman et al. 1973; Aldridge and Trimble 1971; Benchimol et al. 1974; Bourassa et al. 1978; Bousvaros et al. 1972; Frick et al. 1974; Glassman et al. 1974; Griffith et al. 1973; Iscoitz et al. 1975; Levine et al. 1975; Malinow et al. 1973; Maurer et al. 1974; McLaughlin et al. 1977; Nilter-Hauge and Levorstad 1980; Rösch et al. 1972); retrospectively in medically treated patients (Bemis et al. 1973; Ben-Zvi et al. 1974; Bruschke et al. 1981; Gensini and Kelly 1972; Gensini et al. 1974; Henderson and Rowe 1973; Kimbiris et al. 1974; Kramer et al. 1981; Marchandise et al. 1978; Moccetti and Lichtlen 1976; Nash et al. 1977; Rösch et al. 1976; Shub et al. 1981); and with retrospective comparisons of medically and surgically treated patients (Ben-Zvi et al. 1974; Gensini et al. 1974; Henderson and Rowe 1973; Nash et al. 1977). Data from these studies are conflicting because of differing indications for re-examination, nonuniform definitions of progression, and greatly varying intervals between coronary angiograms. There is only one prospective, randomized study comparing progression of the disease in bypassed and medically treated patients after a uniform follow-up (Palac et al. 1981).

The aim of the present study was to estimate the rate of progression of coronary artery disease by repeated coronary angiograms over a 5-year follow-up in randomized bypassed and medically treated patients with stable angina pectoris at entry.

Patients and Methods

From a group of 100 patients with stable angina pectoris meeting specific entry criteria (Varnauskas and Olsson 1977) we randomly selected 50 each for medical therapy or bypass surgery. These patients have been followed up for 5–7 years, with 100% follow-up at 5 years (Fig. 1)

Medical Group

During follow-up two patients in the medical group refused recatheterization, one emigrated to Spain, and one had a severe allergic reaction during the first angiography and was not re-examined. Ten of the remaining 46 patients died during follow-up. Five patients developed drug-resistant, unstable angina and were recatherized and operated on 9, 27, 27, 61 and 61 months after the primary angiography. The remaining patients were recatheterized 61 ± 4.5 (SD) months after the primary study. Thus, 36 of 40 eligible patients (90%) were re-examined.

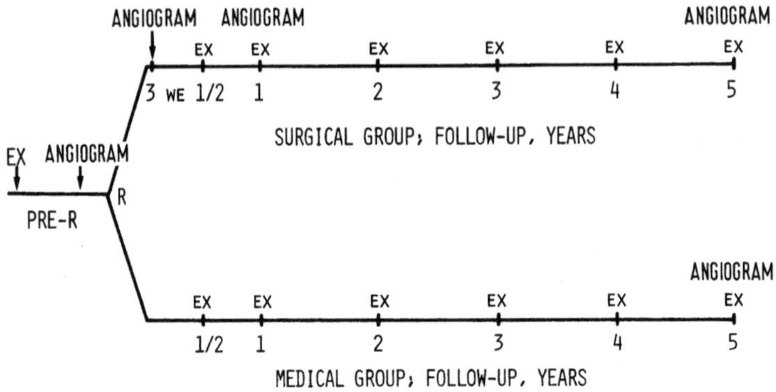

Fig. 1. General design of the study. *R,* randomization; *we,* weeks; *EX,* exercise testing

Surgical Group

Three of the 50 patients assigned for surgery refused to accept the proposed form of treatment and two patients died after randomization but before the scheduled operation. The remaining 45 patients underwent bypass operations without operative mortality and none died during follow-up. All patients had early postoperative angiography (mean, 3 weeks after operation), after which three patients refused further angiographic studies, leaving 42 patients who had postoperative angiograms at 3 weeks, 1 year, and 5 year after the operation (93% adherence rate).

Angiographic Procedures

Left ventricular cineangiograms were made in the right anterior oblique projection. Selective coronary angiograms were made using the Judkins technique as described elsewhere (Frick et al. 1975). Seven coronary arteries were analyzed for each patient: the left main coronary artery, the left anterior descending coronary artery and its diagonal branch, the left circumflex artery, the left obtuse marginal branch, the right coronary artery, and the right ventricular branch. Proximal, middle, and distal segments were analyzed separately as already described (Frick et al. 1975). The coronary lesions were scored on the basis of reduction in luminal diameter as follows: 1 = 0–49%, 2 = 50%–74%, 3 = 75%–90%, 4 = subtotal obstruction, 5 = complete occlusion. Progression of disease was said to have occurred if the degree of narrowing had increased by at least one grade, or if a new lesion had developed at a previously normal site. In the surgical group progression was recorded separately for segments proximal and distal to the graft, and graft patency was taken into account.

Results

The essential data are shown in Table 1. When the progression in either normal or stenosed segments in ungrafted arteries was compared with progression in corresponding segments in the medical group it became evident that the rate of progression in 5 years was similar for both groups. The same was true for progression in segments distal to graft compared with corresponding segments in the medical group. On the other hand, the rates of progression differed when segments proximal to graft were compared with similar segments in the medical group. Both normal segments proximal to graft ($p<0.05$) and stenosed segments proximal to graft ($p<0.01$) progressed at a greater rate than did corresponding segments in the medical group.

Table 1. Progression of coronary artery disease at 5-year angiography

Analyzed segments	Surgical group[a]	Medical group[a]	Significance[b]
Normal segments in ungrafted arteries	5/121 4.1%	14/207 6.7%	n.s.
Diseased segments in ungrafted arteries	7/31 22.6%	43/178 24.2%	n.s.
Normal segments proximal to graft[c]	8/69 11.6%	2/101 1.9%	<0.05
Diseased segments proximal to graft[c]	54/125 43.2%	42/158 26.6%	<0.01
Segments distal to graft[c]	3/97 3.1%	7/181 3.9%	n.s.

[a] Segments progressed/segments at risk
[b] χ^2 test with Yates' correction
[c] For surgical patients-corresponding sites in medical patients

The three postoperative angiograms offered the possibility of studying the timetable of progression, particularly in the segments proximal to graft. At 3 weeks, six of 125 sègments had progressed (Fig. 2); the rate increased to 16% at 1 year and to 43% at 5 years. When the incidence of total occlusions was analyzed in the proximal progression (Fig. 3) is was found to be high in the surgical group, amounting to 69% at 5 years, versus 38% in similarly progressed segments in the medical group ($p<0.01$).

Table 2 gives the rate of proximal progression in the surgical group in relation to graft patency and closure. The rate is significantly higher ($p<0.01$) for patent grafts.

Table 2. Rate of proximal progression in relation to graft patency

	Consecutive angiograms 3 weeks	1 year	5 years
Patent grafts	6/182[a]	21/170	62/162
Occluded grafts	0/12	0/24	4/32

[a] Segments progressed/segments at risk

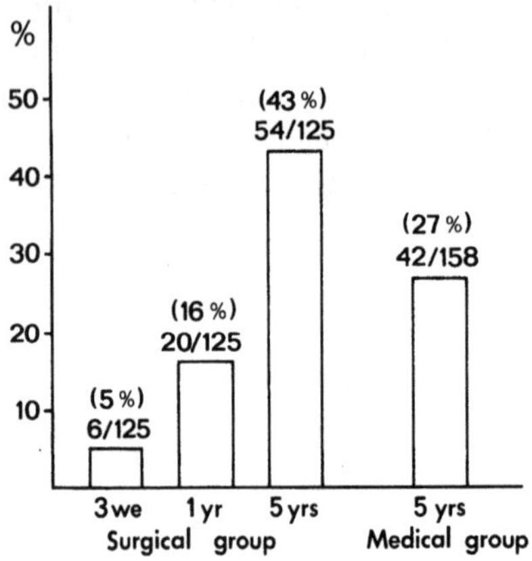

Fig. 2. Cumulative incidence of progression of initially obstructed proximal segments in the surgical group compared with progression of corresponding segments in the medical group

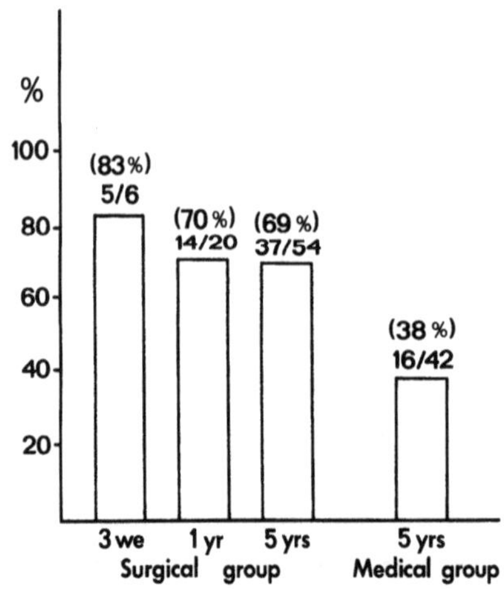

Fig. 3. Rate of total occlusion in progressed proximal segments

Discussion and Conclusion

The highest incidence of progression in the medical group was on previous lesions (Table 1); this is in general agreement with previous reports (Bemis et al. 1973; Palac et al. 1981; Shub et al. 1981). The same general pattern was evident in the ungrafted arteries of the surgical group (Fig. 4), signifying that the events taking place in the ungrafted arteries of surgically treated patients reliably indicate progression of coronary artery disease in general. This hypothesis is further strengthened by the same rate of progression in the distal segments (Table 1).

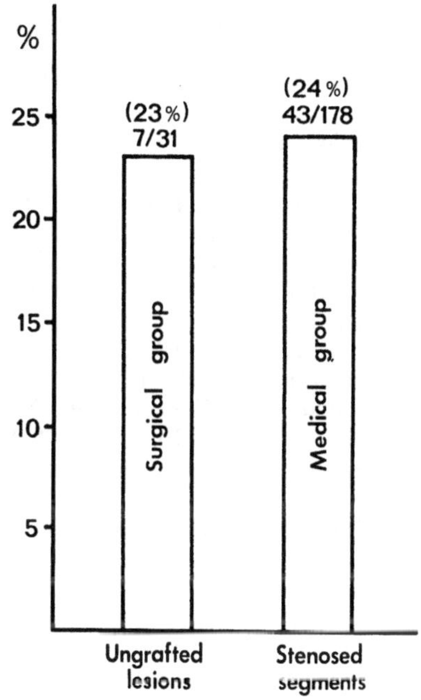

Fig. 4. Incidence of progression in ungrafted segments and stenosed segments in the two study groups

The above reasoning does not seem to apply to segments proximal to graft, where the rate of progression was significantly higher than that for corresponding segments in the medical group (Table 1), and the incidence of total occlusion was also high (Fig. 3). It seems plausible to conclude that a thrombotic component is involved in the progression of coronary atherosclerosis. This line of reasoning is supported by the early occurrence of proximal progression (Fig. 2) and its evident relation to the patency of the grafts (Table 2). The mechanism is presumably the loss of pressure gradient across the stenosis, caused by the patent graft distal to it. The finding of increased rate of progression in segments proximal to graft is at variance with the findings of Palac et al. (1981), who recorded equal rates of progression for segments proximal to graft and for similar segments in medical patients. The explanations for this discrepancy remain speculative.

References

Alderman EL, Matlof HJ, Wexler L, Shumway NE, Harrison DC (1973) Results of direct coronary-artery surgery for the treatment of angina pectoris. N Engl J Med 288:535

Aldridge HE, Trimble AS (1971) Progression of proximal coronary artery lesions to total occlusion after aortocoronary saphenous vein bypass grafting. J Thorac Cardiovasc Surg 62:7

Bemis CE, Gorlin R. Kemp HG, Herman MV (1973) Progression of coronary artery disease. A clinical arteriographic study. Circulation 47:455

Benchimol A, Harris CL, Fleming H, Desser KB (1974) Progression of obstructive coronary artery disease after implantation of aorto-coronary saphenous vein bypass grafts. J Thorac Cardiovasc Surg 68:257

Ben-Zvi J, Hildner FJ, Javier RP, Fester A, Samet P (1974) Progression of coronary artery disease. Cinearteriographic and clinical observations in medically and surgically treated patients. Am J Cardiol 34:295

Bourassa MG, Lesperance J, Saltiel J, Corbara F, Campeau L (1978) Progression of obstructive coronary disease 5 to 7 years after aortocoronary bypass surgery. Circulation 58 [Suppl I]: 100

Bousvaros G, Piracha AR, Chaudhry MA, Grant C, Older TM, Pifarre R (1972) Increase in severity of proximal coronary disease after successful distal aorto-coronary grafts: its nature and effects. Circulation 46:870

Bruschke AVG, Wijers TS, Kolsters W, Landman J (1981) The anatomic evolution of coronary artery disease demonstrated by coronary arteriography in 256 nonoperated patients. Circulation 63:527

Frick MH, Valle M, Harjola P-T, Korhola O (1975) Changes is native coronary arteries after coronary bypass surgery. Am J Cardiol 36:744

Gensini GG, Kelly AE (1972) Incidence and progression of coronary artery disease. Arch Intern Med 129:814

Gensini GG, Esente P, Kelly A (1974) Natural history of coronary disease in patients with and without coronary bypass graft surgery. Circulation 49 and 50 [Suppl II]:98

Glassman E, Spencer FC, Krauss KR, Weisinger B, Isom OW (1974) Changes in the underlying coronary circulation secondary to bypass grafting. Circulation 49 and 50 [Suppl II]:80

Griffith LSC, Achuff SC, Conti CR, Humphries JO, Brawley RK, Gott VL, Ross RS (1973) Changes in intrinsic coronary circulation and segmental ventricular motion after saphenous-vein coronary bypass graft surgery. N Engl J Med 288:589

Henderson RR, Rowe GG (1973) The progression of coronary atherosclerotic disease as assessed by cine-coronary arteriography. Am Heart J 86:165

Itscoitz SB, Redwood DR, Stinson EB, Reis RL, Epstein SE (1975) Saphenous vein bypass grafts: long-term patency and effect on the native coronary circulation. Am J Cardiol 36:739

Kimbiris D, Lavine P, Van Den Broek H, Najmi M, Likoff W (1974) Devolutionary pattern of coronary atherosclerosis in patients with angina pectoris. Am J Cardiol 33:7

Kramer JR, Matsuda Y, Mulligan JC, Aronow M, Proudfit WL (1981) Progression of coronary atherosclerosis. Circulation 63:519

Levine JA, Bechtel SJ, Gorlin R, Cohn PF, Herman MV, Cohn LH, Collins JJ Jr (1975) Coronary artery anatomy before and after direct revascularization surgery: clinical and cine angiographic studies in 67 selected patients. Am Heart J 89:561

Malinow MR, Kremkau EL, Kloster FE, Bronchek LI, Rösch J (1973) Occlusion of coronary arteries after vein bypass. Circulation 47:1211

Marchandise B, Bourassa MG, Chaitman BR, Lesperance J (1978) Angiographic evaluation of the natural history of normal coronary arteries and mild coronary atherosclerosis. Am J Cardiol 41:216

Maurer BJ, Oberman A, Holt JH Jr, Kouchoukos NT, Jones WB, Russel RO Jr, Reeves TJ (1974) Changes in grafted and nongrafted coronary arteries following saphenous vein bypass grafting, Circulation 50:293

McLaughlin PR, Berman ND, Morton BC, Schwartz L, Morch JE (1977) Long-term angiographic assessment of the influence of coronary risk factors on native coronary circulation and saphenous vein aortocoronary grafts. Am Heart J 93:327
Moccetti T, Lichtlen P (1976) Coronary sclerosis: progression on the basis of repeated coronarography. Minerva Med 67:4221
Nash DT, Gensini G, Simon H, Arno T, Nash SD (1977) The Erysichthon syndrome. Progression of coronary atherosclerosis and dietary hyperlipidemia. Circulation 56:363
Nitter-Hauge S, Levorstad K (1980) Does aortocoronary saphenous vein bypass surgery change the native coronary arteries? Acta Med Scand 207:189
Palac RT, Hwang MH, Meadows WR, Croke RP, Pifarre R, Loeb HS, Gunnar RM (1981) Progression of coronary artery disease in medically and surgically treated patients 5 years after randomization. Circulation 64 [Suppl II]: 17
Rösch J, Judkins MP, Green GS, Kidd H (1972) Aortocoronary venous bypass grafts. Radiology 102:567
Rösch J, Antonovic R, Trenouth RS, Rahimtoola SH, Sim DN, Dotter CT (1976) The natural history of coronary artery stenosis. A longitudinal angiographic assessment. Diagn Radiol 119:513
Shub C, Vlietstra RE, Smith HC, Fulton RE, Elveback LR (1981) The unpredictable progression of symptomatic coronary arters disease. A serial clinical-angiographic analysis. Mayo Clin Proc 56:155
Varnauskas E, Olsson B (1977) The European multicenter CABG trial. In: Yu PN, Goodwin JF (eds) Progress in cardiology. Lea and Febiger, Philadelphia, pp 83–89

Quantitative Coronary Angiography: Progression and Regression of Coronary Artery Disease Over 3–5 Year Intervals

W. Rafflenbeul, S. Peters, M. Kreft, and P. R. Lichtlen

Med. Hochschule Hannover, Department für Innere Medizin, Abteilung für Kardiologie, Karl-Wiechert-Allee 9, 3000 Hannover 61, FRG

Evolution of coronary artery disease is characterized by a broad spectrum of pathological patterns identified by means of repeated coronary angiography. An exact classification is difficult for several reasons:

1. Progression of coronary artery disease might very well be different in each patient, or even in each individual coronary artery.
2. Subjective estimation of changes in coronary anatomy from angiograms is fraught with both intra- and interobserver variability.
3. The degree of obstruction might change due to disproportionate vasodilation of the prestenotic and the stenotic segment, either spontaneously or after application of vasodilator drugs.

To overcome some of these pitfalls in the present study, the evolutionary pattern of coronary artery disease was quantitatively evaluated, using morphometric analysis of repeated angiograms.

Material and Methods

Repeated coronary angiograms of 58 patients were quantitatively evaluated. All patients had significant coronary artery disease at the time of the first angiogram, and the second coronary angiogram was performed following aggravation of anginal symptoms in the majority of cases. However, this particular study focused on the anatomical changes during the interval, irrespective of the clinical course. In 29 patients (group I) coronary angiograms were repeated after an average interval of 36 months (range: 30–47 months); in 29 other patients (group II) the average interval was 60 months (range: 50–65 months).

In both the first and the second angiogram of each patient 20 identical coronary artery segments were identified, and their diameters measured with a vernier caliper of high reading accuracy (0.05 mm). To facilitate calculations and corrections for magnification, the caliper was attached to a digitizing unit connected to a programmable calculator (A2D-Prodical).

The diameters of both normal and stenotic segments were measured in as many projections as were available, i.e., in three to five (mean: four) different angiographic projections. Particular care was taken to measure the vessel segments at identical sites in the first and second angiograms. In coronary stenosis, the narrowest diameter was taken. Reference diameters of all 20 segments were assessed in a pilot study including 83 patients with angiographically normal coronary arteries. The degree of area stenosis was calculated with the formula:

$$\% \text{ area stenosis} = \left(1 - \frac{D_{sten}^2}{D_{norm}^2}\right) \times 100$$

where D_{norm} is the diameter of the undiseased, prestenotic vessel and D_{sten} the narrowest diameter in the obstruction.

Taking into account intraobserver variability and variable vascular tone, diameter changes of more or less than 20% were discriminative, allocating the individual coronary artery segment to one of the following subgroups:

1. Unchanged segments
   a) Persistently normal
   b) Stationary obstructions
2. Progressive segments
3. Regressive segments

Results

In group I, 42% of all measured segments remained normal over the 36-month interval. In group II, 42% of segments demonstrated unchanged normal diameters after the 60-month interval. Persisting normal coronary artery segments were distributed almost equally among the three major coronary artery branches - left anterior descending coronary artery, left circumflex, and right coronary artery - in both groups.

Quantitatively, 88% of obstructions measured in the initial coronary angiograms remained at their degree of severity over the 36-month interval and 83% over the 60-month interval.

Overall progressive disease was found in 17% of all measured segments in group I and in 22% in group II. Table 1 depicts the progression rate of selected coronary artery segments in groups I and II.

Table 1. Progression rate of specific coronary artery segments, indicated as percentage of all measurements taken in that particular segment

Vessel	After 36 months (group I)	After 60 months (group II)
Left main coronary artery	8%	10%
Left anterior descending artery	20%	22%
Left circumflex artery	11%	22%
Major posterolateral branch	25%	32%
Right coronary artery	17%	28%

Figure 1 illustrates the characteristics of progressive disease in the three major coronary artery branches. Vessels with progressive disease were subdivided into (a) initially normal segments in which either <50% stenosis or >75% stenosis could be measured in the interval angiogram, and (b) vessel segments with <50% stenosis initially which became >75% stenosis after the interval.

Most progression was from an initially normal segment to a mild-to-moderate stenosis (<50%). As demonstrated in Fig. 1, this type of progressive coronary atherosclerosis was found in 70%, 50%, and 55% of all progressive left anterior descending, left circumflex, and right coronary arteries respectively.

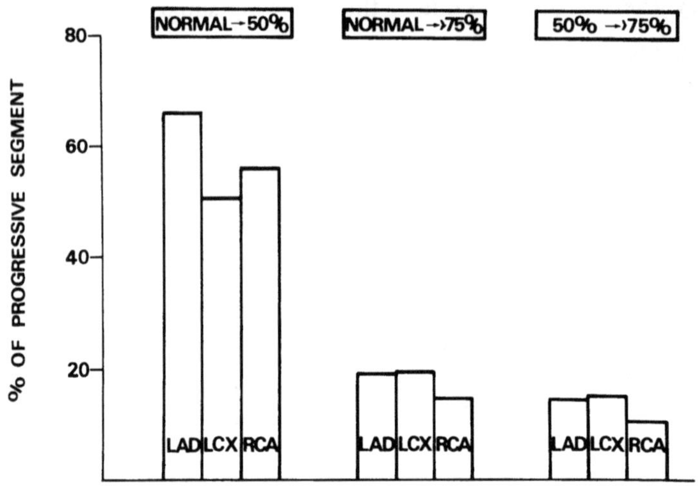

Fig. 1. The pattern of progressive coronary artery disease in different coronary arteries. *LAD*, left anterior descending coronary artery; *LCX*, left circumflex coronary artery; *RCA*, right coronary artery

Regarding regressive coronary artery disease, we measured a diameter increase of more than 20% in nearly 20% of segments. In most cases, however, long-term vasodilator drug treatment and/or spontaneous changes in coronary artery vasomotor tone might have been responsible for the "regression." True regression of lesions beyond any doubt, i.e., a reduction of stenosis severity from >70% to <50%, was measured in only eight lesions, with an average degree of obstruction of 78% initially, 45% at the time of the second angiogram. Figure 2 shows a typical example of a regressive stenosis of the left anterior descending coronary artery.

Discussion

Comparison of coronary angiograms repeated in the same patient with coronary artery disease after a defined intervall of time is appropriate for studying the evolution of coronary artery disease. However, conclusions from repeated angiographic studies may be fraught with substantial errors:

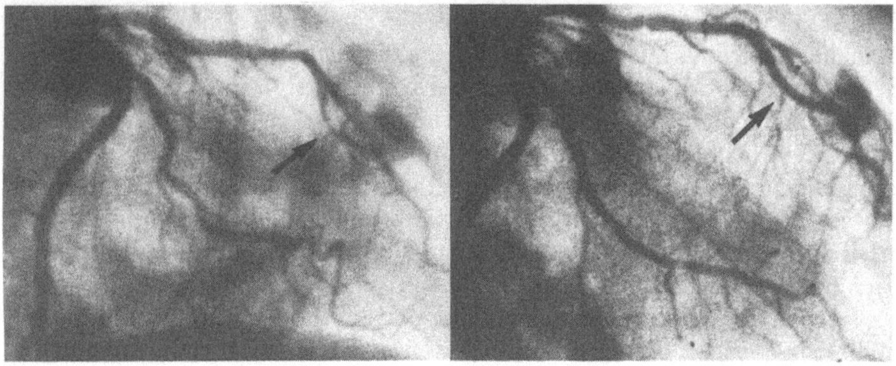

Fig. 2. Typical regressive obstruction of the left anterior descending coronary artery during a 44-month interval. *Arrows* indicate the most obstructed diameter, measured at 1.35 mm and 2.30 mm in the first and the second angiogram respectively

1. Since selection of patients mostly entails persistance or progression of clinical symptoms, the study population might be short on patients with stable disease, and obviously excludes all patients whose disease progression had a fatal course.
2. To include patients with differing severity of coronary artery disease might be inappropriate because the speed of anatomical changes may vary according to the stage of the disease and may be judged differently by the observer.
3. Because in most instances the second angiogram is performed only to reassess suitability for bypass surgery, most studies are designed retrospectively, show a highly variable time interval between angiograms, and are poorly controlled.
4. Long intervals between observations can mean the use of new and upgraded X-ray equipment for the second study, another source of variability.
5. In most studies, progression of coronary artery disease is assessed by qualitative analysis which - despite sophisticated scoring systems - too often is fraught with substantial intra- and interobserver variability (Detre et al. 1975; Zir et al. 1976; Sanmarco et al. 1978). But even when quantitative measurements are taken, as in the present study, the physiological state of the patient during coronary angiography may substantially influence the results. Dynamic changes in luminal diameter due to different vasomotor tone, intramural hemorrhage, platelet aggregation, or thrombolysis may also alter the angiographic appearance of the disease.

Taking into consideration the relatively small number of patients in our study, the percentage of angiograms which met the criteria for progression were found to be similar to the numbers previously presented by Bruschke et al. (1981) and by Kramer et al. (1981).

In this particular study, however, we wanted to focus predominantly on the segmental changes quantified in the major branches of coronary arteries.

Table 1 illustrates the variable progression rate of different coronary artery branches after both intervals. After 3 years distinctive differences were found between the relative numbers of progressive segments. In some vessels, such as the left main coronary artery and the left anterior descending coronary artery, progression is not related to the interval between studies, whereas in the left circumflex and the right coronary artery the length of time seems to be an important determinant of progression. However, the highly variable progression rate indicates an unique velocity of progression for each vessel segment, which even may vary at different times during the course of the disease.

In contrast to researchers using a more qualitative approach, we found the highest incidence of progression in vessel segments with normal diameters measured at the initial study. Almost 60% of progressive segments went from normal at the onset to a mild-to-moderate (<50%) obstruction at the second study. Other studies (Bruschke et al. 1981; Landmann et al. 1978; Roesch et al. 1976) emphasize the increase of stenosis severity in already initially obstructed vessels, a relatively rare finding in our study (Fig. 1). This discrepancy might be explained by a substantial difference between qualitative and quantitative analysis of coronary angiograms: Whereas the expert reader focuses his attention on coronary artery obstructions to classify the severity of the disease, objective measurements are capable of precisely identifying even more subtle changes. Thus, there may be a general underestimation of progression in studies using a subjective method to detect and grade coronary findings.

Repeated angiography proved to be most promising in the detection of regressive coronary artery disease. In a previous study using the same quantitative measurements (Rafflenbeul et al. 1979) we found considerable regression of single lesions in patients with unstable angina pectoris restudied after only 1 year of vigorous medical treatment. Again, in the present study, long-term adequate vasodilator therapy might explain the relatively high incidence of coronary artery vessel segments with substantially increased diameters after the interval. Other factors, such as composition, remodeling, and healing processes of the single stenosis, may contribute to the angiographic appearance of regressive disease. However, our data indicate that the process of regression is more a feature of the individual lesion than of the overall coronary artery disease.

References

Bruschke AVG, Wijers TS, Kolsters W, Landmann J (1981) The anatomic evolution of coronary artery disease demonstrated by coronary arteriography in 256 nonoperated patients. Circulation 63:527–536

Detre KM, Wright E, Murphy ML, Takaro J (1975) Observer agreement in evaluating coronary angiograms. Circulation 52:979–986

Kramer JR, Matsuda Y, Mulligan JC, Aronow M, Proudfit WL (1981) Progression of coronary atherosclerosis. Circulation 63:519–526

Landmann J, Kolsters W, Bruschke AVG (1978) Progression der obstruktiven koronaren Herzkrankheit, dargestellt anhand wiederholter Koronarangiographie. Schweiz Med Wochenschr 108:55

Rafflenbeul W, Smith LR, Rogers WJ, Mantle JA, Rackley CE, Russell RO (1979) Quantitative coronary arteriography: coronary anatomy of unstable angina pectoris one year after optimal medical therapy. Am J Cardiol 43:699

Roesch J, Antonovic R, Trenouth RS, Rahimtoola SH, Sim DN, Dotter CT (1976) The natural history of coronary artery stenosis. Diagn Radiol 119:513–520
Sanmarco ME, Brooks SH, Blankenhorn DH (1978) Reproducibility of a consensus panel in the interpretation of coronary angiograms. Am Heart J 96:430–437
Zir LM, Miller SW, Dinsmore RE, Gilbert JP, Harthorne JW (1976) Interobserver variability in coronary angiography. Circulation 53:627–632

Progression to Complete Coronary Obstruction Without Myocardial Infarction in Patients Who Are Candidates for Percutaneous Transluminal Angioplasty: A 90-Day Angiographic Follow-Up

W. Wijns, P. W. Serruys, M. van den Brand, H. Suryapranata, C. J. Kooijman, J. H. C. Reiber, and P. G. Hugenholtz*

Thoraxcenter, P.O. Box 1738, 3000 DR Rotterdam, The Netherlands

From September 1980 to September 1982, 153 patients were chosen as good candidates for elective percutaneous transluminal coronary angioplasty (PTCA). All had disabling but stable angina pectoris and proximal stenosis of a major coronary artery suitable for balloon dilation.

In ten of these 153 PTCA candidates, the vessel planned for angioplasty was totally occluded at the time of the intervention. The median interval from the previous diagnostic angiogram was 90 days (range, 1–250 days). This clinical observation raised the question of what happened in the interval between diagnostic angiography and the intervention. Do patients suitable for PTCA represent a highly selected subgroup with rapidly progressive atherosclerosis? If not, another mechanism could be responsible for the progression to complete coronary obstruction, presumably a thrombotic process.

The clinical records of the study group were thus retrospectively reviewed and the coronary angiograms analyzed with our computer-based angiographic analysis system. The quantitative data obtained were compared with those available on the remaining PTCA candidates not showing progression to complete obstruction (76 of 143 to date).

Method: The Quantitative Coronary Angiography Analysis System

The procedure for the computer-aided quantitative analysis of selected coronary lesions has been described extensively elsewhere (Reiber et al. 1982; Kooijman et al. 1982).

The cinefilm was mounted on a specially developed cine-video converter, allowing different optical magnifications of regions within the original cineframe. For routine use a magnification with a factor of 2 has been found optimal. Regions of interest in the video-converted magnified portion of the cineframe, encompassing the arterial segment to be analyzed, are digitized and stored in computer memory for subsequent processing. After automated contour detection of the coronary segment using a weighted sum of first and second derivative functions, the diameter function, calibrated in millimeters, was computed. Calibration was achieved by using the intracardiac catheter as a scaling device.

---

* With the technical assistance of I. Broeders

The normal size of the artery over the obstruction was determined by a first-degree least squares polynomial analysis of the diameter function. This first-degree polynomial allows the vessel to taper. From the minimal value of the diameter function (obstruction diameter) and the computed reference diameter at the site of the stenosis, the percentage diameter narrowing (interpolated technique) was calculated as:

$$\% \text{ diameter stenosis} = \left[1 - \frac{\text{obstruction diameter}}{\text{reference diameter}}\right] \times 100$$

The precision and the accuracy of percentage diameter stenosis measurements assessed from Perspex models filled with contrast agent were found to be 1.6% and 1.9% respectively when compared with known true values.

Results

Quantitative Analysis of Coronary Angiograms

In the group of ten patients, the artery showing progression to complete obstruction was the left anterior descending in three cases, the right coronary artery in three others, the left circumflex artery in three, and a bypass graft in the remaining one. The median percentage diameter stenosis assessed from the diagnostic angiograms was 66% (range 45–81).

The average severity of these lesions was not different from that measured in 76 consecutive PTCA candidates; the individual values plotted in Fig. 1 showed an almost complete overlap between the groups. Of these 76 PTCA candidates with the obstructive artery remaining patent, 26 were selected for paired analysis of both diagnostic and therapeutic angiograms.

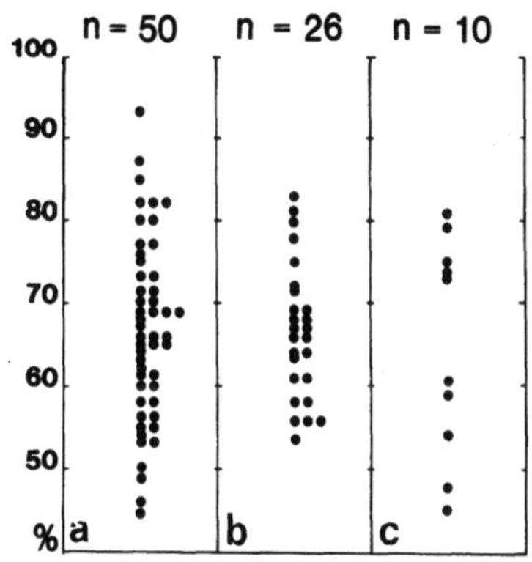

Fig. 1a–c. Individual data for percentage of diameter stenosis from diagnostic angiograms **a** in 50 PTCA candidates not suitable for paired analysis, **b** in 26 patients sequentially studied, and **c** in the ten patients progressing to complete obstruction

To be included in the comparative study, both coronary angiograms had to be performed in the same projection, and of sufficient quality to allow quantitative measurements. In this retrospective analysis no attempt was made to standardize on inspiratory level, volume and rate of injection of contrast material, technical characteristics of the X-ray systems. Most importantly, the vasomotor tone in both conditions was unknown and neglected. The median delay between the diagnostic and the so-called therapeutic angiogram in these patients was 52 days (range 1–300). As shown previously for percentage diameter stenosis, no difference was observed between the study group and the subgroup of 26 patients representative of the remaining PTCA group as far as obstruction and reference diameter were concerned (Fig. 2). Hence, the severity of the stenosis, expressed either as a percentage of luminal narrowing or as an absolute stenosis diameter was not predictive of the subsequent event, namely the progression to complete obstruction.

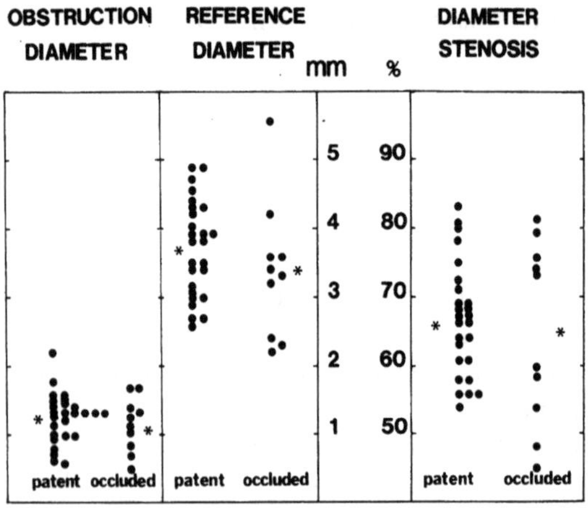

Fig. 2. Comparison between the individual data of obstruction and reference diameters in millimeters and the percentage diameter stenosis from diagnostic angiograms. The values shown on the left side of each pannel represent the 26 patients with a remaining patent artery while those on the right represent the study group of ten. The mean values are indicated by *asterisks*

A comparison of the paired data obtained on the 26 patients with patent PTCA-related arteries during the interval between both angiograms is shown in Fig. 3.

No significant difference was observed in the mean values of obstruction and reference diameters, or in those of percentage diameter stenosis (Table 1). This suggests that no detectable progression or regression of atherosclerotic lesions had occurred.

With Grubbs' estimators used for precision (Grubbs 1948), these paired data provide some insight into the total variability of the cineangiographic procedure and the computer analysis under the worst circumstances, since no special care was taken to reduce the potential sources of variability, such as X-ray geometry and setting, or vasomotor tone (Serruys et al. 1980).

Under these particular conditions, the precision of the method, estimated by the standard deviation of the random component of the total measurement error, was 0.3 mm for the obstruction diameter, 0.5 mm for the reference diameter, and 5% for the percentage of diameter stenosis.

Table 1. Comparison between diagnostic and therapeutic angiography in 26 patients

	Diagnostic angiography	PTCA
Obstruction diameter (mm)	1.2±0.4	1.2±0.4
Reference diameter (mm)	3.7±0.7	3.6±0.8
Diameter stenosis (%)	66±8	64±8

Data are given as mean±SD

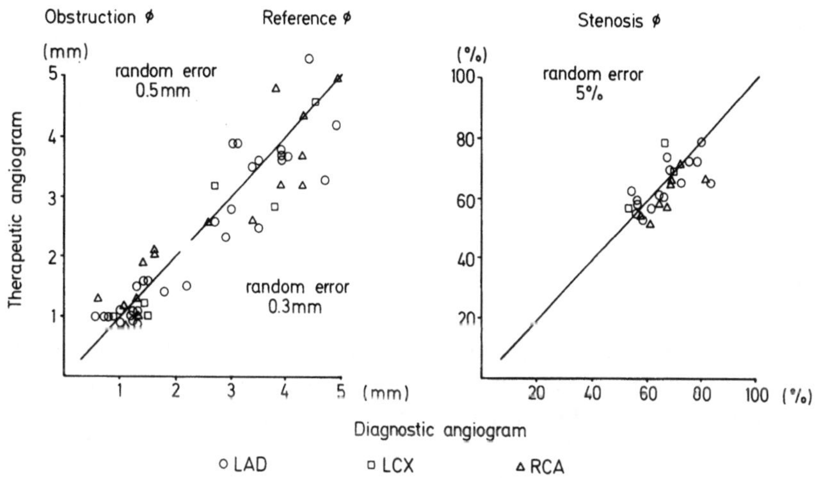

Fig. 3. Comparison between the first (*horizontal axis*) and the second angiogram (*vertical axis*) in 26 patients. *LAD*, left anterior descending; *LCX*, left circumflex; *RCA*, right coronary artery

Clinical Data

A retrospective review of the clinical records in the study group shows that all but two patients experienced exacerbation of their anginal symptoms, sufficiently disabling in three cases to require hospitalization (Table 2).

Despite the fact that recent coronary occlusion had occurred, as evidenced by sequential angiograms, no patient had overt clinical or electrocardiographic signs of acute myocardial infarction. Only one patient with right coronary artery involvement was suspected of having developed a silent myocardial infarction, since a new Q wave (less than 0.04 s long) appeared in the inferior leads of his electrocardiogram. Finally, in nine of the patients the occluded artery was filled by collaterals on the second angiogram. In the remaining patient progression to coronary occlusion was observed one day after diagnostic angiography, and no significant collateral flow appeared during this short period of time.

Table 2. Summary of the clinical and angiographic data in the study group

	Unstable angina	Myocardial infarction	Collateral flow	Interval between angiograms (days)
1	–	–	+	92
2	+	–	+	99
3	+	+	+	42
4	+	–	+	6
5	⊞	–	+	37
6	+	–	+	113
7	⊞	–	+	76
8	–	–	–	1
9	⊞	–	+	171
10	+	–	+	240
Total	8/10	1/10	9/10	Median: 90

⊞, Admission to coronary care unit

Discussion

Unexpected progression to complete obstruction was observed in 5% of all PTCA candidates. When compared with the other patients at the time of diagnostic angiography, this subgroup showed no difference in the severity of the coronary lesions, analyzed quantitatively. Thus, the severity of the coronary stenosis on the diagnostic angiogram was not predictive of progression to complete obstruction.

The proportion of left circumflex and right coronary arteries becoming occluded – six of ten – was surprisingly high, since two-thirds of our PTCA patients had left anterior descending artery disease.

A review of the clinical records shows that progression to complete obstruction was clearly associated with worsening of the anginal symptoms, but without the occurrence of myocardial infarction. Myocardial necrosis could have been prevented by the development of collaterals.

One may speculate that occlusion of the PTCA-related vessel in these patients was not related to rapidly progressive atherosclerosis but was due to a thrombotic process. Evolving coronary thrombosis has been reported in unstable angina (Rentrop et al. 1981). In three of the ten patients the occluded PTCA-related vessel was perforated by a guide wire restoring antegrade blood flow, permitting the subsequently planned balloon dilation (Heyndrickx et al. 1982; Savage et al. 1982).

Conclusion

Progression to complete obstruction of a coronary artery planned for elective PTCA occurred in 5% of patients and was unrelated to the initial severity of the stenosis.

Worsening of the anginal symptoms in PTCA candidates should alert the clinician to evolving disease. In our patients presenting with unexpected complete obstruction, PTCA could be performed after mechanical or pharmacological reopening of the artery. This supports the hypothesis that a thrombotic process was the underlying mechanism of progression.

Acknowledgements. The authors thank A. Wagenaar for her secretarial assistance and R. W. Brower for reviewing the manuscript.

References

Grubbs FE (1948) On estimating precision of measuring instruments and product variability. J Am State Assoc 43:243

Heyndrickx GR, Serruys PW, van den Brand M, Vandormael M, Reiber JHC (1982) Transluminal angioplasty after mechanical recanalisation in patients with chronic occlusion of coronary artery (abstract). Circulation 66 [Suppl II]:5

Kooijman CJ, Reiber JHC, Gerbrands JJ, Schuurbiers JCH, Slager CJ, den Boer A, Serruys PW (1982) Computer-aided quantitation of the severity of coronary obstructions from single view cineangiograms. Proc ISMIII, IEEE cat no 82 CH 1804-4, p 59

Reiber JHC, Gerbrands JJ, Booman F, Troost GJ, den Boer A, Slager CJ, Schuurbiers JCH (1982) Objective characterization of coronary obstructions from monoplane cineangiograms and three-dimensional reconstruction of an arterial segment from two orthogonal views. In: Schwartz MD (cd) Application of computers in medicine. IEEE cat no TH 0095-0, p 93

Rentrop P, Blanke H, Karsch KR, Kaiser H, Kostering H, Leitz K (1981) Selective intra coronary thrombolysis in acute myocardial infarction and unstable angina pectoris. Circulation 61:307

Savage R, Hollman J, Gruentzig AR, King S III, Douglas J, Tankersley R (1982) Can percutaneous transluminal coronary angioplasty be performed in patients with total occlusion (abstract). Circulation 66 [Suppl II]:330

Serruys PW, Steward R, Booman F, Michels R, Reiber JHC, Hugenholtz PG (1980) Can unstable angina pectoris be due to increased coronary vasomotor tone? Eur Heart J [Suppl B] 1:71

The Influence of Physical Rehabilitation and Risk-Factor Control on Long-Term Prognosis of Postinfarction Patients

V. Kallio

The Rehabilitation Research Centre of the Social Insurance Institution,
Peltolantie 3, 20720 Turku 72, Finland

Primary risk factors amenable to intervention even after myocardial infarction include physical inactivity, smoking, hypercholesterolemia, hypertension, personality, and psychosocial stress. In this paper the main emphasis is on measures aimed at intervening on physical inactivity, smoking, and hypercholesterolemia. Recommendations presented are based on those proposed by a recent working group of three councils of the International Society of Cardiology (1980). In addition, some results of a Finnish multifactorial intervention study will be reported (Kallio et al. 1979).

Physical Training

Many nonrandomized controlled studies suggesting that supervised training programs reduce mortality and reinfarction have been published (Bruce 1974; Kellerman 1982). Although these studies have been criticized because of their lack of a randomized control group, they are important sources of data on the effects of physical exercise after myocardial infarction.

The results of five prospective, randomized clinical trials on the secondary preventive effects of physical training are shown in Table 1. The number of patients studied was rather small, ranging from 298 to 733. The control group re-

Table 1. Overall mortality in prospective randomized trials on feasibility and effects of physical training after myocardial infarction (May et al. 1982)

	Number of patients randomized	Mortality (%)		*p*
		Intervention group	Control group	
Wilhelmsen et al. (1975)	315	17.7	22.3	0.38
Kentala (1972)	298	17.1	21.9	0.37
Palatsi (1976)[a]	380	10.0	14.0	0.30
National Exercise and Heart Disease Project (Shaw 1981)	651	4.6	7.3	0.20
Southern Ontario Multicentre Exercise-Heart Trial (Shephard 1980)	733	9.5	7.3	0.36

[a] In the Palatsi study the figures refer to coronary deaths

ceived routine care, or low-intensity exercise. Intervention usually consisted of individualized supervised training. In one of the studies daily home exercise was used. Excepting the Ontario Multicenter Exercise Heart Trial, all the remaining studies showed a favorable trend, but no significant reduction in mortality. In the Canadian study, the mortality in the intervention group was somewhat, but not significantly, higher than in the controls.

The Finnish study (Kallio et al. 1979), which included advised or supervised physical exercise as part of the comprehensive intervention program, will be referred to later in this paper. If the mortality figures observed in this study were included in the analysis of the pooled data shown in Table 1 as proposed by May et al. (1982), the six studies would be consistent with a 19% reduction in total mortality in the intervention group; this is statistically significant ($p<0.05$).

All studies on the secondary preventive effects of exercise training were affected by several problems:

1. High drop-out rate
2. Physical exercise post myocardial infarction applied routinely in many centers, without consideration of individual patient differences
3. Contamination of control group, 'drop-in'
4. Difficulties in influencing one factor only
5. High number of patients is required to show a statistically significant effect on mortality and morbidity

Low compliance with the exercise program formed the major problem in all studies, with drop-out rates usually 40%–60% (Oldridge 1982).

It can be concluded that the studies mentioned above have not provided a definite explanation concerning the effect of an intensive, long-term physical training program on the prognosis after acute myocardial infarction. Physical exercise after myocardial infarction improves the quality of life, however, and has the following preventive effects on risk factors as well (Ehsani et al. 1982; Erkelens et al. 1979; Froelicher et al. 1980; Kallio 1978; Streja and Mymin 1979):

1. Decrease in blood pressure and heart rate at any given work load
2. Increase in blood HDL, i.e., decrease in cholesterol
3. Decrease in blood triglycerides
4. Better weight control
5. Decrease in stress, anxiety, and depression
6. Decrease in catecholamine secretion during exercise

It can thus be recommended as a component of an intervention program after myocardial infarction. The clinical state of the patient and the results of an exercise test will determine what kind of training program, if any, is advisable in the individual case.

Smoking

In spite of controversial results about the role of smoking as a prognostic indicator after myocardial infarction (Mulcahy et al. 1977; The Coronary Drug Project Research Group 1979; Weinblatt et al. 1968), several studies indicate that stopping smoking after myocardial infarction significantly reduces the number of reinfarctions and deaths (Mulcahy et al. 1977; Jenkins et al. 1976; Pohjola et al. 1979; Salonen 1980; Sparrow et al. 1978; Wilhelmsson et al. 1975). The risk of fatal reinfarction or sudden death is reduced by 20%–50%.

Wilhelmsson et al. (1975) showed a significant reduction in nonfatal reinfarctions, cardiovascular deaths, and total deaths (Table 2) in patients who stopped smoking after myocardial infarction.

Table 2. Reinfarctions and deaths during 2 years' follow-up in relation to smoking habits after myocardial infarction (Wilhelmsson et al. 1975)

	Stopped $n=231$ (%)	Continued $n=174$ (%)	p
Reinfarction	9	18	<0.01
Cardiovascular death	5	10	<0.05
Overall mortality	7	13	<0.05

The mortality between 6 months and 3 years after infarction of patients who continued to smoke was compared with that of those who stopped smoking within 6 months after the infarction in a recent Finnish study (Salonen 1980). Total mortality was significantly lower in patients who stopped smoking than in those who continued the habit (Table 3). A clear trend was observed with regard to coronary mortality. There was a dose-response relation between the number of cigarettes smoked daily and mortality. The impact of smoking was greatest in the subgroups of patients with an otherwise good prognosis. It was estimated that 28% of deaths in the entire group of initial smokers could be attributed to continued smoking after infarction.

Table 3. Deaths between 6 months and 3 years after myocardial infarction in relation to smoking habits (Salonen 1980)

	Stopped $n=221$ (%)	Continued $n=302$ (%)	p
Coronary deaths	10	16	0.053
Overall mortality	12	20	0.019

Based on the available scientific evidence, the recommendation is that every physician should vigorously advise all patients to stop smoking after myocardial infarction. In the ISFC Scientific Councils Report (International Society of Cardiology 1980) it is proposed that all health-care personnel be involved in providing advice about smoking, and that such advice be provided from the start of treatment. Information given to spouse and family is important. Printed material and audiovisual aids, important as they are, cannot replace personal advice. Long-term supervision is necessary to prevent the patient from resuming the habit. Weight gain, depression, or irritability sometimes connected with cessation of smoking can usually be prevented by careful counseling.

High Blood Cholesterol

Some studies indicate that serum cholesterol continues to be a risk factor for reinfarction, although a weaker one than for the first attack (Schlant et al. 1982). The results of the majority of intervention trials based on diet modification or drug treatment, however, do not show any reduction in the number of reinfarctions or in mortality (May et al. 1982). The early study by Morrison (1960) using a low-fat diet with 100 patients showed a significant reduction in mortality after 12 years' follow-up. The Oslo Diet-Heart study (Leren 1970) shows that it is possible to reduce serum cholesterol by means of dietary intervention. Total mortality 5 years after myocardial infarction was reduced by 25%, which is not statistically significant. However, there was a reduction in the combined incidence of both fatal and nonfatal reinfarctions and all major coronary heart disease relapses in the intervention group. After 11 years of follow-up there was still a significantly smaller number of fatal myocardial reinfarctions in the intervention group.

While a clear-cut answer to the question of the prognostic significance of lowering high cholesterol values after myocardial infarction is still lacking, the advice to reduce plasma cholesterol level is considered essential on the following theoretical bases, as indicated in the report of the ISFC Scientific Councils (International Society of Cardiology 1980):

1. To limit progression of atherosclerosis and to support regression of existing arterial disease
2. To diminish liability to thrombosis by changing dietary fat intake
3. To provide an educational example to the relatives of the patient, who may as yet be unaffected by overt atherosclerosis but are known to share an enhanced risk of coronary heart disease

The dietary recommendations include caloric restriction in the obese; reduction of saturated fat intake to about 8%–10% of food energy, and of cholesterol intake to less than 300 mg/day, with a ratio of polyunsaturated to saturated fatty acids of about 0.75; increased intake of foods rich in gel-forming fiber, such as pectins; and an increased proportion of dietary protein to be derived from vegetable sources.

Risk Factor Combination and Mortality

Data on the effect of risk factor combinations on mortality were recently presented by the Coronary Drug Research Group (Schlant et al. 1982). Table 4 indicates that overall mortality in patients with low-risk profiles is about ⅓ of that seen in the high-risk patients, as is the rate of sudden death alone. These data may be taken as indirect evidence favoring a comprehensive risk factor modification after myocardial infarction.

Table 4. Five-year percentages of deaths and sudden deaths in post myocardial infarction patients with low- and high-risk profiles (Schlant et al. 1982)

Profile	No. of patients	Deaths (%)	Sudden deaths (%)
Cholesterol <250 Nonsmoker Moderate or vigorous physical activity	292	10.6	5.1
Cholesterol >250 Smoker Light physical activity	383	30.0	14.1

Hypertension

Blood pressure after myocardial infarction is evidently unrelated to survival over the next 5 years (Kannel et al. 1980). No clear-cut evidence has been presented on the effect of treatment of hypertension on the risk of reinfarction. However, recent evidence from trials on patients with even mild hypertension, but without coronary heart disease, has shown the benefits of blood pressure reduction (Hypertension Detection and Follow-up Program Cooperative Group 1982). The available data indicate that the decision to treat hypertensive patients after myocardial infarction should be based on conventional principles. Patients with poor left ventricular function should be treated with caution, but with an aim toward normal levels. Some evidence suggests that an excessive drop in blood pressure may precipitate further cardiovascular events (International Society of Cardiology 1980).

Particular attention should be given to hygienic measures in controlling hypertension, including weight reduction, limitation of salt intake, regular daily exercise, and/or relaxation programs.

Personality and Psychosocial Stress

Some studies indicate that a so-called type-A personality may be particularly liable to myocardial infarction (Friedman 1976; Rosenman 1978). The studies available did not supply any evidence in support of the view that behavior modification or other psychological measures would be effective in reducing morbidity or mortality after myocardial infarction. Psychosocial problems are important with regard to successful rehabilitation, however, and due attention should be paid to them in the comprehensive care of the patient (Thoresen et al. 1981).

Organized Aftercare

Data indicating the importance of organized aftercare in myocardial infarction patients were presented by Vedin et al. (1976). Table 5 shows that the number of reinfarctions was significantly lower in patients who were given treatment at a special myocardial infarction outpatient clinic as compared with those in routine care. No drugs to control risk factors were given to the patients.

Table 5. Effect on nonfatal reinfarctions and deaths of organized aftercare in patients after myocardial infarction (Vedin et al. 1976)

	Intervention group $n=96$ (%)	Reference group $n=85$ (%)	p
Nonfatal reinfarction	11	26	<0.025
Coronary deaths	9	15	Not significant
Total deaths	13	16	Not significant
New coronary events	21	41	<0.05

The Finnish Multifactorial Intervention Trial

Some results of the Finnish study performed under the auspices of a WHO project are reported here with the kind permission of the other Finnish investigators Dr. Hämäläinen, Professor Hakkila, and Dr. Luurila (Kallio et al. 1979). The study was aimed at assessing the effectiveness of comprehensive rehabilitative and preventive programs in reducing recurrent myocardial infarction, cardiovascular diseases, mortality and sudden death, and at contributing to the early physical, psychosocial, and vocational rehabilitation of patients with cardiovascular disease.

The study group consisted of 375 consecutive acute myocardial infarction patients under 65 years, 301 men and 74 women. I would like to point out in particular that the patients were entirely nonselected. On dismissal from the hospital they were randomly allocated, controlling for age and sex, to an intervention group (188 patients) or to a control group (187 patients). No significant differences between the groups existed as regarded the history, heart failure and/or arrhythmias in the hospital, and characteristics at discharge from the hospital.

Five patients refused to participate in the intervention program; three of them died during the first year. All three patients are included in the mortality statistics.

All patients were given general advice in the hospital on rehabilitation and secondary preventive measures. The program for the intervention group was started 2 weeks after discharge from the hospital and consisted of optimal medical care, antismoking advice, dietary intervention, a physical exercise program, and counsel on psychosocial problems.

Medical examination by an internist was performed at least once a month during the first 6 months after acute myocardial infarction, and after that when necessary, or at least at three-month intervals. In addition to the internist, the team included a social worker, a psychologist, a dietician, and a physiotherapist. In Turku the program was based at the local special institute for rehabilitation, with a 10-day residential period at the beginning. In Helsinki the program was executed at the outpatient department of the hospital with less emphasis on supervised physical training sessions. The program of the first year, as applied in Turku, is shown in Fig. 1.

Medical check-up	x	x	x	x	x	x			x			x
Physical exercise	XXXX XXXX XXXX	XXXX XXXX XXXX	XX XX	XX XX	XX XX	XX XX	XX XX	XX XX	XX XX	XX XX	XX XX	XX XX
Dietary advice	XXXX	x				x			x			x
Social work		x	x	x		x	x	x				
Interview by psychologist	x	x	x			x						x
Months	1	2	3	4	5	6	7	8	9	10	11	12

Fig. 1. Intervention program during the first year after myocardial infarction

Patients in the control group were followed up by their own doctors, and they were seen by the study team only once a year during the follow-up.

Body weight, serum cholesterol, serum triglycerides, systolic and diastolic blood pressure, and smoking habits were recorded at the yearly follow-up visits, and the data are presented in Table 6. Differences between the intervention and control groups were most marked 1 year after myocardial infarction, and most of the differences were still significant 3 years after myocardial infarction. There were no significant differences between the groups in smoking. The number of cigarettes smoked daily, however, was significantly reduced in the intervention group.

Table 6. Differences in some risk factors between intervention (I) and control (C) groups one and three years after myocardial infarction (Kallio et al. 1979)

	1 year		3 years	
	I	C	I	C
Weight (kg)	72[b]	75	72[d]	75
Serum cholesterol (mmol/liter)	6.5[c]	7.3	6.5[c]	7.4
Serum triglycerides (mmol/liter)	1.6[b]	2.0	1.6[a]	1.9
Systolic blood pressure (mmHg)	135[b]	143	136[b]	145
Diastolic blood pressure (mmHg)	85[b]	89	85[b]	88
Stopped smoking (%)	50[d]	42	54[d]	51

[a] $p<0.05$
[b] $p<0.01$
[c] $p<0.001$
[d] Not significant

These results indicate that the patients in the intervention group adhered well to the intervention program, and that the risk characteristics chosen for intervention were amenable to treatment after myocardial infarction.

Coronary mortality 3 years after myocardial infarction was significantly lower in the intervention group (18.6%) than in the controls (29.4%, $p=0.02$). This difference was due mainly to the reduction in sudden deaths, the corresponding percentages being 5.8 in the intervention group and 14.4 in the control group ($p<0.01$). The numbers of nonsudden deaths were not significantly different in the two groups. According to preliminary analysis a significant difference between the groups in the number of sudden deaths ($p<0.05$) was still present 6 years after myocardial infarction.

There was a trend to reduced overall mortality in the intervention group 3 years after myocardial infarction ($p=0.093$), with 21.8% in the intervention group and 29.9% in the controls.

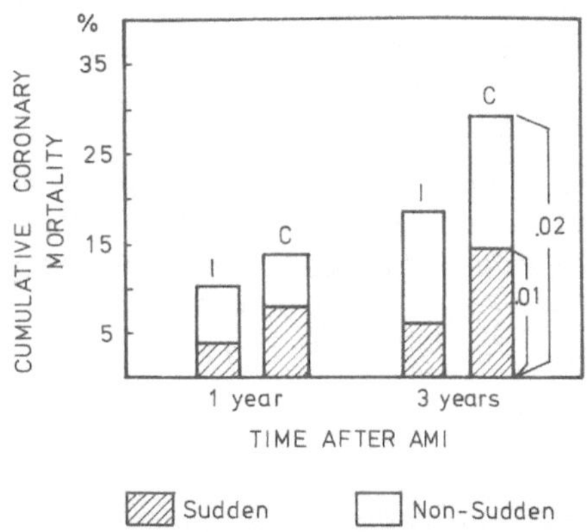

Fig. 2. Cumulative 1- and 3-year coronary mortality and distribution of cases according to sudden and nonsudden deaths in the intervention (*I*) and control (*C*) groups (Kallio et al. 1979)

The rate of reinfarction verified clinically during the 3-year follow-up was somewhat, but not significantly, higher in the intervention group, the percentage being 18.1 as compared with 11.2 in the control group. This may have been due, at least partly, to a better medical supervision of the intervention patients, who were often hospitalized and carefully examined even after a minor pain attack. The number of reinfarctions may have been underestimated clinically in the control group, a hypothesis which is supported by the fact that the numbers of new Q or QS findings were nearly identical in both groups during the follow-up. It should also be noted that five reinfarctions in the intervention group occurred during the first month after myocardial infarction, before the intervention program had begun.

The prognostic significance of various risk characteristics in the intervention group compared with the controls was also examined. The following factors were included: Age, sex, history of myocardial infarction, history of angina pectoris, arterial hypertension, functional class according to NYHA classification, history of diabetes, smoking habits before myocardial infarction, heart failure in hospital, serum ASAT-tertiles[1], and heart size.

It was found that patients below 50 years of age had a significantly lower coronary mortality in the intervention group as compared with the controls. This difference was due mainly to the reduction in nonsudden coronary deaths. As regards sudden deaths, there was a significantly lower mortality in the intervention group than in the controls in patients aged 60 to 64.

History of previous myocardial infarction or angina pectoris had a significantly smaller effect on subsequent mortality in the intervention group than in the controls.

Patients with a history of hypertension, or those diagnosed in the hospital as hypertensives, had a similar 3-year survival rate in both the intervention group and the control group. In contrast, patients with no such history had a significantly better survival rate in the intervention group than in the control group.

Heart failure indicated a severe prognosis in both the intervention and the control group, while patients without heart failure in the intervention group had a significantly better 3-year survival rate than those in the control group. Sudden death, in particular, was quite uncommon in the intervention group patients who had no heart failure in the hospital.

The beneficial effect of belonging to the intervention group was also demonstrated for patients with reasonably good physical working capacity at 1 year after myocardial infarction. Patients tolerating a work load of more than 70 watts had a significantly better prognosis during the following 2 years in the intervention group than the controls.

---

[1] *ASAT,* Aspartate aminotransferase enzyme

Conclusions

There is evidence suggesting that physical inactivity, smoking, hyperlipidemia, and hypertension influence the prognosis even after myocardial infarction.

Cessation of smoking is the most effective single intervention measure after myocardial infarction, and every physician should vigorously advise all patients to stop all forms of smoking.

Coronary mortality, and especially the number of sudden deaths, can be reduced by using a multifactorial intervention program with special emphasis on optimal medical control, physical exercise, and health education, beginning a few weeks after acute myocardial infarction. While the best results are to be expected in relatively low-risk patients, all patients should receive appropriate advice and well-organized care, which should start on dismissal from hospital and be most intensive during the first 6 months after myocardial infarction.

References

Bruce RA (1974) Progress in exercise cardiology. In: Yu, PN, Goodwin JF (eds) Progress in cardiology, vol 3. Lea and Febiger, Philadelphia, pp 113-172

Ehsani AA, Martin WH, Health GW, Coyle EF (1982) Cardiac effects of prolonged and intense exercise training in patients with coronary artery disease. Am J Cardiol 50:246-254

Erkelens DW, Albers JJ, Hazzard WR, Frederick RC, Bierman EL (1979) High-density lipoprotein-cholesterol in survivors of myocardial infarction. JAMA 20:2185-2189

Friedman EH (1976) Psychosocial factors in coronary risk and rehabilitation. In: Stocksmeier U (ed) Psychological approach to the rehabilitation of coronary patients. Springer, Berlin Heidelberg New York

Froelicher V, Jensen D, Atwood JE, McKirnan MD, Gerber K, Slutsky R, Battler A, Ashburn W, Ross J (1980) Cardiac rehabilitation: evidence for improvement in myocardial perfusion and function. Arch Phys Med Rehabil 61:517-522

Hypertension Detection and Follow-up Program Cooperative Group (1982) The effect of treatment on mortality in "mild" hypertension. Results of the hypertension detection and follow-up program. N Engl J Med 16:976-980

International Society of Cardiology (1980) Secondary prevention in myocardial infarction survivors. Heart Beat 3:1-3

Jenkins CD, Zyzanski SJ, Rosenmann RH (1976) Risk of new myocardial infarction in middle-aged men with manifest coronary heart disease. Circulation 53:342

Kallio V (1978) Results of rehabilitation in coronary patients. Adv Cardiol 24:153-163

Kallio V, Hämäläinen H, Hakkila J, Luurila OJ (1979) Reduction in sudden deaths by a multifactorial intervention programme after acute myocardial infarction. Lancet II:1091-1094

Kannel WB, Sorlie P, Castelli WP, McGee D (1980) Blood pressure and survival after myocardial infarction: the Framingham study. Am J Cardiol 45:326-330

Kellerman JJ (1982) Can we improve the prognosis of coronary heart disease? In: Mathes P, Halhuber MJ (eds) Controversies in cardiac rehabilitation. Springer, Berlin Heidelberg New York, pp 121-127

Kentala E (1972) Physical fitness and feasibility of physical rehabilitation after myocardial infarction in men of working age. Ann Clin Res 4 [Suppl 9]: 1-84

Leren P (1970) The Oslo Diet-Heart Study: eleven-year report. Circulation 42:935

May GS, Eberlein KA, Furberg CD, Passamani ER, DeMets DL (1982) Secondary prevention after myocardial infarction: a review of long-term trials. Prog Cardiovasc Dis 4:331-352

Morrison LM (1960) Diet in coronary atherosclerosis. JAMA 173:884

Mulcahy R, Hickey N, Graham IM, MacAirt J (1977) Factors affecting the 5-year survival rate of men following acute coronary heart disease. Am Heart J 93:556-559

Oldridge NB (1982) Compliance and exercise in primary and secondary prevention of coronary heart disease: a review. Prev Med 11:56–70
Palatsi I (1976) Feasibility of physical training after myocardial infarction and its effect on return to work, morbidity and mortality. Kaleva, Oulu
Pohjola S, Siltanen P, Romo M, Haapakoski J (1979) Effect of quitting smoking on the long-term survival after myocardial infarction. Proc 2nd Sci Meeting Working Group on Epidem and Prev Eur Society of Cardiol no 033
Rosenman RH (1978) Role of type A behavior pattern in the pathogenesis of ischemic heart disease and modification for prevention. Adv Cardiol 25:35–46
Salonen JT (1980) Stopping smoking and long-term mortality after acute myocardial infarction. Br Heart J 43:463–469
Schlant RC, Forman S, Stamler J, Canner PL (1982) The natural history of coronary heart disease: prognostic factors after recovery from myocardial infarction in 2789 men, the 5-year findings of the Coronary Drug Project. Circulation 66 [Suppl 2]:401–414
Shaw LW (1981) Effects of a prescribed supervised exercise program on mortality and cardiovascular morbidity in patients after a myocardial infarction. The National Exercise and Heart Disease Project. Am J Cardiol 48:39–46
Shephard RJ (1980) Recurrence of myocardial infarction. Observations on patients participating in the Ontario Multicentre Exercise-Heart Trial. Eur J Cardiol 11:147–157
Sparrow D, Dawber TR, Colton T (1978) The influence of cigarette smoking on prognosis after a first myocardial infarction. J Chron Dis 31:425–432
Streja D, Mymin D (1979) Moderate exercise and high-density lipoprotein-cholesterol. Observation during a cardiac rehabilitation program. JAMA 20:2190–2192
The Coronary Drug Project Research Group (1979) Cigarette smoking as a risk factor in men with a prior history of myocardial infarction. J Chron Dis 32:415–425
Thoresen CE, Telch MJ, Eagleston JR (1981) Approaches to altering the type A behaviour pattern. Psychosomatics 22:6
Vedin JA, Wilhelmsson C, Tibblin G, Wilhelmsen L (1976) The postinfarction clinic in Göteborg, Sweden. A controlled trial of a therapeutic organization. Acta Med Scand 200:453
Weinblatt E, Shapiro S, Frank CW et al. (1968) Prognosis of men after first myocardial infarction: mortality and first recurrence in relation to selected parameters. Am J Public Health 58:1329–1347
Wilhelmsen L, Sanne H, Elmfeldt D, Grimby G, Tibblin G, Wedek H (1975) A controlled trial of physical training after myocardial infarction, effects on risk factors, nonfatal reinfarction and death. Prev Med 4:491–508
Wilhelmsson C, Vedin JA, Elmfeldt D, Tibblin G, Wilhelmsen L (1975) Smoking and myocardial infarction. Lancet I:415–419

The Influence of Beta-Blockers on Long-Term Prognosis in Postinfarction Patients

Å. Hjalmarson and L. Wilhelmsen

Department of Medicine, Sahlgren's Hospital and Östra Hospital, University of Göteborg, Göteborg, Sweden

Since the first report, by Snow, in 1965 that propranolol reduced mortality in patients with acute myocardial infarction, a number of studies have been performed to evaluate the role of beta-blockade. Despite the large number of studies the positive results from 1965 have not proved easy to reproduce. The purpose of this presentation is to review the randomized and double-blind trials with beta-blockers in patients with acute myocardial infarction and in post-infarction.

Inconclusive Trials

All studies published between 1965 and 1974 failed to demonstrate any positive effect of beta-blockade on mortality. All were characterized by relatively low numbers of patients, and too few end points to demonstrate any effect on mortality. Several such inconclusive studies have also been reported during the past 10 years (Table 1). As will be discussed later, taking into consideration all randomized trials of various types of beta-blockers started a week or more after myocardial infarction, there is about a 25% reduction in mortality. Several thousand patients are needed to demonstrate that such a reduction – from a placebo mortality of 10%–15% – is due to a beneficial effect of the treatment. It is therefore not very surprising that the trials listed in Table 1, with relatively low numbers of patients and end points, were all inconclusive.

Table 1. Inconclusive trials

Author	Year	No. of patients	No. of deaths	Compound
Reynolds and Whitlock	1972	87	6	Alprenolol
Barber et al.	1975	484	87	Practolol
Andersen et al. (>65 yrs)	1979	198	83	Alprenolol
Wilcox et al.	1980	388	55	Atenolol Propranolol
Wilcox et al.	1980	315	24	Oxprenolol
Baber et al.	1980	720	55	Propranolol
Coronary Prevention Research Group	1981	313	23	Oxprenolol
McIlmoyle et al.	1982	391	35	Metoprolol

Reduction of Overall Mortality by Beta-Blockade

All randomized double-blind trials which have produced any positive effects on mortality by the administration of a beta-blocker are listed in Table 2. It can be seen that five of the eight listed included more than 1300 patients and three of these five were studies which showed a significant reduction of overall mortality (The Norwegian Multicentre Study Group 1981; Hjalmarson et al. 1981; Beta-Blocker Heart Attack Study Group 1981; Beta-Blocker Heart Attack Trial Research Group 1982). Although overall mortality was reduced by as much as 50% in two of the other studies (Andersen et al. 1979; Wilhelmsson et al. 1974), due to the low numbers of deaths statistical significance was not reached. Despite the fact that 3053 patients were included in the practolol trial (Multicentre International Study 1975, 1977) and 1456 in the sotalol trial (Julian et al. 1982), a 20% reduction in overall mortality achieved in the studies was also statistically insignificant. Several thousand more patients are needed in a study such as these two, where the placebo mortality was less than 10%, in order to obtain a statistically significant reduction if the true reduction is 20%. Of the studies which did not demonstrate a significant reduction in overall mortality (Andersen et al. 1979; Wilhelmsson et al. 1974; Multicentre International Study 1975, 1977; Hansteen et al. 1982; Julian et al. 1982), all but one (Julian et al. 1982) reported a significant reduction in sudden death and/or cardiac death.

Table 2. Reduction of total mortality by long-term beta-blockade

Author	Year	Beta-blocker	No. of patients	Reduction in overall mortality (%)
Wilhelmsson et al.	1974	Alprenolol	230	50[a]
Multicentre International Study	1975, 1977	Practolol	3053	20[a]
Andersen et al. (≤65 yrs)	1979	Alprenolol	282	55[a]
Norwegian Multicentre Study Group	1981	Timolol	1884	36
Hjalmarson et al.	1981	Metoprolol	1395	36
BHAT	1982	Propranolol	3837	26
Hansteen et al.	1982	Propranolol	560	32[a]
Julian et al.	1982	Sotalol	1456	18[a]

[a] Not statistically significant

As can be seen from Tables 1 and 2, in the alprenolol study from Copenhagen (Andersen et al. 1979) the patients were divided into two age-groups. These age-groups were formed prospectively and the positive effect on mortality was obtained by alprenolol in patients ≤65 years of age, while a trend towards a higher mortality in the alprenolol group was found for patients older than 65. As will be discussed later, the negative results in the older age-group might be due to a poor selection of patients, including acute myocardial infarction patients with marked hypotension and heart failure as well. Treatment was administered intravenously, then orally, and began shortly after the arrival of the patient at the hospital in only two of the eight studies listed in Table 2 (Andersen et al. 1979; Hjalmarson et al. 1981). All others were late-entry studies where treatment was begun 1–6 weeks after onset of infarction. The treatment period ranged from 3 months to 3 years.

The first really convincing study showing a reduction in overall mortality for all randomized patients after myocardial infarction was the timolol trial of the Norwegian Multicentre Study Group, published in 1981. This study achieved a 36% reduction among all randomized patients, and, calculated per protocol, counting only deaths within 28 days after blind tablet withdrawal, total mortality was reduced by 39% (Fig. 1). The effect on witnessed sudden death was even more marked. In contrast to the findings in the early intervention trial on alprenolol in Copenhagen (Andersen et al. 1979), similar reductions in mortality were found for patients above and below 65 years of age. The total number of patients randomized in this study was 1884, with 152 deaths in the placebo group and 98 in the timolol group ($p < 0.001$). Timolol (10 mg twice daily) or placebo was given to patients surviving acute myocardial infarction, with treatment beginning 7–28 days after infarction and covering a period of 12–33 months (mean, 17 months).

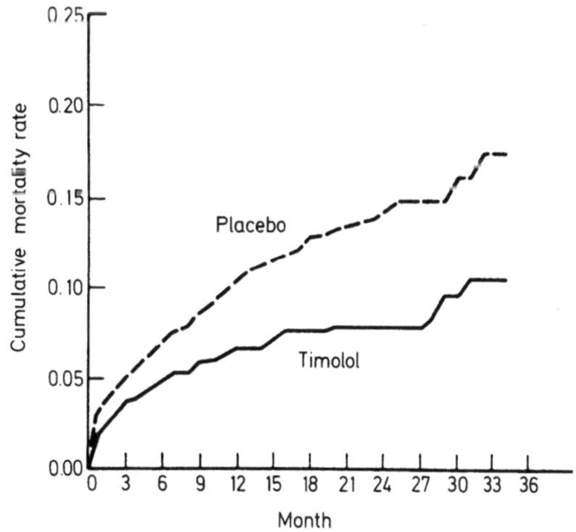

Fig. 1. Cumulative mortality in the Norwegian timolol trial (The Norwegian Multicentre Study Group 1981)

A second study showing a reduction in overall mortality for all randomized patients was the Swedish metoprolol trial, also published in 1981 by Hjalmarson et al. (Fig. 2). This study showed similar reductions in patients above and below 65 years of age, in agreement with the Norwegian timolol study. In contrast to the timolol study, however, this was an early-entry trial, with start of treatment shortly after arrival at the hospital (mean delay, 11 h). Metoprolol was given i.v. (15 mg), followed by 200 mg daily for 3 months, and placebo was given in a similar manner over a the same treatment period. The treatment was started in 1395 patients with suspected acute myocardial infarction, 809 of whom developed a definite infarction and 169 a probable myocardial infarction during the follow-up period. After the double-blind treatment period of 90 days, open treatment with 100 mg metoprolol twice daily was recommended, and long-term follow-up continued thereafter. During the 90-day double-blind phase 62 patients from this placebo group died, compared with 40 from the metoprolol group ($p<0.03$). The difference in mortality between the two groups was maintained after 1 year of follow-up ($p=0.016$).

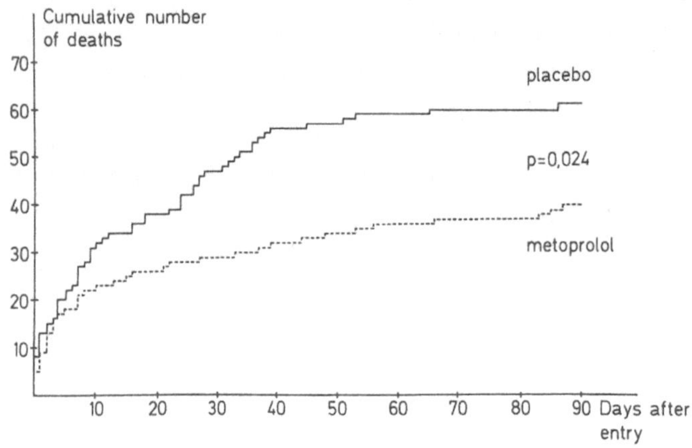

Fig. 2. Cumulative number of deaths in the Göteborg metoprolol trial (Hjalmarson et al. 1981)

The American propranolol trial (BHAT) (Beta-Blocker Heart Attack Study Group 1981; Beta-Blocker Heart Attack Trial Research Group 1982) was also published in 1981, and showed a significant reduction in cumulative mortality of 26% (Table 3). Similar to the Norwegian timolol trial, this was a late-entry trial, with start of treatment 5–21 days after infarction. A similar reduction in mortality with propranolol was seen for all age groups. Medication was begun with 20 mg propranolol or placebo, followed by 40 mg propranolol or placebo over 8 h for at least 48 h. Based upon the serum propranolol level, the dose was further adjusted. Of the 3837 patients enrolled, 82% were assigned to the 180 mg per day regimen and 18% were assigned to the 240 mg per day regimen. The trial was stopped 9 months ahead of schedule and the follow-up period was 3–36 months (mean, 25 months). A total of 3837 patients were randomized, and there were 188 deaths in the placebo group, 138 in the propranolol group ($p<0.01$).

Table 3. Life tables for propranolol and placebo groups (Beta-Blocker Heart Attack Trial Research Group 1982)

Period (months)	Propranolol			Placebo		
	No. alive at beginning of interval	Deaths	Cumulative mortality (%)	No. alive at beginning of interval	Deaths	Cumulative mortality (%)
1-3	1916	37	1.93	1921	50	2.60
4-6	1878	10	2.45	1869	31	4.22
7-12	1868	23	3.66	1838	34	5.99
13-18	1844	24	5.03	1803	30	7.69
19-24	1501	29	7.13	1458	20	9.15
25-36	1087	14	9.00	107	22	12.52
36+	202	1	10.26	204	1	13.29
Total	-	138	-	-	188	-

Reduction of Reinfarctions by Long-term Beta-Blockade

A number of studies have been published reporting a reduction in the incidence of reinfarction by prophylactic administration of beta-blockers compared with placebo (Table 4). The incidence of reinfarction seems to have been reduced by at least 25%, which is comparable to the average reduction in mortality in postinfarction trials. For three of the studies (The Norwegian Multicentre Study Group 1981; Hjalmarson et al. 1981; Julian et al. 1982) significant reduction in reinfarctions was obtained when fatal and nonfatal reinfarctions were calculated. For the other three studies in Table 4, the figures given refer to the reduction of nonfatal reinfarctions only. In the American propranolol trial (Beta-Blocker Heart Attack Study Group 1981; Beta-Blocker Heart Attack Trial Research Group 1982), a nonsignificant 15% reduction in the incidence of reinfarctions has been obtained (C. Furberg, personal communication).

Table 4. Reduction in reinfarctions by long-term beta-blockade

Author	Year	Beta-blocker	No. of patients	Reduction in reinfarctions (%)
Wilhelmsson et al.	1974	Alprenolol	230	11[a]
Multicentre International Study	1975, 1977	Practolol	3053	23[a]
Norwegian Multicentre Study Group	1981	Timolol	1884	28
Hjalmarson et al.	1981	Metoprolol	1395	35
Hansteen et al.	1982	Propranolol	560	24[a]
Julian et al.	1982	Sotalol	1456	41

[a] Nonfatal reinfarctions only; not statistically significant

Selection of Patients

An important question is whether the results from the reported trials can be generalized and are valid for most postinfarction patients. In Table 5, the population base from which the trial patients were selected is reported for four of the five largest randomized beta-blocker trials; for the multicenter international study on practolol the population base is not known. For the BHAT studies and those of timolol and sotalol, about 50% of the eligible patients were included in the trial. Furthermore, about 20% of the eligible patients in these studies had true contraindications to beta-blockade. Considering the other criteria for inclusion, it seems reasonable to believe that the results obtained are valid and representative for 80% of the patient population with infarction. Only 23% of the eligible patients were included in the American propranolol trial (BHAT). The placebo mortality was much lower in this trial than in other long-term trials. Obviously, mainly low-risk patients were included. The results of this trial might therefore not be valid for high-risk postinfarction patients. However, the timolol study from Norway reported a 36% reduction in overall mortality where high-risk patients were included.

Table 5. Comparison of trials

	Timolol (The Norwegian Multicentre Study Group 1981)	BHAT (1971, 1982)	Metoprolol (Hjalmarson et al. 1981)	Sotalol (Julian et al. 1982)	Practolol (Multicentre International Study 1975, 1977)
No. of patients evaluated	3647	16400	2619	3234	–
No. of patients randomized	1884	3837	1395	1456	3038
Patients included (%)	52	23	53	45	–
Duration of follow-up (months)	12–33	12–39	3	12	1–24
Reduction in mortality (%)	36	26	36	18	20

Using various prognostic models, such as the one by Vedin et al. (1977), it is possible to identify patients at particularly high risk of death. Aiming at reducing mortality, a prophylactic treatment with beta-blockade could be instituted only in patients at higher mortality risk. However, the fact that the beta-blockers which have been reported to reduce mortality were also found to reduce the incidence of nonfatal reinfarction makes it more difficult to limit the treatment only to patients at high mortality risk. There is no good method at present to predict which patients will suffer nonfatal reinfarctions. A patient who does suffer a nonfatal reinfarction will be transferred to a higher mortality risk group. It seems reasonable, therefore, to recommend long-term treatment with beta-blockers to all postinfarction patients without contraindications. The prophylactic treatment also seems valuable for all ages up to 75 years. The deleterious effects of alprenolol in patients above 65 years of age in the Copenhagen study (Andersen et al. 1979) seem to be due to incorrect selection of patients.

Start and Duration of Treatment

Among the studies reporting a positive effect of beta-blockers on survival, only two (Andersen et al. 1979; Hjalmarson et al. 1981) began with i.v. administration of treatment shortly after the patients' arrival in hospital, followed by oral treatment. In the Copenhagen alprenolol study (Andersen et al. 1979) a positive effect was obtained only in patients 65 years of age or younger, while deleterious effects seem to be induced by alprenolol in patients above 65 years of age. Thus, there is only one early-entry trial in which the beta-blocking therapy caused a significant reduction in mortality for all randomized patients (Hjalmarson et al. 1981). According to a preliminary report by McIlmoyle et al. (1982), using the same doses of metoprolol as in the Göteborg trial (Hjalmarson et al. 1981) no conclusive results were obtained. This raises a question as to whether the findings of the Göteborg group can be generalized to other settings (Furberg et al. 1982). However, it is not very likely that a study as small as the one reported by McIlmoyle and co-workers should give any conclusive results. The Göteborg metoprolol trial is the only large one among the randomized placebo-controlled trials where intravenous treatment was started on admission and followed by oral treatment. Five other such studies all proved inconclusive, most likely due to very few end points (Andersen et al. 1979; Evemy and Pentecost 1978; Johansson 1980; Yusuf et al. 1980; McJlmoyle et al. 1982). Besides the positive effect on mortality and development of infarction in the Göteborg metoprolol trial, the early institution of metoprolol had a number of beneficial clinical effects. There were decreases in the incidence of ventricular fibrillation, ventricular tachycardia, chest pain, and severity of congestive heart failure, and the treatment meant a shorter hospital stay for the patients (Hjalmarson et al. 1983). Furthermore, there are reasons to believe that the property of the beta-blocking agent that reduces mortality in the late postinfarction phase is the same one that reduces mortality in the very early postinfarction phase. In the Göteborg metoprolol trial there was a reduction in all conditions which can cause death, including arrhythmias, congestive heart failure, rupture of ventricular wall, heart failure, and fresh infarct development (Hjalmarson et al. 1983). These are the causes of death during late postinfarction follow-up as well (up to 3 years). Mortality is known to be highest during the very early phase of acute myocardial infarction. It therefore seems logical to institute prophylactic treatment with beta-blockade as early as possible, taking into account proper selection of patients, tolerance data for the beta-blocker used, and personal history of the patient.

Concerning the duration of treatment, several studies have demonstrated that a period of up to 3 years is indicated. Since mortality falls during the years after myocardial infarction, the relative importance of prophylactic treatment therefore declines with time. Unless there are other indications for continued treatment with beta-blockers, such as angina pectoris or hypertension, the treatment may be withdrawn after 2–3 years.

Selection of Beta-Blocking Agents

The properties of the beta-blocking agents are listed in Table 6, which includes all beta-blockers with positive effects on survival after myocardial infarction. The only property in common for these beta-blockers is the $beta_1$-receptor blockade. It seems unlikely that the other properties – including $beta_2$-receptor blockade, intrinsic stimulatory activity and membrane-stabilizing activity – play an important role in postinfarction prophylaxis against death and reinfarction. It is well known that the $beta_1$-receptor blockade is the property responsible for all other important positive effects of the beta-blockers in hypertension, angina pectoris, and tachyrhythmias.

Table 6. Properties of beta-blockers shown to reduce mortality in myocardial infarction

Beta-blocker	$Beta_1$	$Beta_2$	ISA	MSA
Alprenolol	+	+	+	+
Practolol	+	–	+	–
Timolol	+	+	–	–
Metoprolol	+	–	–	–
Propranolol	+	+	–	+

ISA, intrinsic stimulatory activity; *MSA*, membrane stabilizing activity

Aspects of Tolerance

Based upon the experience gained from the larger trials in particular (The Norwegian Multicentre Study Group 1981; Hjalmarson et al. 1981; Beta-Blocker Heart Attack Study Group 1981; Beta-Blocker Heart Attack Trial Research Group 1982; Julian et al. 1982), the overall tolerance to beta-blockade after myocardial infarction is very good. This is also true for the early-entry trial where metoprolol was given from the first day in the hospital (Hjalmarson et al. 1981). As can be expected, there are somewhat more adverse cardiovascular reactions in the beta-blocker groups than in the placebo groups. However, these reactions – mainly bradycardia and hypotension – are benign. A significant aggravation of heart failure in the larger trials has not been reported (The Norwegian Multicentre Study Group 1981; Hjalmarson et al. 1981; Beta-Blocker Heart Attack Study Group 1981; Beta-Blocker Heart Attack Trial Research Group 1982). On the contrary, in the early-entry trial from Göteborg (Hjalmarson et al. 1981), metoprolol had a prophylactic effect against development of severe congestive heart failure. Among other side-effects, asthenia and fatigue are more frequent in the beta-blocker group, as are cold hands and feet and bronchial obstruction in some of the trials using nonselective blocking agents (The Norwegian Multicentre Study Group 1981; Beta-Blocker Heart Attack Trial Research Group 1982). Cardioselectivity might be of importance with regard to these side-effects. In all the larger trials, angina pectoris and tachyrhythmias were more common in the placebo groups, as expected.

Conclusion

In the early phase of acute myocardial infarction mortality is very high (15%–20% in nonselected patients during the hospital stay); it declines during the next few years. Most important for the short- and long-term prognosis is the severity of myocardial ischemic damage. In order to improve the prognosis it is justified to institute prophylactic treatment as soon as possible after onset of symptoms. It would most likely be best to institute treatment before onset of symptoms if the patients at risk for infarction could be identified. Prophylactic treatment should be aimed at both mortality and development of myocardial infarction.

A number of large randomized double-blind trials have convincingly demonstrated a reduction in mortality and in incidence of infarction by about 25%. No other medical treatment has been as convincing in this respect. When selecting a drug for prophylactic treatment it seems right to recommend one of the agents that has been shown to have a significant effect on mortality and on the incidence of infarction. This is true for three beta-blocking agents, namely timolol, metoprolol, and propranolol. It remains to be clarified whether these effects can be generalized to other beta-blockers. For treatment of patients during the very early phase of myocardial infarction the use of metoprolol is recommended. This drug has been found to be both effective and safe during the very early phase. In the trials with timolol (The Norwegian Multicentre Study Group 1981) and propranolol (Beta-Blocker Heart Attack Study Group 1981; Beta-Blocker Heart Attack Trial Research Group 1982) treatment was begun about 2 weeks after onset of infarction, and there are no data on the efficacy or safety of these drugs during the first 2 weeks after infarction. About 20% of patients had contraindications to beta-blockade in the three trials with timolol (The Norwegian Multicentre Study Group 1981), metoprolol (Hjalmarson et al. 1981) and propranolol (Beta-Blocker Heart Attack Study Group 1981; Beta-Blocker Heart Attack Trial Research Group 1982), which means that about 80% of all infarctions can be safely treated with a selective beta-blocker during the early phase (valid for metoprolol) and during long-term follow-up (valid for timolol, metoprolol, and propranolol). The aim of prophylactic treatment is to prevent death and reduce the possibility of reinfarction. Since it cannot be predicted which patients are at risk for reinfarction all patients with myocardial infarction – contraindications taken into account – should be recommended for long-term treatment of 2–3 years.

References

Andersen MP, Bechsgaard P, Frederiksen J, Hansen DA, Jürgensen HJ, Nielsen B, Pedersen F, Pedersen-Bjergaard O, Rasmussen SL (1979) Effect of alprenolol on mortality among patients with definite or suspected acute myocardial infarction. Lancet II:865–867

Barber JM, Boyle D McC, Chaturvedi NC, Singh N, Walsh MJ (1975) Practolol in acute myocardial infarction. Acta Med Scand [Suppl] 587:213–219

Baber NS, Wainwright Evans D, Howitt G, Thomas M, Wilson C, Lewis JA, Dawes PM, Handler K, Tuson R (1980) Multicentre postinfarction trial of propranolol in 49 hospitals in the United Kingdom, Italy, and Yugoslavia. Br Heart J 44:96–100

Beta-Blocker Heart Attack Study Group (1981) The Beta-Blocker Heart Attack Trial preliminary report. JAMA 246:2073–2074

Beta-Blocker Heart Attack Trial Research Group (1982) A randomized trial of propranolol in patients with acute myocardial infarction. I. Mortality results. JAMA 247:1707–1714

Coronary Prevention Research Group (1981) An early intervention secondary prevention study with oxprenolol following myocardial infarction. Eur Heart J 2:389–393

Evemy KL, Pentecost BL (1978) Intravenous and oral practolol in the acute stages of myocardial infarction. Eur J Cardiol 7:391–398

Furberg C, Friedman L, Cutler J (1982) Should every survivor of a heart attack be given a beta-blocker? (letter to the editor). Br Med J 285:738–739

Hansteen V, Møinichen E, Lorentsen E, Andersen A, Strøm O, Søiland K, Dyrbekk D, Refsum A-M, Tromsdal A, Knudsen K, Eika C, Bakken J jr, Smith P, Hoff PI (1982) One year's treatment with propranolol after myocardial infarction: preliminary report of Norwegian multicentre trial. Br Med J 284:155–161

Hjalmarson Å, Elmfeldt D, Herlitz J, Holmberg S, Málek I, Nyberg G, Rydén L, Swedberg K, Vedin A, Waagstein F, Waldenström A, Waldenström J, Wedel H, Wilhelmsen L, Wilhelmsson C (1981) Effect on mortality of metoprolol in acute myocardial infarction. A double-blind randomised trial. Lancet II:823–827

Hjalmarson Å, Herlitz J, Holmberg S, Rydén L, Swedberg K, Vedin A, Waagstein F, Waldenström A, Waldenström J, Wedel H, Wilhelmsen L, Wilhelmsson C (1983) The Göteborg metoprolol trial. Effects on mortality and morbidity in acute myocardial infarction. Circulation (in press)

Johansson BW (1980) Comparative study of cardioselective beta-blockade and diazepam in patients with acute myocardial infarction and tachycardia. Acta Med Scand 207:47–53

Julian DG, Prescott RJ, Jackson FS, Szekely P (1982) Controlled trial of sotalol for one year after myocardial infarction. Lancet II:1142–1147

McIlmoyle L, Evans A, Boyle D McC, Cran G, Barber JM, Elwood H, Salathia K, Shanks R (1982) Early intervention in myocardial ischaemia. Br Heart J 47:189

Multicentre International Study (1975) Improvement in prognosis of myocardial infarction by long-term beta-adrenoceptor blockade using practolol. Br Med J I:735–740

Multicentre International Study (1977) Supplementary report. Reduction in mortality after myocardial infarction with long-term beta-adrenoceptor blockade. Br Med J III:419–421

Reynolds JL, Whitlock RMI (1972) Effects of a beta-adrenergic receptor blocker in myocardial infarction treated for one year from onset. Br Heart J 34:252–259

Snow PJD (1965) Effect of propranolol in myocardial infarction. Lancet II:551–553

The Norwegian Multicentre Study Group (1981) Timolol-induced reduction in mortality and reinfarction in patients surviving acute myocardial infarction. Lancet II:865–872

Vedin A, Wilhelmsen L, Wedel H, Pettersson B, Wilhelmsson C, Elmfeldt D, Tibblin G (1977) Prediction of deaths and reinfarctions after initial myocardial infarction. Acta Med Scand 201:309–316

Wilhelmsson C, Vedin A, Wilhelmsen L, Tibblin G, Werkö L (1974) Reduction of sudden deaths after myocardial infarction by treatment with alprenolol. Lancet II:1157–1160

Wilcox RG, Roland JM, Banks DC, Hampton JR, Mitchell JRA (1980a) Randomised trial comparing propranolol with atenolol in immediate treatment of suspected myocardial infarction. Br Med J 280:885–888

Wilcox RG, Rowley JM, Hampton JR, Mitchell JRA, Roland JM, Banks DC (1980b) Randomised placebo-controlled trial comparing oxprenolol with disopyramide phosphate in immediate treatment of suspected myocardial infarction. Lancet II:765-769
Yusuf S, Peto R, Bennett D, Ramsdale D, Furse L, Bray C, Sleight P (1980) Early intravenous atenolol treatment in suspected acute myocardial infarction. Lancet II:273-276

Secondary Prevention of Myocardial Infarction with Antiplatelet Drugs

C. R. Klimt and S. A. Forman

University of Maryland and Maryland Medical Research Institute Inc., 600 Wyndhurst Avenue, Baltimore, MD 21210, USA

Nine trials qualified for this limited review of antiplatelet drugs used in secondary prevention of myocardial infarction. The criterion for inclusion was a placebo-controlled, randomized trial with a sample size of at least 100 (May et al. 1982). Six of these trials involved asprin alone, one aspirin plus Persantin (dipyridimole), and two Anturan (sulfinpyrazone).

The first trial by Elwood et al. (1974), conducted in and around Cardiff in 1974, randomized 1239 patients to aspirin and placebo; the entry window was less than 6 months and the dose of aspirin was one 300-mg tablet per day. The average length of follow-up was 12 months. That study was favorable in its overall mortality trend, but a closer look shows that the favorable results pertained to Cardiff alone and only to the subgroup which was treated 6 weeks after the myocardial infarct. Varying accuracy of reporting was considered to be the cause of the discrepancies by location.

Stimulated by these encouraging findings - to which was added a case control study from the Boston Collaborative Surveillance Group (1974) - the Coronary Drug Project rerandomized the suitable and willing patients discontinued from three "negative" treatment groups (two estrogen groups and a dextrothyroxine group) to aspirin and placebo. This new project was called the Coronary Drug Project Aspiring Project (The Coronary Drug Project Research Group 1976), in which 1529 patients were randomized to either three tablets of methylcellulose-coated aspirin a day for a total of 972 mg, or a corresponding placebo regimen. Mean length of follwo-up was 22 months, but it varied considerable according to when the patients became available from the Coronary Drug Project. In February 1975 the study was discontinued, although the results came as close to significance as those of any of the aspirin studies. For total mortality the *p* value was .07, corresponding to a reduction of 30% in mortality. The reasons for the premature discontinuation were nonhomogeneity of results for the previous treatment group in the Coronary Drug Project and the special selection of these patients.

The German-Austrian Study Group Multicenter Trial (Breddin et al. 1979) also tested aspirin, with 1.5 g Colfarit given in three divided doses of .5 g each per day. The entry window was 28–42 days, and a total of 626 patients were randomized, 309 to placebo and 317 to aspirin. The average observation period was 24 months. Aspirin gave more favorable findigs than placebo, but again, significance was not achieved. The study had a relatively large number of dropouts, and several of the participating clinics had to be excluded for noncompliance with the protocol.

The second study, of Elwood and Sweetnam (1979), randomized 1725 patients, increasing the aspirin dose this time from 300 to 900 mg per day; the average follow-up was 12 months. That study showed a favorable trend, short of statistical significance, for the end point overall mortality.

From England first, and now from Boston, two primary prevention studies have been initiated, giving one tablet of aspirin every other day to high-risk male physicians who are otherwise healthy and have not suffered a myocardial infarction. As many as 12000 are expected to participate in these primary prevention studies, which will not be discussed in greater detail here.

We now come to the largest aspirin study, the US Aspirin Myocardial Infarction Study, or AMIS, which terminated in 1980 (Aspirin Myocardial Infarction Study Research Group 1980). There were 4524 patients randomized to either placebo or 1 g aspirin per day, given in two divided doses of 500 mg each. The doses were contained in special capsules and appropriate bioavailability studies on this formulation have only now been performed. The entry window was 2 months to 5 years after myocardial infarction (MI), and the mean follow-up was 39 months. Baseline differences in this large study were surprisingly frequent. Seven factors showed a significantly different distribution between treatment groups, and four of these seven can be considered independent risk factors. After adjustment for baseline differences had been performed by Cox analysis, the −11% difference in total mortality was reduced to zero, a small favorable difference for coronary mortality and a slightly larger one for coronary incidence (i.e., the combination of coronary mortality and definite, nonfatal MI) were observed. None of the differences even approached significance, in spite of the size of the study. The recommendations from this study are clear, namely that aspirin is not suitable for the secondary prevention of myocardial infarction. This is the only such study which has gone to such extremes.

Next is the PARIS, or the Persantin-Aspirin Reinfarction Study, also published in 1980, in which 2027 patients were randomized into three groups: 972 mg aspirin plus 225 mg dipyridamole per day; 972 mg per day of aspirin alone, plus a dipyridamole placebo; and a double-placebo control group. Figure 1 presents the mortality findings as two separate studies, although the placebo group was the same for both. The entrance window was again 2–60 months after a qualifying MI, and the mean length of follow-up was 41 months. PARIS was quite encouraging for all three major end points: the 2-year mortality difference between aspirin and placebo was 27%, and for the first 2 years the coronary incidence for the combination of aspirin and dipyridamole was significantly less than that for placebo. However, at the end of the study, the aspirin group and the combination treatment groups were equal with regard to the main end points, and statistical significance had been lost.

The multiplicity of aspirin studies is unparalleled in the history of clinical trials. For this reason varios attempts have been undertaken to pool these results. Canner (1983) compared the results of the six trials of aspirin alone to determine whether a consistent pattern emerged. He used the procedure of combining log odds ratios (Woolf 1955; Fleiss 1973) to asses homogeneity in the trials and to determine the relationship of aspirin to various response variables

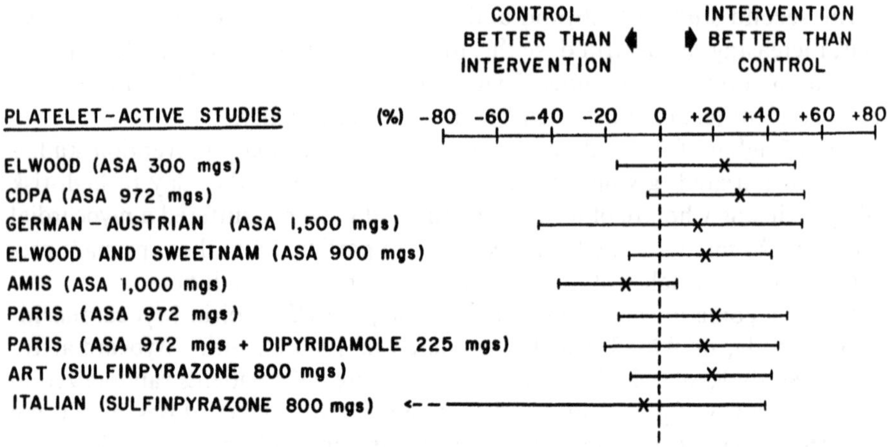

Fig. 1. Relative mortality differences and 95% confidence limits for studies on the prevention of myocardial infarction. *Elwood,* (Elwood et al. 1974); *CDPA,* Coronary Drug Project Research Group (Tick et al. 1974); *ASA,* aspirin (acetylsalicylic acid); *German-Austrian,* Breddin et al. (1979); Elwood and Sweetnam (1979); *AMIS,* Aspirin Myocardial Infarction Study Research Group (1980); *PARIS,* Persantian-Aspirin Reinfarction Trial Research Group (1980); *ART,* Anturan Reinfarction Trial Research Group (1978, 1980); *Italian,* Anturan Reinfarction Italian Study (1982)

in all trials. In an editorial Richard Peto (1980) of Oxford presented a somewhat different statistical approach to the problem, but arrived at basically similar conclusions. He used the procedure of comparing (a) the number of events observed among aspirin takers with the number expected, on the basis of the numbers of patients assigned to the aspirin and placebo groups, (b) the total number of events in both groups, and (c) the null hypothesis of equal event rates in the two groups. Canner's combining the findings from the six trials using log odds ratios revealed a 10% reduction in overall mortality by aspirin, a p value equal to .04. The results of the six trials were not found to be heterogeneous, even including the AMIS Study ($p = 0.2$), thus justifying the combining of results from the six trials. Also confirmed were the undesirable side-effects of aspirin, with even higher significance levels.

In spite of these reassuring attempts at statistically combining six major aspirin trials, one cannot help feeling insecure about the conclusions. Doses ranged from 300 to 1500 mg. The entry of patients into the studies varied over a tremendously long span, a few hours to 5 years. The reversal of the favorable trends of years 1 and 2 in subsequent years makes one pause to think. In addition, of course, the question of benefit-risk ratios has to be considered, and aspirin is by no means a harmless drug.

We now move away from aspirin and the combination of aspirin and Persantin and consider the North American Anturan Reinfarction Trial, abbreviated ART. A first report was published in 1978 (The Anturan Reinfarction Trial Research Group 1978), claiming an overwhelming success after an average observation period of only 4.5 months. The willing and suitable patients were continued in the study, which is astonishing, from an ethical point of view, once success has been claimed. In 1980 the final report claims (The Anturan Reinfarction Trial Research Group 1980) were much more modest, an the investigators had changed the primary end point to "sudden death not due to reinfarction within four months of the qualifying infarct." The classification method was questioned, but the most important criticism is contained in a paper by Dr. Robert Temple of the FDA in the New England Journal of Medicine (Temple and Pledger 1980) and in the Drug Bulletin of the Food an Drug Administration (FDA Drug Bulletin 1978). The prime objection was the exclusion of patients after randomization. Deaths occuring within 7 days after randomization were not counted. Not counted as well were deaths in patients who supposedly had not taken their medication for 7 days prior to death (how that was determined remains obscure). In any case, the total number of deaths - 74 versus 89 in favor of Anturan - is far from being statistically significant. Such a difference would occur one in four times by chance alone.

In January, 1982, yet another Anturan study was published in the Lancet (Anturan Reinfarction Italian Study 1982). This study was conducted in Italy, with 727 patients randomized to either sulfinpyrazone or placebo, and followed up for an average period of 19.2 months. Patients entered the study 15–25 days after their qualifying infarct. The paper does not deal with overall mortality; however, this can be ascertained and the figures have been plotted in Fig. 1. They were slightly negative for Anturan. Not only was there no difference in overall mortality, but cardiovascular mortality, according to the paper, was also almost equal. The only differences found were among nonfatal events, and these were rather "soft" end points.

In the platelet-deaggregating field another drug is being widely investigated - ticlopidine hydrochloride. In the United States, the first study of aspirin versus ticlopidine in transient ischemia attack patients is in its infancy. Fatal and nonfatal stroke are the end points selected.

A follow-up study to the first PARIS is also underway, in which approximately 3000 patients will have been randomly assigned either to placebo or to Asasantin (225 mg Persantin and 972 mg aspirin, divided into three equal doses per day). In this study, patients are entered 4 weeks to 4 months after their qualifying MI. Because of the results of the AMIS a pure aspirin group has been omitted in this trial design. The results of this study will become known in 1984.

Another interesting study from France, called EPSIM (The EPSIM Research Group 1982), has recently been published. It is remarkable in that it compares aspirin with the standard treatment in France, namely oral anticoagulants. In none of the end points has there been any difference between the two treatments, and since placebo treatment was not included we are none the wiser about whether any of these treatments are either effective, neutral, or possibly negative with regard to mortality.

In summary, while we have encouraging findings in this particular drug group, no individual drug has yet been statistically, unequivocally positive, and the combination of results of aspirin studies is favorable but, because of differences in study design, not entirely convincing either.

References

Anturane Reinfarction Italian Study (1982) Sulphinpyrazone in post-myocardial infarction. Lancet 1:237–242

The Anturan Reinfarction Trial Research Group (1978) Sulfinpyrazone in the prevention of cardiac death after myocardial infarction. N Engl. J Med 298:289–295

The Anturan Reinfarction Trial Research Group (1980) Sulfinpyrazone in the prevention of sudden death after myocardial infarction. N Engl J Med 302:250–256

Aspirin Myocardial Infarction Study Research Group (1980) A randomized controlled trial of persons recovered from myocardial infarction. JAMA 243:661

Breddin K, Loew D, Lechner K, Uberla K, Walter E (1979) Secondary prevention of myocardial infarction. Comparison of acetylsalicylic acid, phenprocoumon and placebo. A multicenter two-year prospective study. Thromb Haemost 40:225

Canner PL (1982) Aspirin in coronary heart disease: comparison of six clinical trials. Presented at the fourth international symposium of clinical trials (Beer-Sheva, January 1982) Isr J Med Sci 5:1983

The Coronary Drug Project Research Group (1976) Aspirin in coronary heart disease. J Chron Dis 29:625

Elwood PC, Sweetnam PM (1979) Aspirin and secondary mortality after myocardial infarction. Lancet 2:1313

Elwood PC, Cochrane Al, Bur ML, Sweetnam PM, Williams G, Welsby E, Hughes SJ, Renton R (1974) A randomized controlled trial of acetylaslicylic acid in the secondary prevention of mortality from myocardial infarction. Br Med J 1:436

The EPSIM Research Group (1982) A controlled comparison of aspirin and oral anticoagulants in prevention of death after myocardial infarction. N Engl J Med 307:701–708

FDA Drug Bulletin (1978) Sulfinpyrazone and prevention of myocardial infarction, May–July 1978, pp 19–20

Fleiss JL (1973) Statistical methods for rates and proportions. Wiley, New York, pp 115–117

Boston Collaborative Drug Surveillance Group (1974) Regular aspirin intake and acute myocardial infarction. Med J 1:440

May GS, Eberlein KA, Furberg CD, et al. (1982) Secondary prevention after myocardial infarction: a review of long-term trials. Prog Cardiovasc Dis 24:349

The Persantin-Aspirin Reinfarction Trial Research Group (1980) Persantine and aspirin in coronary heart disease. Circulation 62:449

Peto R (1980) Editorial: Aspirin after myocardial infarction. Lancet 1:1172–1173

Temple R, Pledger GW (1980) The FDA's critique of the anturan reinfarction trial. N Engl J Med 303:1488–1492

Woolf B (1955) On estimating the relation between blood group and disease. Ann Hum Genet 19:251–253

Oral Anticoagulants and/or Aspirin

E. A. Loeliger
Interne Geneeskunde, Academisch Ziekenhuis, Leiden, The Netherlands

Important progress has been made during the past few years in the understanding of putative successes and failures of oral anticoagulation (OAC) in general, and in the secondary prevention of myocardial infarction in particular. Not only did the conception of thrombotic pathogenesis of the transmural type of myocardial infarction revive after successful removal of acute coronary obstruction by the use of streptokinase, a thrombolytic agent (Loeliger 1981); the results of the Dutch Sixty-Plus Reinfarction Study, which showed a significantly better prognosis for patients given continued oral anticoagulant therapy (Sixty-Plus Reinfarction Study Research Group 1980), reopened the discussion about oral anticoagulants in myocardial infarction (Mitchell 1981). It became clear that strict adherence to a well-defined therapeutic range (Poller 1982), therapeutic quality control (Duxbury 1982), and standardization of the prothrombin time (Loeliger and Lewis 1982) were essential for successful anticoagulation; in their absence such treatment is doomed to failure (Loeliger 1981).

In spite of extensive discussion in widely read medical weeklies, these constructive developments in oral anticoagulant control have received insufficient attention. Only 4 weeks ago, the *New England Journal of Medicine* published without comment the report of the French *Enquête de Prévention Secondaire de l'Infarctus du Myocarde* (called the EPSIM Research Group), which concluded that "aspirin in the dosage used (0.5 g, three times a day) is probably not different from oral anticoagulants in affecting mortality and morbidity after a major infarction" (EPSIM Research Group 1982), a conclusion which, however, lacked validation by data on the quality of anticoagulation achieved. Considered more closely, the figures presented by the EPSIM group strongly suggest that more than half of the patients were underdosed (Loeliger 1983). At most, only about 35% of the prothrombin times measured in patients of the anticoagulant group are likely to have been within the recommended therapeutic range. Table 1 summarizes the results of the French study. These figures certainly do not preclude the possibility that oral anticoagulants, if properly administered, offer powerful protection against recurrent myocardial infarction, or, on the other hand, that conventional-dose aspirin prevents a small proportion of such events. The benefit of aspirin found by the Aspirin Myocardial Infarction Study (AMIS) Research Group (Table 2) amounted to an 18% lower rate of reinfarction in the aspirin group as compared with the placebo group. This marginal beneficial effect on morbidity was not reflected by any lowering of the mortality among the patients in this trial (AMIS Research Group 1980).

Table 1. Results of EPSIM study on aspirin and oral anticoagulants (EPSIM Research Group 1982)

	OAC	ASA	Difference (OAC–ASA)
RMI	20	32	−37.5%[a]
Death	65	72	−10%[a]

RMI, recurrent myocardial infarction; *OAC*, oral anticoagulant; *ASA*, aspirin
[a] Not significant

Table 2. Results of the Aspirin Myocardial Infarction Study (AMIS Research Group 1980)

	Placebo	ASA	Difference (placebo–ASA)
RMI	262	215	−18%[a]
Death	219	245	+12%[a]

[a] Not significant

The only study thus far performed that convincingly demonstrates a mild antithrombotic action of aspirin in preventing the formation of apposition thrombi is the well-controlled prospective randomized trial performed by Norwegian investigators in patients with an aortic ball-valve prosthesis (Dale 1976, 1977). The results of a similar study done in Argentina are of no contributive value as long as the levels of anticoagulation achieved in the comparison groups are not known (Altman et al. 1976). In contradistinction to the Argentine investigators, those in Norway meticulously defined these levels in terms of an internationally standardized thromboplastin. Figure 1 illustrates the quality of anticoagulation achieved by the Norwegians as compared with that obtained by the Leiden Thrombosis Center: whereas in Leiden about 80% of the

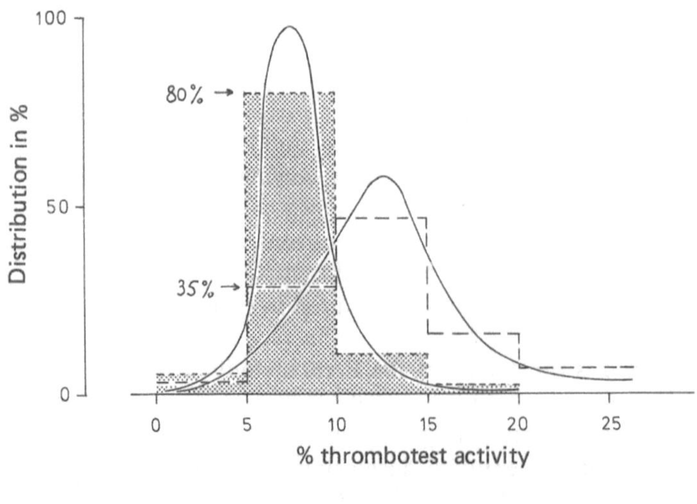

Fig. 1. Distribution of the prothrombin times over the scale of clotting activity (as obtained with Thrombotest) found in patients treated with oral anticoagulants in the Norwegian study and in patients of the Leiden Thrombosis Centre. While in the Norwegian study only 35% of the prothrombin times complied with the therapeutic range of 5%–10% Thrombotest, more than twice the number of prothrombin times were in the optimal range for patients in the Dutch study

prothrombin times are maintained within therapeutic limits of 5%–10% Thrombotest, this was the case for only 35% in Norway. This explains why the incidence of arterial thromboembolism remained high in the Norwegian study. Table 3 summarizes, under the headings "mild OAC" and "mild OAC+ASA," the clinical results of the Norwegian study; those obtained in The Netherlands are presented under the third heading, "adequate OAC". It is clear that the addition of aspirin to mild anticoagulants induced a significant reduction in thromboembolic events, i.e., from 9.3% to 1.8% but at the same time an - in my view - inacceptably high incidence of severe gastrointestinal bleeding. The third column presents data on thromboembolic events as registered in the Leiden Thrombosis Centre and on bleeding complications as observed in the six Dutch Thrombosis Centers which participated in the Sixty-Plus Reinfarction Study (Sixty-Plus Reinfarction Study Research Group 1982), all seven centers applying similarly intensive treatment. These figures unequivocally demonstrate that well-controlled and adequately intensive anticoagulation safely protects the patient with an artificial heart valve against systemic thromboemboli.

Table 3. Incidence (% per year) of thromboembolic events or bleeding complications during well-defined oral anticoagulation (OAC) without and with aspirin (ASA)

		Mild OAC[a] (72% of INR<2.8)		Mild OAC+ASA[a] (67% of INR<2.8)		Adequate OAC (70%–85% of INR>2.8)	
Thromboembolic events		9.3		1.8		±1[b]	
Bleeding complications	GI	1.6	4.7	9.6	13.1	1.5	5.9[c]
	Intracran.	2.3		0.9		1.8	
	Others	0.8		2.6		2.6	

INR, International Normalized Ratio
[a] Dale et al. (1977)
[b] Leiden Thrombosis Center (unpublished retrospective data)
[c] Sixty-Plus Reinfarction Study Research Group (1980)

In terms of these fundamental considerations the results of the Dutch Sixty-Plus Reinfarction Study are easily understood (Sixty-Plus Reinfarction Study Research Group 1980; Mitchell 1981). Table 4 summarizes the statistics on morbidity and mortality in this study, based on efficacy. The reinfarction rate was much lower in the anticoagulant group than in the placebo group ($p<0.001$). Figure 2 illustrates the development of the difference in reinfarctions observed in the two groups over the chosen observation period of 2 years. There was no obvious indication of rebound. Furthermore, the occurrence of reinfarction was not correlated with the duration of anticoagulation of the patients prior to the trial, a period ranging from 6 months to more than 10 years (average, 6 years). These results suggest that adequate long-term oral anticoagulation leads to an impressive lowering (by about 65%) of the incidence of recurrent myocardial infarction, for an unlimited period. This benefit must be weighed against the risks of long-term oral anticoagulation, however, the major risk being intracranial bleeding. Considered on an intention-to-treat basis, the Sixty-Plus Reinfarction Study showed (Table 5) that although the incidence of bleeding increased significantly, fatal as well as nonfatal cerebrovascular accidents tended to occur less frequently in the anticoagulant group than in the placebo group (Sixty-Plus Reinfarction Study Research Group 1982).

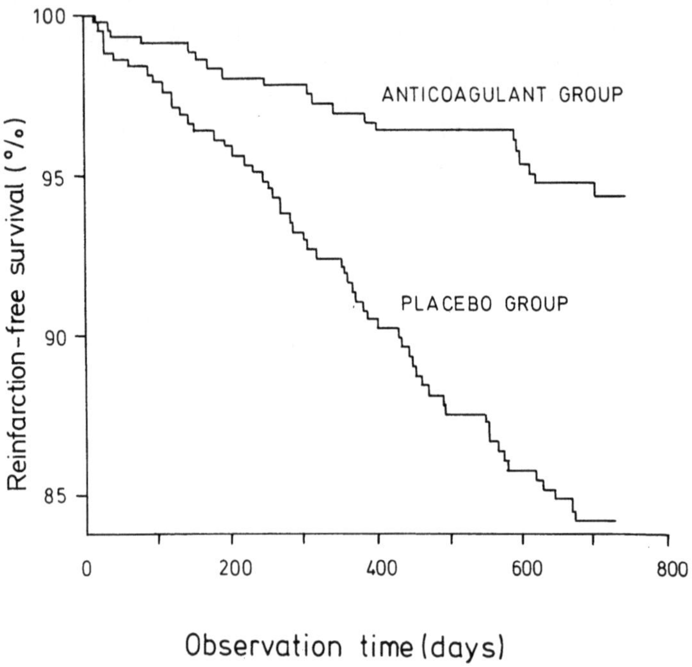

Fig. 2. Curves showing reinfarction-free survival for patients of the two groups studied by the Sixty-Plus Reinfarction Study Group, based on events observed under treatment. The 2-year incidence of recurrent infarction was 5.7% in the anticoagulant-treated group as against 15.9% in the placebo group ($p = 0.001$)

Table 4. Events in Patients of the Sixty-Plus Reinfarction Study (efficacy basis)

	Placebo	OAC
Reinfarction		
(lethal)	58 (24)	20 (4)
Sudden death	14	14
Lethal intracranial		
events	5	6
Other lethal events	6	4

OAC, oral anticoagulant

Table 5. Intracranial events in the Sixty-Plus Reinfarction Study. (), fatal events

	OAC	Placebo
Hemorrhage	8 (6)	1 (1)
Infarction	0	3 (3)
Brain tumor	0	1 (1)
Nature uncertain	4 (3)	15 (7)
Total	12 (9)	20 (12)

OAC, oral anticoagulant

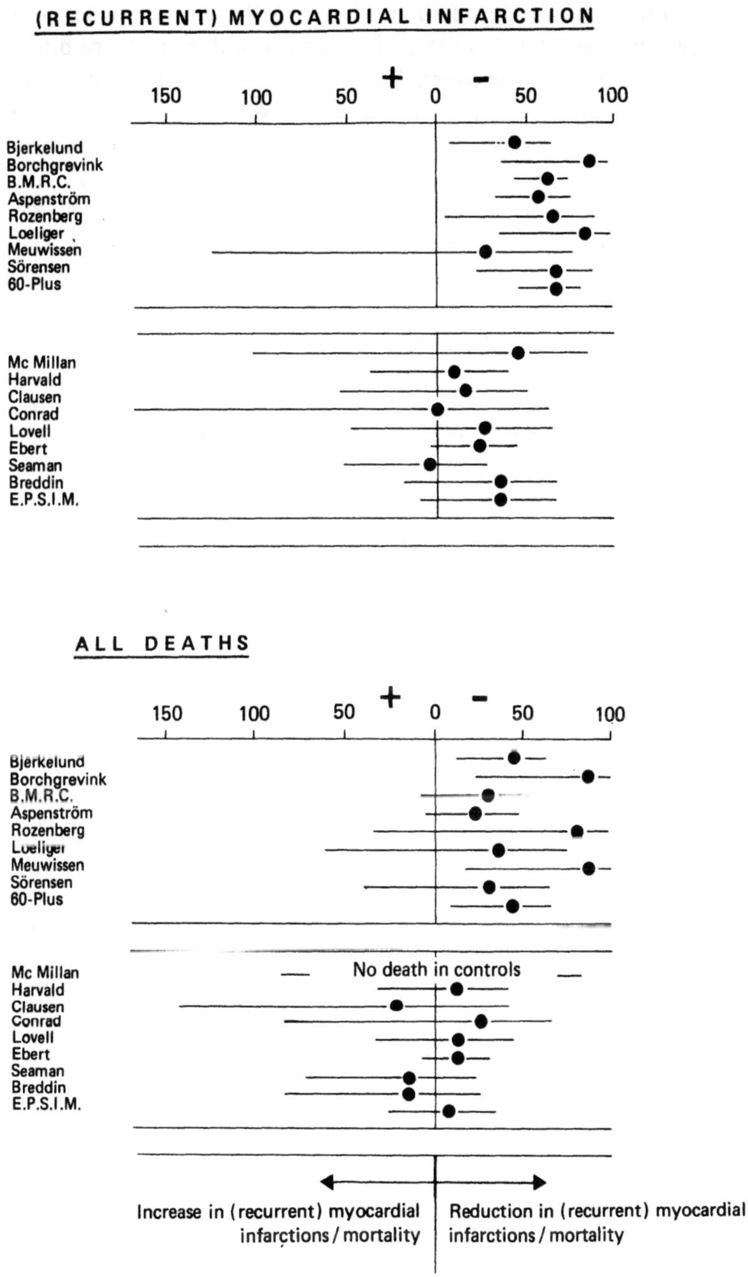

Fig. 3. Schematic representation of the beneficial effect of long-term oral anticoagulant therapy as observed in the 18 published prospective comparative trials in patients with coronary atherothrombosis. In the E.P.S.I.M. study, the controls were on Aspirin. The relative differences in (recurrent) myocardial infarction and total mortality were determined mainly on an efficacy basis. The 9 trials in which levels of anticoagulation were largely *in*side target range 2.5–5 INR (Loeliger and Lewis 1982) are listed in the upper parts of the figure, while those with prothrombin times largely *out*side target range or unknown are presented in the lower parts. 95% confidence limits are based on odd ratio considerations (Baptista and Pike 1977; Thomas and Gast 1977)

Figure 3 shows my personal views on the data provided thus far by prospective clinical trials. On the basis of prothrombin times, published or obtained on request from the authors, I was able to divide the studies into a group of nine likely to have administered levels of anticoagulation sufficient to produce favorable results, and nine who either under- or overtreated, or did not define the levels of anticoagulation. From the data shown in Table 6 and Fig. 3, one must conclude that the group of investigators who administered adequately controlled therapy achieved benefits almost equal to those obtained in the Sixty-Plus Study. Unfortunately, the vast majority of trials did not fulfill the criteria to be met by the type of trial whose results will be considered valid (i.e., true) and generalizable (i.e., widely applicable). A well-designed and well-controlled study, with anticoagulation started at the time of the first myocardial attack and continued, is still lacking. There is good reason to hope, however, that two large-scale studies now in preparation, one in the Netherlands and the other in Norway, will provide the data so badly needed to definitely end the persisting and unfortunate controversy concering the value of long-term oral anticoagulation in the secondary prevention of myocardial infarction.

Table 6. Decrease in events (%) under OAC in 18 trials as compared with the Sixty-Plus Study

	Sixty-Plus study	Trials	
		With adequate OAC ($n=9$)	With insufficiently defined OAC ($n=9$)
Reinfarction	66	60	27
Death	43	42	−1

Three conclusions may be drawn from the data published to date. First, the lowering of the incidence of myocardial reinfarction by long-term prophylaxis with conventional-dose aspirin is, at most, marginal. Second, the postulation of the mild antithrombotic action of aspirin is strongly influenced by the results obtained in patients with heart valve prostheses, in whom aspirin combined with mild oral anticoagulants proved to develop significantly better protection against systemic thromboembolism than did mild oral anticoagulants alone, a benefit for which the price of a high rate of severe gastrointestinal bleeding had to be paid. In such patients, adequately controlled intensive oral anticoagulation alone provides at least equally effective protection with fewer bleeding complications. Third, there is good reason to believe that adequately controlled, intensive long-term oral anticoagulation lowers the risk of reinfarction in patients with transmural myocardial infarction by approximately 65% and, consequently, of overall mortality by about 40%. Such treatment increases the incidence of intracranial bleeding, a risk which is compensated for by the prevention of cerebral thromboembolic events.

References

Altman R, Boullon F, Raca R, et al. (1976) Aspirin and prophylaxis of thromboembolic complications in patients with substitute heart valves. J Thorac Cardiovasc Surg 72:127
AMIS Research Group (1980) A randomized, controlled trial of aspirin in persons recovered from myocardial infarction. JAMA 243:661
Aspenstrøm G, Korsan-Bengtsen K (1964) A double blind study of dicumarol prophylaxis in coronary heart disease. Acta Med Scand 176:563
Baptista J and Pike MC (1977) Exact two-sided confidence limits for the odds ratio in a 2 × 2 table. Applied Stat 26: 214–220
Bjerkelund CJ (1957) The effect of long-term treatment with dicoumarol in myocardial infarction. Acta Med Scand 158 [Suppl 330]:
Borchgrevink CF (1960) Long-term anticoagulant therapy in angina pectoris and myocardial infarction. Acta Med Scand [Suppl 359]
Breddin K, Loew D, Lechner K et al. (1980) Secondary prevention of myocardial infarction: a comparison of acetylsalicylic acid, placebo and phenprocoumon. Haemostasis 9:325
British Medical Research Council (1964) An assessment of long-term anticoagulant administration after cardiac infarction. Br Med J 2:837
Clausen J, Andersen PE, Andresen P, et al. (1961) Langtids-antikoagulansbehandling efter akut hjerteinfarkt. Ugeskr Laeger 123:987
Conrad LL, Kyriacopoulos JD, Wiggins CW et al. (1964) Prevention of recurrences of myocardial infarction. Arch Intern Med 114:348
Dale J (1976) Arterial thromboembolic complications in patients with Starr-Edwards aortic ball balve prostheses. Am Heart J 91:653
Dale J (1977) Arterial thromboembolic complications in patients with Björk-Shiley and Lillehei-Kaster aortic disc valve prostheses. Am Heart J 93:715
Dale J, Myhre E, Storstein O, et al. (1977) Prevention of arterial thromboembolism with acetylalicylic acid. A controlled clinical study in patients with aortic ball valves. Am Heart J 94:101
Duxbury BMcD (1982) Therapeutic control of anticoagulant treatment. Br Med J 284:702
Ebert RV, Borden CW, Hipp HR et al. (1969) Long-term anticoagulant therapy after myocardial infarction. JAMA 207:2263
EPSIM Research Group (1982) A controlled comparison of aspirin and oral anticoagulants in prevention of death after myocardial infarction. N Engl J Med 307:701
Harvald B, Hilden T, Lund E (1962) Long-term anticoagulant therapy after myocardial infarction. Lancet II:626
Loeliger EA (1981) Oral anticoagulation in the secondary prevention of myocardial infarction. Acta Med Scand 210 [Suppl. 651]:3
Loeliger EA (1983) A controlled comparison of aspirin and oral anticoagulants in prevention of death after myocardial infarction. N Engl J Med 308:282
Loeliger EA, Lewis SM (1982) Progress in laboratory control of oral anticoagulants. Lancet 2:318
Loeliger EA, Hensen A, Kroes F, et al. (1967) A double-blind trial of long-term anticoagulant treatment after myocardial infarction. Acta Med Scand 182:549
Lovell RHH, Denborough MA, Nestel PJ et al. (1967) A controlled trial of long-term treatment with anticoagulants after myocardial infarction in 412 male patients. Med J Aust 2:97
MacMillan RL, Brown KWG, Watt DL (1960) Long-term anticoagulant therapy after myocardial infarction. Can Med Assoc J 83:567
Meuwissen OJAT, Vervoorn AC, Cohen O, et al. (1969) Double-blind trial of long-term anticoagulant treatment after myocardial infarction. Acta Med Scand 186:361
Mitchell JRA (1981) Anticoagulants in coronary heart disease – retrospect and prospect. Lancet 1:257
Poller L (1982) Anticoagulants reassessed. Br Med J 284:1425
Rozenberg MC, Kronenberg H, Firkin BG (1965) "Thrombotest" and prothrombin time: a controlled clinical trial. Aust Ann Med 14:3

Seaman AJ, Griswold HE, Reaume RB et al. (1969) Long-term anticoagulant prophylaxis after myocardial infarction. N Engl J Med 281:115
Sixty-Plus Reinfarction Study Research Group (1980) A double-blind trial to assess long-term oral anticoagulant therapy in elderly patients after myocardial infarction. Lancet 2:989
Sixty-Plus Reinfarction Study Research Group (1982) Risks of longterm oral anticoagulant therapy in elderly patients after myocardial infarction Lancet 1:64
Sørensen OH, Friis T, Jørgensen AW, et al. (1969) Anticoagulant treatment of acute coronary thrombosis. Acta Med Scand 185:65
Thomas DG and Gart JJ (1977) A table of exact confidence limits for differences and ratios of two proportions and their odds ratio. J Am Stat Assoc 72:73

The Influence of Verapamil Treatment During Acute Myocardial Infarction on Long-Term Prognosis

J. F. Hansen

Medical Department B, Frederiksborg Country Hospital, 3400 Hillerød, Denmark

A double-blind study comparing verapamil with placebo was conducted in 16 Danish medical departments of internal medicine with coronary care units (CCU). All patients below 75 years of age admitted to the CCU with a suspicion of acute myocardial infarction (AMI) were evaluated. Of 7415 patients, 3917 were excluded at admission because of heart failure, heart block, other severely disabling diseases, or treatment with beta-blockers or Ca^{++}-antagonists.

Treatment was started in 3498 patients with 0.1 mg/kg verapamil i.v. and 120 mg perorally at admission followed by 120 mg t.i.d., or matched placebo. Treatment was continued for 6 months for patients verified to have had an AMI according to all three WHO criteria. Treatment was stopped in patients for whom AMI was ruled out. Of 1436 patients with AMI, 717 were treated with verapamil and 719 with placcbo.

After 6 months, 92 patients (12.8%) in the verapamil group and 100 patients (13.9%) in the placebo group were dead. There were a total of 50 reinfarctions (7.0%) in the verapamil group and 60 (8.3%) in the placebo group.

The Possible Influence of Nitrates on Prognosis in Patients with Coronary Heart Disease

W.-D. Bussmann

Klinikum der Johann Wolfgang Goethe-Universität, Zentrum der Inneren Medizin
Abteilung für Kardiologie, Theodor-Stern-Kai 7, 6000 Frankfurt 70, FRG

The question whether nitrates influence prognosis in patients with coronary heart disease cannot be answered from the tentative data available to date from a small group of researchers (Bussmann 1980a; Bussmann et al. 1980a; Bussmann and Giebeler 1983; Bussmann and Haller 1983; Chatterjee et al. 1976; Chiche et al. 1929; Derrida et al. 1978; Flaherty et al. 1980; D. Bennett, 1982, personal communication). At best, these pilot studies can serve to stimulate new trials with larger patient populations.

The first part of this report is concerned with the use of nitrates during acute myocardial infarction (see Bussmann 1980b, 1981; Bussmann et al. 1974, 1976, 1979a, 1980a, b, 1981b; Flaherty et al. 1980). Can intravenous nitroglycerin influence morbidity and mortality in such patients? The second part considers the effect on prognosis when patients with coronary artery disease are treated with nitrates on a long-term basis. Only two studies are available on this topic (Bussmann et al. 1980a, 1981a, 1982; Bussmann and Giebeler 1983; Bussmann and Haller 1983).

Acute Myocardial Infarction

What is known about the early phase following acute myocardial infarction when nitroglycerin is administered intravenously? We evaluated 60 patients in a prospective randomized trial (Bussmann et al. 1981b); 31 received nitroglycerin for 2–4 days, 29 patients served as controls. Both groups were comparable as to age, site of myocardial infarction, and baseline hemodynamics. Diastolic pulmonary artery pressure was about 20 mmHg in both groups.

Morbidity was favorably influenced in the nitroglycerin-treated patients. They had less pain, less dyspnea and fewer ventricular arrhythmias. Bradycardia was less frequent, and there was evidence for less ischemia and reduced infarct size (Bussmann 1981). Ventricular ectopic beats and ventricular fibrillation were also less frequent in patients treated with nitroglycerin than in the control group (Bussmann et al. 1980b).

Frequent ventricular ectopic beats were present in 20% of nitroglycerin-treated patients, as compared with 50% of the control group. The need for lidocaine was reduced as well. The effect on ventricular arrhythmias may have prognostic significance for patients with reinfraction or recurrent myocardial ischemia.

There was less ischemia with nitroglycerin treatment, as evidenced by the reduction in ST-segment elevation during acute intervention, and infarct size was reduced by 30% (Bussmann et al. 1979b, 1981b). CK and CK-MB were used as indices of infarct size.

The development of Q waves was much smaller in patients who received nitroglycerin. Compared with day 1, smaller Q waves were present on day 5 and day 30 (Dowinsky et al. 1982). Chiche and coworkers reported similar results: R-wave reduction following treatment was half of that in the control group (Chiche et al. 1929; Derrida et al. 1978).

Mortality

If morbidity is apparently lower in treated patients, does this imply reduced mortality? During our study five control patients died (see Fig. 1). Only one of the nitroglycerin patients died, during emergency bypass surgery for severe angina pectoris (Bussmann et al. 1980a; Bussmann and Haller 1983).

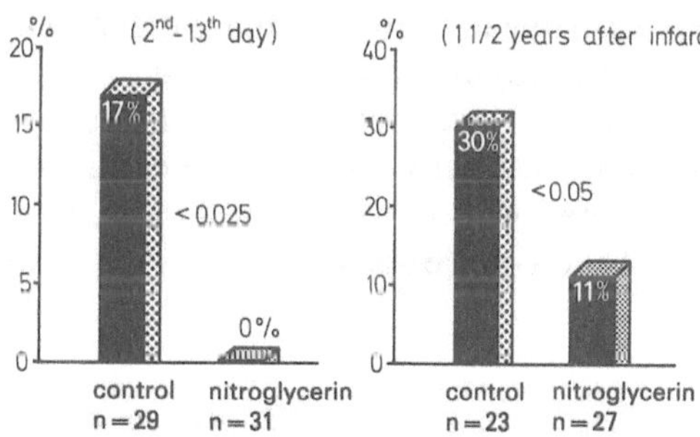

Fig. 1. Early and late cardiac mortality in patients whose myocardial infarctions were treated with nitroglycerin during the acute phase and in controls. Only one nitroglycerin-treated patient died, during emergency bypass surgery on the 6th day postinfarction (*asterisk*). In the control group five patients died (17%)

In Chiche's randomized study seven of 35 controls and two of 35 nitroglycerin-treated patients died (Chiche et al. 1929). David Bennett of St. George's Hospital, London, conducted a double-blind study on the effect of intravenous nitroglycerin on 140 patients with acute myocardial infarction. Nine in the control group died, compared with five during nitroglycerin treatment (D. Bennet 1980, personal communication). Bennett found a 30% reduction in cumulative CK-MB values as well. Flaherty and coworkers had results pointing in the same direction: less mortality and less congestive failure were present in the group treated with nitroglycerin (Flaherty et al. 1980).

It is interesting to note that there was a higher incidence of reinfarction as a cause of death in our cohort during the first few days. The current patient population, however – and this is important – is too small to allow for any definite conclusions. These preliminary data must be confirmed by future studies of larger patient populations.

Postinfarction Period

Obtaining conclusive data for the postinfarction period with respect to the possible influence of nitrates appears to be even more difficult. We evaluated our own patients up to 2 years after the acute myocardial event (Fig. 1). The mortality was 11% in patients initially treated with nitroglycerin and 27% in untreated patients (Bussmann et al. 1980a; Bussmann and Haller 1983).

One important difference between the groups was in the severity of angina pectoris. The nitroglycerin-treated patients had less necrosis, as mentioned before, and consequently more angina during follow-up. Patients with complete extension of their infarction had less severe angina pectoris during follow-up. The dose of nitrates used in these patients correlated with the severity of angina. The daily dose was 38 mg isosorbide dinitrate, as compared with 21 mg/day in the control group (Bussmann et al. 1980a; Busmann and Haller 1983). On the other hand, reduced late mortality may be due primarily to the higher dose of nitrates.

The only paradox, then, is that patients with severe angina pectoris seem to have a better prognosis than those with a less severe type of angina. Reduced infarct size due to nitroglycerin treatment may also contribute to the better outcome in this group, since some fatalities were related to heart failure.

In our study we found a large difference between the groups (Fig. 1 and 2) there being less early and less late cardiac mortality in patients who were initially treated with nitroglycerin and were on sustained high doses of nitrates during follow-up (Bussmann et al. 1980a, Bussmann and Haller 1983).

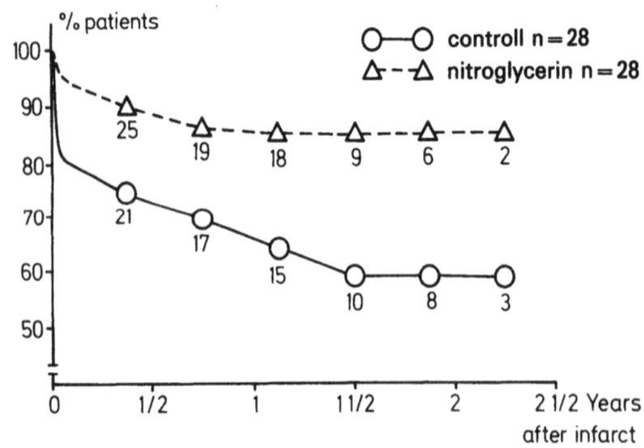

Fig. 2. Early and late cardiac mortality in controls and nitroglycerin-treated patients

Again, however, this result should be viewed with scepticism, since the number of patients randomized is not large enough to make the data statistically convincing. We then evaluated the causes for death during acute myocardial infarction and during follow-up. The incidence of sudden death and reinfarction with or without death was 39% for the control patients, but only 11% for the nitroglycerin-treated group (Fig. 3). Thus, sudden death and reinfarc-

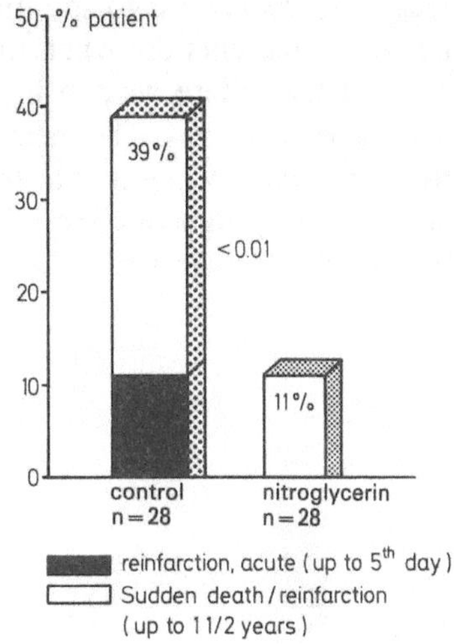

Fig. 3. Incidence of sudden death, and reinfarction with or without death, in the treated and untreated groups. Nitroglycerin-treated patients had three events, as compared with 11 events in the control group

tion seem to be reduced when nitroglycerin is given during the acute phase and an effective dose of isosorbide dinitrate is used during follow-up.

Patients with Coronary Heart Disease: Longterm Effects

The study just reviewed was related to patients undergoing nitrate therapy during the acute and chronic phase. Another study was carried out exclusively on patients with coronary heart disease receiving nitrates during the chronic phase (Bussmann et al. 1981a; Bussmann and Giebeler 1983). There are at least some similarities between the two.

A questionnaire was filled out by those patients still living of 293 who had undergone coronary angiography and ventriculography 7 years earlier. Data on those who had died during the intervening period were culled from medical records and information supplied by family physicians.

It was ascertained that 168 of the patients had received daily doses of nitrates (isosorbide dinitrate, Pharma Schwarz, Monheim). Of these 168, 112 were survivors and 56 had died. The patients who had received nitrates formed two groups - those on a daily dose of <40 mg isosorbide dinitrate (group 1), and those on a daily dose of >40 mg (group 2).

Two-thirds of the case fatalities occurred in patients taking the low dose - less than 40 mg - and only one-third following intake of the higher dose. In the survivors' group, half of the patients were on a low dose of nitrates and half were on a high dose (Fig. 4).

Left ventricular function was assessed by scoring hypo-, a-, and dyskinesis in six different wall segments. Mean values of 6.2 and 6.3 respectively were present in the groups on high and low doses of nitrates. Since this important prognostic parameter is nearly identical in both groups, the difference in mortality may be related to the nitrate dose. Again, this result seems to indicate that fewer patients die when they are on a high-dose regimen.

With time there was an increasing separation between the high- and low-dose survival curves. The mean dose of isosorbide dinitrate was 55 mg/day in the upper and 14 mg/day in the lower curve (Fig. 5). Patients on a high dose have a better prognosis. Mortality was reduced by 30%, compared with the rate for the low-dose group.

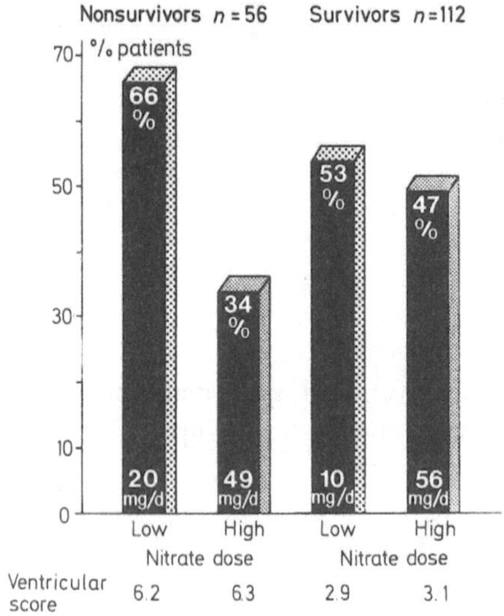

Fig. 4. Less patients died on a high dose of nitrates

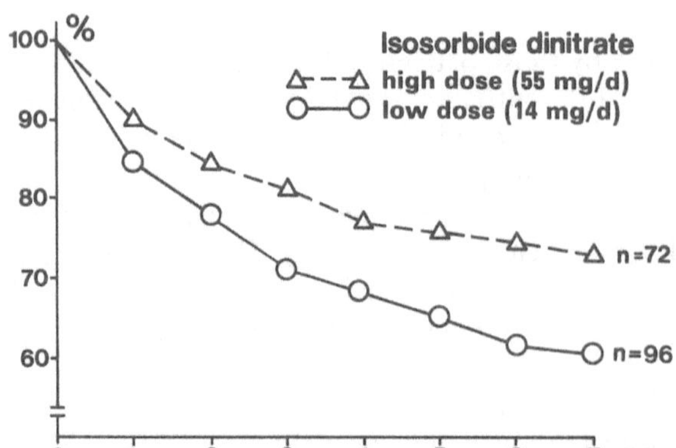

Fig. 5. Seven-year survival rate for 168 patients with coronary heart disease, treated with low and high doses of isosorbide dinitrate.
Mortality in patients on a high dose of isosorbide dinitrate was reduced by 30%–40% in comparison with the low-dose group. The probability of surviving was significantly higher in the high-dose group ($p < 0.06$, Gehan test)

Both groups were compared with regard to the extent of coronary lesions and of ventricular dysfunction, using a score. Ventricular and coronary score were the same in both groups. The heart volume determined by X-ray did not differ significantly. Thus, based on these parameters the groups were comparable.

However, angina pectoris was more severe in patients receiving high doses, and ST-segment depression in the exercise ECG was significantly more extensive in this group. There was no major difference in the use of beta-blockers, calcium-antagonists, or aggregation inhibitors.

In addition to the fact that this is the first study to evaluate this important item, the design of the study itself has several important limitations:

1. The study was carried out retrospectively in a limited number of patients; prospective studies are warranted. However, the first study showing the beneficial effect of beta-blockers on prognosis was also retrospective (Snow 1965).
2. The sources of information on survivors and nonsurvivors were different. Survivors had to fill out a questionnaire; for nonsurvivors charts were consulted or the family physicians were interviewed.
3. The dose amounts used for analysis are the dose taken at the end of the 7-year observation period by survivors and the last dose taken by nonsurvivors. It is not known whether patients took these doses regularly over the entire period.
4. Ventricular and coronary score and heart volume were nearly identical in both groups. However, the severity of angina pectoris and the ST-segment depression during exercise differed: Patients on high doses had more angina and a more pronounced ischemia during exercise than did those on low doses.
5. Patients with more angina pectoris may develop better collaterals, which in turn relates to a better prognosis. Thus, the higher dose of nitrates may be an indicator for the group but not a clear causal factor (Schneider et al. 1982).

Due to these limiting circumstances a conclusion should be drawn with caution: This retrospective study seems to give some evidence for a favorable influence of a higher dose of nitrates on the prognosis in patients with coronary heart disease.

In Februar 1980 we initiated a double-blind, multicenter study in the Frankfurt area. A total of 1000 patients will be randomized to low- and high-dose groups. The high-dose group receives 200 mg isosorbide dinitrate per day, the low-dose group, 12.5 mg. Our objective is to determine ultimate mortality and morbidity in the two collectives. This will take 3–5 years.

Conclusions

In conclusion, there seems to be at least some evidence that nitrates favorably influence early and late mortality in patients who have suffered acute myocardial infarction, or in those with coronary heart disease. Preliminary findings are encouraging enough to warrant additional investigation into this aspect of nitrate therapy in the future.

References

Bussmann W-D (1980a) Do nitrates influence prognosis? European Congress of Cardiology, Paris

Bussmann W-D (1980b) Nitroglycerin bei Herzinfarkt - Von der Kontraindikation zur Indikation. Dtsch Med Wochenschr 105:1551

Bussmann W-D (1981) Nitroglycerin in the treatment of acute myocardial infarction. Acta Med Scand 210 [Suppl 651]:165

Bussmann W-D, Giebeler B (1983) Beeinflußt eine Dauertherapie mit hochdosierten Nitraten die Prognose bei koronarer Herzkrankheit? Klin Wochenschr 61:423

Bussmann W-D, Haller M (1983) Hinweis auf eine Abnahme der Früh- und Spätmortalität beim frischen Herzinfarkt unter Nitroglycerintherapie. Klin Wochenschr 61:417

Bussmann W-D, Vachalowa J, Kaltenbach M (1974) Wirkung von Nitroglycerin beim frischen Herzinfarkt. Z Kardiol [Suppl] I:25 (abstract)

Bussmann W-D, Schöfer H, Kaltenbach M (1976) Wirkung von Nitroglycerin beim akuten Myokardinfarkt. II. Intravenöse Dauerinfusion von Nitroglycerin bei Patienten mit und ohne Linksinsuffizienz und Auswirkung auf die Infarktgröße. Dtsch Med Wochenschr 101:642

Bussmann W-D, Barthe G, Klepzig H Jr, Kaltenbach M (1979a) Nitroglycerindauertherapie beim frischen Herzinfarkt im Vergleich zu einer nicht behandelten Kontrollgruppe. Med Klin 74:191

Bussmann W-D, Schöfer H, Kurita H, Ganz W (1979b) Nitroglycerin in acute myocardial infarction. X. Effect of small and large doses of i.v. nitroglycerin on ST-segment deviation; experimental and clinical results. Clin Cardiol 2:106

Bussmann W-D, Haller M, Kaltenbach M (1980a) Nitroglycerin bei frischem Herzinfarkt. Einfluß auf spätere Angina pectoris. Beeinflussung der Prognose? Z Kardiol 69:201

Bussmann W-D, Neumann K, Kaltenbach M (1980b) Die Wirkung von Nitroglycerin auf die ventrikuläre Extrasystolie beim frischen Herzinfarkt. Dtsch Med Wochenschr 105:369

Bussmann W-D, Giebeler B, Kaltenbach M (1981a) Beeinflussen hochdosierte Nitrate die Prognose bei koronarer Herzkrankheit? Z Kardiol 69:201 (abstract)

Bussmann W-D, Passek D, Seidel W, Kaltenbach M (1981b) Reduction of CK and CK-MP indexes of infarct size by intravenous nitroglycerin. Circulation 63:615

Bussmann W-D, Schneider W, Kaltenbach M (1982) Anfalls- und Langzeittherapie der koronaren Herzkrankheit mit Nitraten. Z Kardiol 71:583 (abstract)

Chatterjee K, Swan HJC, Kaushik VS, Jobin DMG, Magnusson P, Forrester JS (1976) Effects of vasodilatator therapy for severe pump failure in acute myocardial infarction on short-term and late prognosis. Circulation 53:797

Chiche P, Baligadoo SJ, Derrida JP (1979) A randomized trial of prolonged nitroglycerin infusion in acute myocardial infarction. Circulation 59+60 [Suppl II]: 165

Derrida JP, Sal R, Chiche P (1978) Favorable effects of prolonged nitroglycerin infusion in patients with acute myocardial infarction. Am Heart J 96:833 (annotation)

Dowinsky S, Rose D-M, Bussmann W-D (1982) Abnahme von QRS-Nekrosezeichen unter Nitroglyerintherapie beim frischen Herzinfarkt. Z Kardiol 71:252 (Abstrakt)

Flaherty JT, Becker LC, Weisfeldt ML, Weiss JL, Gerstenblith G, Kallman CH, Bulkley BH (1980) Results of prospective randomized clinical trial of intravenous nitroglycerin in acute myocardial infarction. Circulation 62 [Suppl III] 82 (abstract)

Schneider W, Stahl B, Kaltenbach M, Bussmann W-D (1982) Dosis-Wirkungs-Beziehungen bei der Behandlung der Angina pectoris mit Isosorbiddinitrat. Dtsch Med Wochenschr 107:771

Snow PJD (1965) Effect of propranolol in myocardial infarction. Lancet 551

Selection of Patients for Coronary Bypass Surgery

E. Varnauskas

Department of Cardiology, Medical Clinic I, Sahlgrenska Hospital, 41345 Göteborg, Sweden

Most patients who suffer from angina pectoris resistant to medical therapy experience dramatic relief of pain following bypass surgery. Since the introduction of this spectacular method of treatment into cardiological practice, unacceptably severe angina has been considered an indisputable indication for coronary bypass surgery. Although the definition of what is "unacceptable" angina may vary considerably with local medical practices, coronary angiography is the only investigation needed to assess whether bypass operation has a reasonable chance of curing the symptom.

Quite another question arises when coronary bypass surgery is considered for the purpose of preventing premature death. Although two large prospective studies (Takaro et al. 1982a; European Coronary Surgery Study Group 1982) have convincingly demonstrated that surgery prolongs life in patients with stable angina, and one of them (European Coronary Surgery Study Group 1982) actually showed that this advantage is achieved in patients not requiring operation for pain relief, the question regarding more precise definition of candidates for preventive surgery is still unsettled.

The main purpose of this report is to summarize the results of the European Coronary Surgery Study Group (1982) regarding survival, and to focus the attention on the problem of selecting patients likely to experience significantly improved survival with coronary bypass surgery.

The European Coronary Surgery Study Group (1982) performed a prospective, randomized study on a well-defined patient population sample to test the hypothesis that surgery prolongs life. The study included men aged less than 65 years, with stable angina controlled by medical therapy, at least 50% stenosis in two or more major coronary arteries, and good left ventricular function (ejection fraction ≥ 0.5). Patients with intractable angina were not included. The randomization procedure assured equal distribution of prognostically important variables between the two treatment groups, making them comparable. Operative mortality, the number of inserted grafts, and graft patency were on the same order of magnitude as reported by major centers for the corresponding period of time (1973–1976). The proportion of patients experiencing immediate postoperative relief from agnina was in excellent agreement with data reported in the literature. Both treatment groups received high-level medical care, including measures of rehabilitation and secondary prevention, from the beginning of the study. Treatment with antianginal drugs – beta-blockers and nitrates – was maintained as long as medically indicated; in the vast majority of surgically treated patients this treatment was discontinued because of postoperative relief from angina. Coronary bypass surgery was done as soon as possible after randomization in patients assigned to the surgical group. If at any time a patient in the medical group had unacceptable symptoms despite adequate medical therapy, he was eligible for surgery. The minimum followup time was 5 years and the maximum 8. The group of patients randomized to medical treatment was compared with the group randomized to coronary bypass surgery, regardless of what happened to them after randomization. By retaining all patients in their original randomly allocated groups, and by not censoring medical patients who eventually received coronary bypass surgery or excluding surgical patients who were never operated on, this study actually compares the policy of conservative management (medical treatment being the treatment of choice) with the policy of early surgery (coronary bypass surgery being the treatment of first choice).

The following 27 variables were tested for incidence to identify those independently predictive of survival:

1. Mode of treatment
2. Smoking
3. Diabetes mellitus
4. Arterial hypertension
5. Peripheral arterial disease
6. Angina pectoris
7. Length of history of angina
8. History of previous MI
9. Use of digitalis drugs
10. Use of diuretic drugs
11. Use of beta-blocking drugs
12. Resting heart rate
13. Heart rhythm
14. Apical systolic murmur
15. Systolic arterial blood pressure
16. Diastolic arterial blood pressure
17. Resting ECG
18. Serum Cholesterol
19. Heart size (chest roentgenogram)
20. Exercise ECG: ST-segment response
21. Maximum exercise load achieved
22. LV end-diastolic pressure
23. LV ejection fraction
24. Segmental LV wall movements
25. Number of vessels with stenosis
26. Proximal LAD stenosis
27. Age

Seven proved to be indepentently predictive: (a) mode of treatment; (b) number of vessels with stenosis; (c) stenosis in the proximal third of the left anterior descending artery (proximal LAD) as a component of either two- or three-vessel disease; (d) resting ECG showing signs suggestive of previous myocardial infarction and/or specified abnormalities according to the criteria of the HIP Study (Frank et al. 1963); (e) ischemic ST-segment response, predominantly in lead V_5, during maximum level of multistage symptom/sign limited bicycle exercise; (f) peripheral arterial disease diagnosed from history and physical examination; (g) age. In Table 1 survival is compared for the two modes of treatment in the total patient population and in the subsets of patients defined by each of the other six independent predictors. These comparisons convincingly demonstrate significant improvement of long-term survival with the policy of early surgery, the improvement being related to the variables predictive of risk for poor survival.

To evaluate the preventive effect of coronary bypass surgery in patients with various sets of prognostic predictors a probability of surviving 5 years

Table 1. Survival data from the European Coronary Surgery Study (1982)

	Survival at					
	5-year follow-up			8-year follow-up		
	M (%)	S (%)	*p* value[b]	M (%)	S (%)	*p* value[b]
Total population	84	92	.00025	80	89	.0013
Three-vesse disease	82	94	.0003	77	92	.00015
Left main disease	68	86	.11	64	82	.12
Two-vessel disease	88	91	>.20	87	85	>.20
Proximal LAD stenosis[a]	82	93	.0004	79	88	.003
No proximal LAD stenosis	92	93	>.20	88	92	>.20
Exertional ST>1.5 mm	79	92	.0003	77	90	.0003
Exertional ST 0–1 mm	90	95	>.20	85	88	>.20
Resting ECG abnormal	79	90	.0052	73	86	.0049
Resting ECG normal	88	95	.02	87	91	.10
Peripheral artery disease	82	93	.0004	79	88	.003
No peripheral artery disease	92	93	>.20	88	92	>.20
Age >50 years	80	91	.0023	74	84	.17
Age ≤50 years	87	94	.040	85	93	.030

M, medical group; *S*, surgical group

[a] Stenosis in the proximal third of the left anterior descending artery as a component of two- or three-vessel disease.

[b] *p* value represents significance level of survival differences between the two policies of treatment tested by incidence.

with either of the two modes of treatment was estimated by Cox's regression analysis, adjusting for independent predictors of survival (Fig. 1). The figure demonstrates that the estimated 5-year survival with the policy of conservative management decreases with an increasing number of prognostic predictors. It also shows that the policy of early surgery eliminates this predictor effect; survival with the policy of early surgery is estimated at 93%, irrespective of the number of predictors present. While it is highly probable that coronary bypass grafting strongly improves 5-year survival in patients having all predictors of poor prognosis, surgery is unlikely to produce any significant survival benefit over a 5-year period in relatively young symptomatic patients (under 50 years of age) having a normal resting ECG, less than 1.5 mm exertional ST-segment depression, and no peripheral arterial disease.

It might appear surprising that variables related to left ventricular function (ejection fraction, end-diastolic pressure, segmental wall motion abnormalities) were not independently predictive of survival in the European Study. However, this is readily explained by the fact that patients with manifest left ventricular failure, ejection fraction less than 0.5, and left ventricular aneurysm requiring surgery were not included in the study. Likewise, patients with uncontrolled arterial hypertension were not admitted. Recent survival studies comprising patients with ejection fraction down to ≤0.3 have conformed that left ventricular ejection fraction is a powerful predictor in medically treated patients (Mock et al. 1982; Hammermeister et al. 1982), as well as being a potent predictor in surgical series (Hammermeister et al. 1982). The exact border value for left ventricular ejection fraction, below which coronary bypass surgery fails to improve survival, has not been conclusively established. Ejection fraction of 0.3 is considered by many to be such a limit.

Noninvasive predictors of improved survival with coronary bypass surgery proposed by other studies (Takaro et al. 1982a, b; Hammermeister et al. 1982) differ slightly from those of the European Study. This is most likely explained by differences in selecting study population, design of study, surgical experience, and baseline variables tested.

It seems highly justified and necessary that noninvasive variables predictive of improved survival with surgery should be taken into consideration before submitting a patient for coronary angiography. Such predictors emerging from the three studies are here summarized.

Predictors in the European Study (European Coronary Surgery Study Group 1982) were: (a) resting ECG suggestive of possible or probable old myocardial infarction and/or with specified abnormalities according to the criteria of the HIP study (Frank et al. 1963); (b) exertional ST-segment depression of 1.5 mm or more; (c) peripheral arterial disease diagnosed from history and physical examination; (d) increasing age.

Predictors in the Veterans Administration Cooperative Study (Takaro et al. 1982a, b) were: (a) New York Heart Association functional class III or IV; (b) a

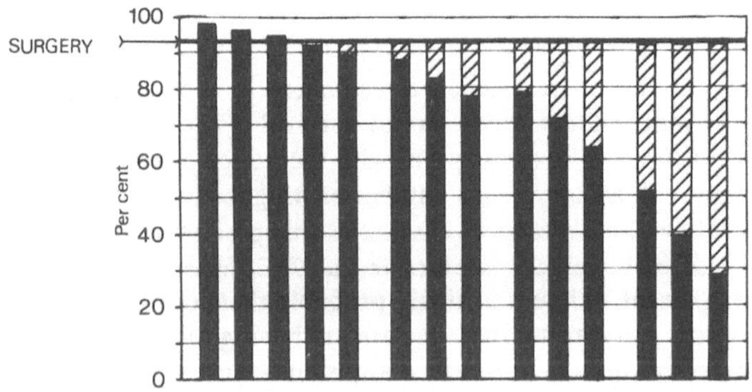

PERIPH. ART. DIS.	0	0	0	0	0	0	0	0	0	0	0	+	+	+
ABNORM. REST. ECG.	0	0	0	0	0	0	0	0	+	+	+	+	+	+
EX. ST. DEPR. ≥ 1.5	0	0	0	0	0	+	+	+	+	+	+	+	+	+
Px LAD STENOSIS	0	0	+	+	–	+	+	–	+	+	–	+	+	–
VESSEL DISEASE	2	3	2	3	LM	2	3	LM	2	3	LM	2	3	LM

Fig. 1. European CS Study (1982)
Estimated 5-year survival (%) by means of Cox's regression analysis in relation to variables predictive of survival. Age is 50 years in all instances. The decreasing survival with increasing number of predictors is present only with the policy of conservative management = ■. With the policy of early surgery the estimated 5-year survival is 93% (⤚), irrespective of presence or absence of prognostic predictors.
▨, estimated survival improvement with the policy of early surgery; *O*, absent; +, present; –, irrelevant; *LM*, left main disease; *Px*, proximal

history of myocardial infarction; (c) a history of hypertension; (d) ST-segment depression on the baseline resting ECG as defined by the Minnesota code. Low-, middle-, and high-risk groups were created on the basis of these four predictors.

Predictors in the Seattle Heart Watch Nonrandomized Study (Hammermeister et al. 1982) were: (a) age ≥48 years; (b) no history of congestive heart failure (corresponding invasive criterion is ejection fraction ≥0.3); (c) no cardiomegaly; (d) no ventricular arrhythmias on resting ECG; (e) no diuretic use; (f) no heart murmur.

It should be noted that there is not much disagreement between these three sets of selection criteria. The criteria derived from the European Study are not in conflict with those derived from Seattle Heart Watch Nonrandomized Study since the European Study by design did not include patients having manifest congestive failure, cardiomegaly, or systolic murmur suggestive of significant mitral regurgitation. Actually, three important predictors in the European Study - signs of myocardial ischemia in resting ECG, markedly positive exercise ECG, and coexisting peripheral arterial disease - supplement rather than contradict the selection ciriteria of the Seattle Study.

The finding of the VA Study that history of arterial hypertension is predictive of improved survival with surgery is in contrast to the finding of the European Study. However, this is readily explained by the fact that patients in whom arterial hypertension was not controlled by medical treatment were not included in the European Study. Another factor of discrepancy is a history of myocardial infarction, which had predictive power in the VA Study but not in the Eurpean Study. A possible explanation is that in the European Study old myocardial infarction was efficiently disclosed by the analysis of the resting ECG, and a history of myocardial infarction had no independent predictive power. New York Heart Association functional class III or IV is generally accepted as a strong indication for coronary bypass surgery solely to relieve pain and has little relevance in this discussion regarding selection of candidates for preventive coronary bypass surgery.

In summary, coronary angiography is strongly indicated in symptomatic patients 50 years of age or younger who have at least two of the three criteria listed below, and in older patients who have at least a positive exercise test according to point 2.

1. Abnormal resting ECG: Signs suggestive of previous possible or probable myocardial infarction and/or specified abnormalities according to the criteria of the HIP Study (Frank et al. 1963)
2. Positive exercise test: ST-segment depression of 1.5 mm or more during maximum level of exercise
3. Peripheral arterial disease diagnosed from history and physical examination

In addition, the patient should not have symptoms or signs of (a) manifest congestive heart failure; (b) cardiomegaly; (c) heart murmur suggestive of significant mitral regurgitation; (d) insufficiently controlled arterial hypertension;

(e) diabetes mellitus requiring insulin; (f) diseases and conditions capable of shortening 5-year survival.

Coronary angiography provides the basis for making the final decision regarding surgery. Assuming that at least 20% improvement of the estimated 5-year survival is a resonable condition, early coronary bypass surgery should be seriously considered in the presence of 50% stenosis and LV ejection fraction ≥0.3 in the following categoris of patients:

1. Patients with left main disease who are 50 years of age or younger and have at least a positive exercise test and an abnormal resting ECG. In patients who are older than 50 a positive exercise test alone is sufficient to indicate surgery.
2. Patients with three-vessel disease including stenosis in the proximal third of the LAD (proximal LAD) who meet the same criteria as patients with left main disease (see 1).
3. Patients with three-vessel disease without proximal LAD stenosis who are 50 or younger and have all three noninvasive variables (positive exercise test, abnormal resting ECG, and peripheral arterial disease). In patients who are older than 50, at least a positive exercise test and peripheral arterial disease are required (this combination has higher predictive value than a combination of a positive exercise test and an abnormal resting ECG).
4. Patients with two-vessel disease including proximal LAD stenosis who are 50 or younger and have at least a positive exercise test and peripheral arterial disease. Patients who are older than 50 should have at least a positive exercise test and an abnormal resting ECG.
5. Patients with two-vessel disease without proximal LAD stenosis who are 50 or younger should have all three noninvasive predictors. In older patients at least a positive exercise test and peripheral arterial disease should be present.

The above selection criteria are based on the estimated values for 5-year survival and are valid only if used together with a sound clinical judgement. For instance, a markedly positive exercise test (ST depression ≥1.5 mm, low level of maximum exercise performed, insufficient increase in systolic blood pressure) carries heavier prognostic weight than a positive exercise test.

It is recognized that desires and anxiety of patients, local interest and medical practices, local "results" of diagnostic tests, and management strategies influence clinical decision making (Friesinger 1982).

References

European Coronary Surgery Study Group (1982) Long-term results of prospective randomized study of coronary artery bypass surgery in stable angina pectoris. Lancet II:1173

Frank CW, Weinblatt E, Shapiro S, Seiden GE, Sager RV (1963) The HIP Study of incidence and prognosis of coronary heart disease: criteria for diagnosis. J Chron Dis 16:1239

Friesinger GC (1982) The reasonable workup before recommending medical or surgical therapy: an overall strategy. Circulation 65 [Suppl II]:25

Hammermeister KE, DeRouen TA, Dodge HT (1982) Comparison of survival of medically and surgically treated coronary disease patients in Seattle Heart Watch: a non-randomized study. Circulation 65 [Suppl II]: 53

Mock MB, Ringqvist I, Fisher LD, et al. (1982) Survival of medically treated patients in the coronary artery surgery study (CASS) registry. Circulation 66: 562

Takaro T, Peduzzi P, Detre KM, Hultgren HN, et al. (1982a) Survival in subgroups of patients with left main coronary artery disease. Veterans Administration cooperative study of surgery for coronary arterial occlusive disease. Circulation 66: 14

Takaro T, Hultgren HN, Detre KM, Peduzzi P (1982b) The Veterans Administration Cooperative Study of Stable Angina: current status. Circulation 65 [Suppl II]: 60

[illegible]

Subject Index

MIX
Papier aus verantwortungsvollen Quellen
Paper from responsible sources
FSC® C105338

If you have any concerns about our products,
you can contact us on
ProductSafety@springernature.com

In case Publisher is established outside the EU,
the EU authorized representative is:
Springer Nature Customer Service Center GmbH
Europaplatz 3, 69115 Heidelberg, Germany

Printed by Libri Plureos GmbH
in Hamburg, Germany